The Cultural Politics of COVID-19

COVID-19 isn't simply a viral pathogen nor is it, strictly speaking, the trigger of a global pandemic. Since the outbreak began in late-2019, an outpouring of clinical and scientific research, together with an array of public health initiatives, have sought to understand, mitigate, or even eradicate the virus. This book represents a snapshot of critical responses by researchers from 10 countries and 4 continents, in a collective effort to explore how Cultural Studies can contribute to our struggle to persevere in a "no normal" horizon, with no clear end in sight. Together, the essays address important questions at the intersection of culture, power, politics, and public health: What are the possible outlines for the panic-pandemic complex? How has the pandemic been endowed with meanings and affective registers, often at the tipping points where existing social relations and medical understanding were being rapidly displaced by new ones? How can societies discover ways of living with, through, and against COVID that do not simply reproduce existing hierarchies and power relations?

The 30 essays comprising this collection, along with the editors' introduction, explore the formative period of the COVID pandemic, from mid-2020 to mid-2021. They are grouped into three sections – 'Racializations,' 'Media, Data, and Fragments of the Popular,' and 'Un/knowing the Pandemic' – themes that animate, but do not exhaust, the complex cultural and political life of COVID-19 with respect to identity, technology, and epistemology. No doubt, readers will chart their own pathway as the pandemic continues to rage on, based on their own unique circumstances. This book provides critical-intellectual guideposts for the way forward – toward an uncertain future, without guarantees.

The chapters in this book were originally published as a special issue of the journal, *Cultural Studies*.

John Nguyet Erni is Dean of Humanities and Chair Professor of Cultural Studies at The Education University of Hong Kong. Previously, he was Fung Hon Chu Endowed Chair of Humanics at Hong Kong Baptist University. His most recent book is *Law and Cultural Studies: A Critical Rearticulation of Human Rights*.

Ted Striphas, Coeditor of the journal *Cultural Studies*, is Associate Professor of Media Studies, University of Colorado Boulder, USA. He is author of *The Late Age of Print* and of the upcoming monograph *Algorithmic Culture*. Twitter: @striphas

The Cultural Politics of COVID-19

Edited by
John Nguyet Erni and Ted Striphas

Routledge
Taylor & Francis Group

LONDON AND NEW YORK

First published 2023
by Routledge
4 Park Square, Milton Park, Abingdon, Oxon OX14 4RN

and by Routledge
605 Third Avenue, New York, NY 10158

Routledge is an imprint of the Taylor & Francis Group, an informa business

Chapters 1, 2 and 4–31 © 2023 Taylor & Francis
Chapter 3 © 2021 John Clarke. Originally published as Open Access.

British Library Cataloguing in Publication Data
A catalogue record for this book is available from the British Library

ISBN13: 978-1-032-30186-0 (hbk)
ISBN13: 978-1-032-31585-0 (pbk)
ISBN13: 978-1-003-31041-9 (ebk)

DOI: 10.4324/9781003310419

Typeset in Myriad Pro
by Newgen Publishing UK

Publisher's Note
The publisher accepts responsibility for any inconsistencies that may have arisen
during the conversion of this book from journal articles to book chapters, namely
the inclusion of journal terminology.

Disclaimer
Every effort has been made to contact copyright holders for their permission to
reprint material in this book. The publishers would be grateful to hear from any
copyright holder who is not here acknowledged and will undertake to rectify any
errors or omissions in future editions of this book.

Contents

Citation Information

The chapters in this book were originally published in the journal *Cultural Studies*, volume 35, issue 2–3 (2021). When citing this material, please use the original page numbering for each article, as follows:

Chapter 1
> *Introduction: COVID-19, the multiplier*
> John Nguyet Erni and Ted Striphas
> *Cultural Studies*, volume 35, issue 2–3 (2021), pp. 211–237

Chapter 2
> *Covid-19 and the mundane practices of privilege*
> Kumarini Silva
> *Cultural Studies*, volume 35, issue 2–3 (2021), pp. 238–247

Chapter 3
> *Following the science? Covid-19, 'race' and the politics of knowing*
> John Clarke
> *Cultural Studies*, volume 35, issue 2–3 (2021), pp. 248–256

Chapter 4
> *'Give me liberty or give me Covid!': Anti-lockdown protests as necropopulist downsurgency*
> Jack Bratich
> *Cultural Studies*, volume 35, issue 2–3 (2021), pp. 257–265

Chapter 5
> *Racism is a public health crisis! Black Power in the COVID-19 pandemic*
> Lisa B. Y. Calvente
> *Cultural Studies*, volume 35, issue 2–3 (2021), pp. 266–278

For any permission-related enquiries please visit:
www.tandfonline.com/page/help/permissions

Notes on Contributors

Charles R. Acland is Distinguished University Research Professor in the Department of Communication Studies, Concordia University, Montreal. His most recent book is *American blockbuster: movies, technology, and wonder* (2020).

Rebecca A. Adelman is Professor and Chair of Media and Communication Studies at the University of Maryland Baltimore County. She is the author of *Beyond the Checkpoint: Visual Practices in America's Global War on Terror* (2014), *Figuring Violence: Affective Investments in Perpetual War* (2019), and the co-editor of *Remote Warfare: New Cultures of Violence* (2020).

Ien Ang is Distinguished Professor of Cultural Studies at the Institute for Culture and Society, Western Sydney University (Australia) and the author of numerous books, including *Desperately Seeking the Audience* (1991), *On Not Speaking Chinese: Living Between Asia and the West* (2001) and, most recently, the co-authored *Chinatown Unbound: Trans-Asian Urbanism in the Age of China* (2019).

Muhammad Azam is a development practitioner. His areas of interest include urban governance, social policy, and digital geographies.

Jeffrey A. Bennett is Professor and Chair of Communication Studies at Vanderbilt University. He is the author of *Managing Diabetes: The Cultural Politics of Disease* (2019) and *Banning Queer Blood: Rhetorics of Citizenship, Contagion, and Resistance* (2009).

Christiaan De Beukelaer is Senior Lecturer at the University of Melbourne. His research explores two distinct topics: the revival or sailing vessels as a means of zero-emission cargo transport and the role of UNESCO in global cultural policy-making processes. His books include *Global Cultural Economy* and *Cultural Policies for Sustainable Development*.

Jack Bratich is Associate Professor in the journalism and media studies department at Rutgers University, USA. He takes a critical approach to the intersection of popular culture and political culture. His work applies autonomist social theory to such topics as craft media, reality television, social movement media, and the cultural politics of war.

Lisa B. Y. Calvente is Communication and Black Studies scholar. Her interests lie in the critical interrogation of anti-black and brown racism and the experiences, representations and theories of the Black Diaspora, and coloniality.

Allen Chun is Research Fellow Emeritus in the Institute of Ethnology, Academia Sinica, Taipei, Taiwan. From August 2019, he has been Chair Professor in the Institute for Social Research and Cultural Studies, National Chiao Tung University, Hsinchu, Taiwan. His interests involve cultural theory, nation-state formation, transnationalism and identity, and his research has focused mostly on Taiwan, Hong Kong, and Singapore.

John Clarke is Emeritus Professor at the UK's Open University and a Leverhulme Emeritus Fellow. He is currently working on the turbulent times marked by the rise of nationalist, populist, and authoritarian politics.

John Nguyet Erni is Dean of Humanities and Chair Professor of Cultural Studies at The Education University of Hong Kong. Previously, he was Fung Hon Chu Endowed Chair of Humanics at Hong Kong Baptist University. His most recent book is *Law and Cultural Studies: A Critical Rearticulation of Human Rights*.

James N. Gilmore is Assistant Professor of Media & Technology Studies in the Department of Communication at Clemson University. He researches the cultural politics of technology and daily life.

Elmo Gonzaga is Assistant Professor of Cultural Studies at the Chinese University of Hong Kong. He writes on political aesthetics and popular culture. His most recent publications include articles on bureaucratic boredom in *New formations* (2020) and popular critique in *Cultural studies* (2020). His most recent monograph is *Humour as politics* (2017).

Leon Gurevitch is Associate Professor and Associate Dean of Research at Victoria University of Wellington's Faculty of Architecture and Design. Leon's work focuses on design sociology, labour and the global creative industries, transformative technologies, and complex systems design. Leon is a member of the Visual Effects Society and has published research and exhibited design work around the world.

Sajjad Hasnain is a development practitioner. He works with the themes centred around religion, environment, and public affairs.

James Hay is Research Professor in the Institute of Communications Research and the Department of Media & Cinema Studies in the College of Media at the University of Illinois-Urbana-Champaign. He is the ex-Director of the Institute of Communications Research and the ex-Editor-in-Chief of the journal, *Communication & Critical/Cultural Studies*.

Mette Hjort is Professor of Film and Screen Studies at the University of Lincoln and Head of the Lincoln School of Film and Media. She is also Chair Professor of Humanities at the Hong Kong Baptist University, Affiliate Professor of Scandinavian Studies at the University of Washington, and Visiting Professor of Cultural Industries at the University of South Wales. Mette's publications include the monograph *Small Nation, Global Cinema* (2005) and the two-volume edited work, *The Education of the Filmmaker* (2013).

Nicholas Holm is Senior Lecturer in Media Studies at Massey University, New Zealand. He writes on political aesthetics and popular culture. His most recent publications include articles on bureaucratic boredom in *New Formations* (2020) and popular critique in *Cultural Studies* (2020). His most recent monograph is *Humour as Politics* (2017).

Chris Ingraham is Assistant Professor of Communication and core faculty member in the Environmental Humanities graduate program at the University of Utah. Alongside various articles in the areas of media, cultural, and rhetorical studies, he is the author of *Gestures of Concern* (2020).

Rimi Khan is Lecturer in the School of Communication and Design at RMIT University Vietnam. Her research is broadly concerned with creativity, diverse citizenship, and cultural economy. Her most recent work examines creative labour and ethical fashion economies in Asia. Her book, *Art in Community: The Provisional Citizen* (2016), examines the institutional, aesthetic, and economic agendas that make communities creative, cohesive, and productive.

Sukhmani Khorana is Vice Chancellor's Senior Research Fellow at the Young and Resilient Research Centre at Western Sydney University. Previously, she was a Senior Lecturer in Cultural Studies and Academic Program Leader at the University of Wollongong. Sukhmani has published extensively on diasporic cultures, multi-platform refugee narratives, and the politics of empathy.

Yeran Kim is Professor in the School of Communications, Kwangwoon University, Seoul, South Korea. She has published a number of papers and books, including '*Idol Republic: Global Emergence of Girl Industries and Commercialization of Girl Bodies*'. Her current research focuses on the cultural intersection of affect, communication, and society in the contemporary digital media ecology.

Madhavi Mallapragada is Associate Professor in the Department of Radio-Television-Film at the University of Texas at Austin. Her research focuses on cultural studies of online media; immigration and Asian American popular culture; and race and media industries.

Alexander J. Means is Associate Professor of Educational Policy with Global Perspectives in the Department of Educational Foundations at the University of Hawai'i at Mānoa. His research draws on scholarly traditions in sociology and critical theory to examine educational policy and governance in relation to political, economic, cultural, technological, and social change.

Asif Mehmood is a doctoral student at the State University of New York, College of Environmental Sciences and Forestry (SUNY-ESF), Syracuse, NY, USA. He is interested in questions of urban political ecology, infrastructure, land, and nonhuman ecologies.

Ravindra N. Mohabeer holds a PhD in Communication and Culture and is a faculty member and Chair of the Department of Media Studies at Vancouver Island University, Canada. His research focuses on a multidimensional social theory of invisibility, the intersections of digital expression, do-it-yourself and everyday culture, and on belonging bisected by race, class, and non-urbanity.

Elspeth Probyn is Professor of Gender & Cultural Studies at the University of Sydney. She has published several ground-breaking monographs including *Sexing the Self* (1993), *Outside Belongings* (1996), *Carnal Appetites* (2000), *Blush: Faces of Shame* (2006), and *Eating the Ocean* (2016). Her current research focuses on fishing as extraction, fish markets as gendered spaces of labour, and anthropocentric oceanic change.

Harriette Richards is Honorary Fellow in the School of Culture and Communication and Research Associate in the School of Social and Political Sciences at the University of Melbourne. She is currently working on research investigating radical transparency in the fashion industry and gendered dynamics in the innovation sector as well as a monograph about fashion and the settler colonial imagination.

Raka Shome is Professor and Harron Family Endowed Chair in the Department of Communication at Villanova University, Pennsylvania. She has published numerous essays and special issues of journals on topics such as postcolonial media studies, Cultural Studies and the Global South, Asian Modernities, Asian mobilities, gender and transnationalism and Whiteness (in particular white femininity).

Kumarini Silva is Associate Professor of Communication at the University of North Carolina-Chapel Hill. Her research is at the intersection of identity, politics, post-colonial studies, cultural studies, and popular culture.

Her current research looks at how affective relationships, especially calls to and of love, animate regulatory practices that are deeply cruel and alienating.

Graham B. Slater is an independent scholar based in Reno, Nevada (USA). He studies the relationship between critical theory, ecology, culture, and the politics of education. His recent work appears in *Educational Philosophy and Theory; Policy Futures in Education; Educational Studies;* and *Discourse: Studies in the Cultural Politics of Education.*

Josh Smicker is Assistant Professor of Communication and Chair of the Department of Communication at Catawba College, and is a former associate editor of the journal *Cultural Studies.* His work is primarily focused on the intersections of new media technologies and experiences and management of trauma and violence, both in terms of the use of technologies as therapeutics as well as platforms for mobilizing new forms of violence and horror often organized around race, gender, and sexuality.

Jon Stratton is an adjunct professor at the University of South Australia. Jon has published widely in *Cultural Studies, Media Studies, Jewish Studies, Australian Studies* and on race and multiculturalism. Jon's most recent books are *Multiculturalism, Whiteness and Otherness in Australia* (2020) and, coedited with Jon Dale and with Tony Mitchell, *An Anthology of Australian Albums: Critical Engagement* (2020).

Ted Striphas, Coeditor of the journal *Cultural Studies*, is Associate Professor of Media Studies, University of Colorado Boulder, USA. He is author of *The Late Age of Print* and of the upcoming monograph *Algorithmic Culture.* Twitter: @striphas.

Fan Yang is Associate Professor in the Department of Media and Communication Studies at the University of Maryland, Baltimore County (UMBC). She is the author of *Faked in China: Nation Branding, Counterfeit Culture, and Globalization* (2016). Yang's scholarship lies at the intersection of transnational media/cultural studies, globalization and communication, postcolonial studies, and contemporary China.

Sheng Zou is a postdoctoral research fellow at the University of Michigan's International Institute. He received his Ph.D. in Communication from Stanford University. His research interests include global media industries, digital media and society, platform economy and labor, and digital journalism. His current work explores the intersection of governance, politics, and popular culture in digital China, particularly statesociety interactions through new media platforms.

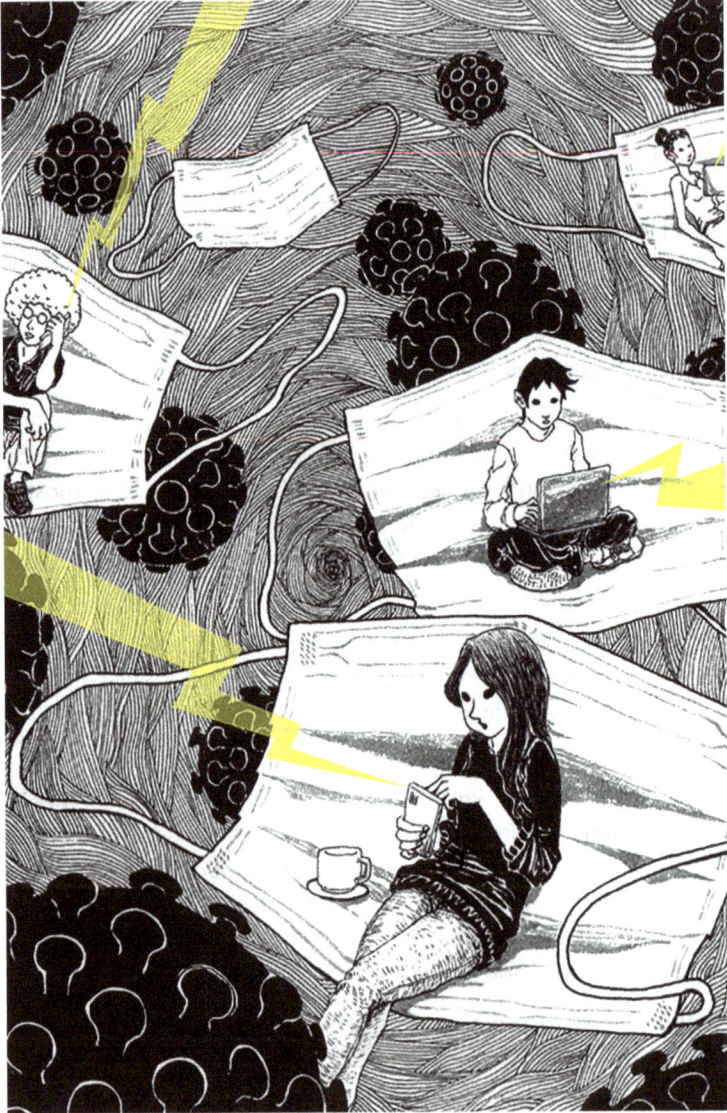

"Face Masks Connect Us," Hirofumi Ito (@hiro_bouzu) - 2021

Introduction: COVID-19, the multiplier

John Nguyet Erni and Ted Striphas

ABSTRACT
The global COVID-19 pandemic has robbed us of normal life, however 'normal' may be defined. Yet it has also (re)activated certain strands of cultural research that attempt to steer a path parallel to that of biomedical research. Why do we need Cultural Studies in the midst of this nightmarish period? Aside from reactivating and thinking with disciplinary specificities, the COVID crisis has fairly quickly prompted a realization from the early days of the pandemic that a situation far exceeding public health has emerged, with frightening epidemiological, social, cultural, and geopolitical implications. We issued a call for critical, short, and punchy thought pieces in May 2020 and received an overwhelming number of responses globally. In this Introduction, we attempt to outline a certain 'grid of intelligibility' that can be conferred upon three specific frames unique to the sort of response that Cultural Studies can make to COVID, frames that are shared in different ways among the contributors to this volume. The frames that we focus on include: the articulation of a cultural lifeworld of the pandemic (in a conscious attempt to connect with the lessons about the force of signification and public political deliberation learned from other pandemics, especially global AIDS); the manner in which COVID has been weaponized in government manoeuvres and in virulent forms of racialization; and the affective and bodily registers that mark our collective vulnerability. In this mapping, COVID multiplies semantically, politically, and corporeally. It is hoped that this Special Issue provides not only a sort of memory archive for what the world has gone through in 2020–21, but also hopefully some intellectual guidance for the way forward.

The panic pandemic

Where even to begin with COVID-19?

On its own, a debilitating and deadly global pandemic is enough to over-whelm – physically, psychologically, spiritually, and intellectually. As of this writing, 117 million COVID cases have been recorded worldwide, and of those cases, more than 2.6 million people have died. Let that sink in for a moment: 2.6 million people, *gone* – and not just 'people' in the abstract, but family members, friends, lovers, mentors, colleagues, acquaintances, public figures, personal connections, and total strangers. Never mind the untold numbers of COVID 'long-haulers' whose bodies, seemingly unable to overcome infection, endure protracted suffering; or the billions of people whose daily lives have been turned upside down and inside out socially, professionally, and financially. Who doesn't long for a day when *it* will finally be over? And yet, as vaccines finally begin rolling out in the early spring of 2021, we hear *it* might never get back to normal as the virus continues to mutate, as we struggle with the awful truth that we can still spread COVID despite inoculation, and as new, compensatory habits estrange us, maybe permanently, from once familiar people, places, objects, and practices.

Yes, it is enough to overwhelm, but the COVID pandemic hardly exists in isolation. The world first caught wind of novel coronavirus (2019-nCoV), a.k.a SARS-CoV-2, a.k.a., COVID-19 in early 2020 as summer wildfires, stoked by climate change, decimated 18.5 million hectares of Australian bush. Ten months later, large portions of the American West similarly went up in flames, the acrid smoke so pervasive that one of COVID's few pleasures – seeking refuge outdoors – became its own public health hazard. In between, the senseless murders of Breonna Taylor, George Floyd, Rayshard Brooks, and scores of other Black persons at the hands of U.S. law enforcement reinforced long-standing fears about whether, within cultures of white supremacy, Black lives mattered at all, and if so, how.

The specificity of the U.S. national context should not, however, obscure the linkages between these instances of state-sanctioned violence and those happening in Hong Kong SAR, Brazil, China, India, and elsewhere, nor the broader attacks on democratic processes wrought by reactionary authoritarian regimes across the globe. The deadly insurrection at the United States Capitol on January 6, 2021, inflamed by former President Donald J. Trump, is perhaps the most spectacular manifestation of this tendency, an event that left many observers wondering if the existential dread of 2020 would ever finally lift.

The point here is to recognize the *multiplicity* of the COVID-19 pandemic – that is, to refuse to accept it as a public health crisis primarily, as though it were somehow separable from these highly charged events; or, in a different vein, to reject the idea that these events were merely the backdrop against which COVID unfolded. COVID-19 was and remains so overwhelming because it is not one thing but many things simultaneously; or rather, because it refers to a series of crises superimposed with such pressure as to leave one wondering where even to begin at all. When we conceived of this project around May 2020, we were fully aware of the importance of a collective endeavour, involving people with varying experiences of COVID-19, to tell us what important social, cultural, political, and discursive markers were emerging to form a sense of the global crisis. In the ten months of preparing this Special Issue, the panic has grown deeper in epidemiological *and* cultural terms. What is a possible outline of the panic-pandemic complex, with what immediate and longer-term, knowable and unfathomable, consequences? This is an enormous intellectual task for cultural researchers, because as Paula A. Treichler (1999) in her groundbreaking book *How to Have Theory in an Epidemic* has emphasized, understanding and moving with analytical precision with the complexity of an epidemic – i.e. alongside a biomedical crisis lies the multifarious and disorienting discourses that form a wild 'epidemic of signification' – is paramount for any kind of useful cultural research.

At one level, we take stock of the fragile 'certainties' that have been circulating since the onset of the COVID global pandemic (Klingsberg 2020). By fragile certainties, we are pointing to the peculiar discursive handles that somehow endow panic with meanings, often at the tipping points where existing social relations were rapidly, and shockingly, being displaced by new ones. The inventory below may easily be dismissed as myths and urban legends, silly stuff held by feeble minds. Yet these fragile certainties, however fleeting and outlandish, help us to trace the contour of a certain popular archive about COVID:

(1) COVID-19 is chemical warfare unleashed from a Wuhan lab.
(2) A psychic predicted the pandemic in her 2008 book.
(3) A COVID infection turns the patient into a zombie.
(4) Holding your breath for 10 seconds can act as a test for COVID-19, a test proven valid among elderly persons.
(5) U.S. colleges hold 'COVID-19 parties' so that students will deliberately get infected.
(6) Some churches hold 'release parties' for their congregation to gather with food, drinks, and music without observing social distancing rules and without wearing masks.
(7) Dean Koontz, in his 1981 novel *The Eyes of Darkness*, writes of a 'perfect weapon' called 'Wuhan-400,' which was the 400th visible strain of man-made microorganisms created at the RDNA labs outside of the city of Wuhan.
(8) The coronavirus crisis was deliberately created by telecommunication companies in order to keep people at home while their engineers install 5G technology everywhere.
(9) A super-chain in the U.S. recalled a brand of toilet paper because it was contaminated with the virus, as it was made in China.
(10) Various theories about how to prevent the virus include avoiding spicy food, eating garlic, and drinking bleach.

(11) A 'miracle mineral solution,' which is 28 percent sodium chlorite mixed in distilled water, is said to prevent infection. There are reports that it's being sold online for US$900 per gallon.
(12) Because the COVID vaccine injects a small piece of bio-sensing genetic material into our bodies, teaching our cells how to identify the coronavirus and produce antibodies to fight it, the vaccine will alter our DNA and control our minds.
(13) Pets will spread the disease since a dog in Hong Kong was alleged to have been infected with the virus (the world's first such reported case).
(14) A COVID-19 vaccine will use microchip surveillance technology created by Bill Gates-funded research.
(15) COVID-19 vaccines contain aborted human fetal tissue and will cause female infertility.
(16) A vaccine contains animal products and is not halal, causing vaccination hesitation especially among some South Asian communities.

To us, marking the vernacular cultural lifeworld of COVID in this way is useful for pointing out the obvious: much of the pandemic is utterly unknowable and prone to mystification. But more, the unknowable is no laughing matter. Thinking of how this deadly serious issue of knowing/unknowing has spawned a certain landmark tradition in cultural research of public health and epidemics, we recall the work on the cultural politics of HIV/AIDS since some three decades ago, of important voices such as those of Paula A. Treichler, Douglas Crimp, Cindy Patton, Simon Watney, Jan Zita Grover, Gina Corea, Steven Epstein, Leo Bersani, and many more.

In much of the critical scholarship on HIV/AIDS, realizing that a pandemic is 'cultural' is far from adequate, because lurking underneath, above, and around the cultural forces is epidemiological work claiming to speak the 'ultimate truth.' What is needed is a profound understanding of the imperative to keep deliberating and fighting over the very *uncertainties and contradictions* in epidemiological work, and how to actively keep alive, even agitate, public debates. Paula A. Treichler (cited in Gates and Leger 2000, p. 393) emphasizes that when fear and confusion reigned in the early stages of the AIDS epidemic, patients and activists fought not only on the medical front, but also against the authorities and the media working to foreclose public debates:

An epidemic of a fatal infectious disease is like a war, or a natural disaster, or a huge pile-up on the highway: it cries out for immediate action. In an epidemic, the public health approach also calls for prevention or eradication now to prevent even more cases in the future. Or maybe you're one of its victims, and see others sick and dying as well. The pressure's on to do something, make the epidemic stop, right here, right now. There's an incredible sense of crisis and urgency, whether or not you know how it's transmitted or who's at risk, whether or not you've identified its cause. With AIDS/HIV, the centrality of sex, homosexuality, and other taboo stuff definitely complicated the sense of urgency and delayed action; but I think those factors also made it even harder to clear a space for deliberation, for really thinking about, "What's going on here? What do we believe? What does this epidemic mean?"

'Theory' matters in the AIDS crisis, Treichler notes, because theory is the very real task of going through the messy processes through which those living with the crisis establish a semblance of certainty, sort things out, and continuously revise their treatment options and the political actions appropriate for the moment. Vitally, as a cultural researcher, Treichler (cited in Gates and Leger 2000, p. 394) has had to

> identify a wide spectrum of responses to the urgency of finding treatment, and many different ways of balancing urgency with deliberation—what I'm equating here with "theory." Often these responses are very sophisticated, which is a lot to ask if you have this thing that's killing you. For some, it meant saying, "I would rather take this medication than nothing. I'm willing to take that risk. I don't know if it works, but I would rather do that. And if it turns out that it hasn't worked, I accept that." They found a way of dealing with profound uncertainty. Others could not; it was too difficult not to believe that these drugs were going to help. Living with such quandaries is part of what theory means. For me, that's what the notion of an "epidemic of signification" did. It gave me a handle on the way that different people were producing meanings of the epidemic, quite apart from what might be true or false.

Morbidity and mortality are undeniable, but the struggle for 'signification' can steer alternative discursive paths away from dangerously fatal ones, albeit without guarantees. Minimally, calling a pandemic 'cultural' requires steadfast diagnostic work and real political conversation about just how medical realities, crises, and even 'cures' are publicly produced, not 'discovered' in any teleological sense (see also Sterne 2017).

In public debates, therefore, what repertoire of key ideas with which to speak and think about a pandemic crisis, and what gets obscured, has always been part of the necessary intellectual work. In 1987, in the throes of the first decade of the AIDS epidemic, Jan Zita Grover published the landmark essay, 'AIDS: Keywords.' The piece endeavoured to extend Raymond Williams' (1983) unique approach to cultural semantics, 'keywords,' to the linguistic territory that at once defined and was defined by this seemingly new disease complex. Significantly, 'AIDS: Keywords' was out front in recognizing that the bodily and biomedical dimensions of HIV/AIDS could not be bracketed from the terminology conventionally used by the medical establishment, pharmaceutical companies, journalists, activists, lay people, and, of course, persons living with AIDS. 'The advent of AIDS as a socially meaningful fact in the West,' Grover observed (1987, p. 17), 'has generated an enormous outpouring of words' including *AIDS, bisexual, gay community, heterosexual community, patient zero, person with AIDS (PWA), risk, victim,* and more.

Importantly, words were not an end in themselves. Grover challenged readers to consider how the vocabulary of HIV/AIDS indexed deeper, existential changes to societies beset by the epidemic: 'The kinds of words that Williams traces were invented or reimagined at the straining points where old social relations were giving way to new ones' (Grover 1987, p. 17). And so it was for the entries appearing on Grover's list which, similarly, embodied the tensions, contradictions, confusions, obfuscations, hopes, dreams, fears, desires, and pleasures of living – and perhaps dying – in a world where AIDS had become an inescapable fact of existence. Ultimately, the goal of 'AIDS: Keywords' was hopeful, driven by a belief that a close examination of words at the crux of AIDS discourse might one day provoke semantic changes and other adaptations to better 'fit … reality,' rather than mere acquiescence to 'an already authorized tradition' (Grover 1987, p. 18).

We return to 'AIDS: Keywords' inspired by a similar hope: that of identifying, however provisionally, some of the key terms that have come to be associated with the COVID pandemic, terms that may trigger new ways of understanding the human/virus/science/sociality complex. And we turn to it, with Williams' (1983) work, with due acknowledgment of how a *global* pandemic stretches the limits of keywords as an interpretive framework. Indeed, it is critical to understand that keywords are neither transcontextual nor translinguistic; the vocabularies identified by both Grover and Williams are bounded in important ways. If nothing else, it is not lost on us that, like this journal, both authors operated exclusively in the English language as a tool and a paradigm, which exerts an undeniable global dominance, even as it hardly exhausts the range of possible cultural-semantic responses to COVID. We offer the following list with that caveat in mind and in recognition, then, of the need to make keywords a more inclusive project moving forward. All this is to say we are keenly aware that there are many excellent analyses out there in other languages, locales, and cultural disciplines that our volume does not capture (cf. Chen and Chua 2020). That said, many of the candidate 'COVID keywords,' below, are drawn from the contributions to this volume, whose authors' collective footprint traverses four continents, multiple languages, and numerous speech communities: *antibodies; Asians; asymptomatic; balcony; Black; border; boredom; care; China; conspiracy; climate change; contact tracing; community; coronavirus; cross-species transmission; droplets; essential; flattening the curve; freedom; gym etiquette; hate speech; herd; home; immunity; isolation; isopropyl alcohol; lockdown; long COVID; mask; N95/KN95; pandemic; personal protective equipment; police; quarantine; rapid testing; race/racism; remote; resilience; r-naught (R0); SARS-COV-2; shame; social distancing; solidarity; superspreader; supply chain fragility; toilet rolls; touch; vaccine (nationalism); variant; ventilator; virus; wet market; work from home; Zoom; zoonosis.* Let us continue to extend this inventory, in order to keep public deliberations a living process.

COVID is not, in any simple sense, a parallel moment to the HIV/AIDS crisis, nor to the SARS and MERS outbreaks. Intellectual resources produced in and for an earlier time should inspire, yet they should not be approached as if they provided adequate answers to the myriad questions surrounding COVID-19 today. But neither should the current crisis be taken unreflectively as 'unprecedented' (cf. Kane 2020). There have been so many assertions of how the world has not seen anything like it. Yet strangely, the unprecedented is often placed alongside the comparable, the manageable, and the familiar. Even if there is no common horizon for these pandemic episodes, there are shared lessons, overlapping tendencies, and eerily similar states of exception.

Our COVID localities

In the vast disorienting space of the pandemic, let us begin again, by remarking on where we have been, locally. At least for us, marking one's 'COVID locality' is one way to sketch some meaning into the world we now live in. One of us resides in Hong Kong. Aside from the disruptions of work, the imminent collapse of the public health system, the restrictions on travel, the rising job losses, the fear of falling ill – and yes, the mortal anxiety of running out of toilet rolls at home, too – the experience of battling the epidemic in Hong Kong has been uniquely overlaid by another battle. COVID-19 came to the city at the heels of months of intense protest, which has been widely reported and discussed as the Anti-extradition Law Movement, against a proposed bill by the government to transfer fugitives to the Mainland. Protesters, as well as the legal profession, journalist organizations, foreign governments, and even business groups feared the erosion of Hong Kong's legal system and its built-in safeguards, and they warned of the sinister impact of the bill to stifle and arrest voices of political dissent (see Lee et al. 2019, Tai et al. 2019, Chung 2020, Purbrick 2020).

In early 2020, the considerable level of preparedness among Hong Kong residents when facing the coming of COVID harks back to the deep memory of how the city was plagued by the SARS outbreak in 2003. When news of a potentially fast-spreading respiratory disease hit Hong Kong in early 2020, a social habitus with common practices of personal hygiene and other public preventive measures was already in place. Social activities dropped, frequent handwashing was exercised, and masks worn. But in a rather peculiar way, that deep memory contains not only the formation of a public health consciousness, but also that of a public culture of protest. In 2003, just when the SARS outbreak that afflicted the city began to subside by mid-year, the political tension that had been brewing for some time over the government's attempt to enact Article 23 of the Basic Law – the infamous law that would criminalize treason, sedition, and subversion against the Central People's government – erupted into a mass demonstration on July 1, 2003, resulting in the government's withdrawal of the proposed bill. In other words, SARS of 2003 was experienced as a double affliction to Hong Kong. Few of us who lived through it forget the profound sense of a diminishing city marked by the intersection of a biological pathogen and a political disease. This feeling would be repeated in 2020 by another intersection of a protest and an epidemic.

The intervening years between SARS of 2003 and COVID of 2020 were marked by increasing volatility of public dissatisfaction with the government. Democratic fervour gave hope to the local residents after the show of unity in the massive demonstration on July 1, 2003 successfully forced the government to back down on Article 23. Since then, an annual July 1 mass street protest in Hong Kong has become a powerful symbolic event (see Cheng 2005). The small and large-scale protest experience had accompanied the younger generation, who slowly developed a sense of political purpose for resisting what they viewed as suppression of freedom and other social injustices (Erni 2015, Law 2018, Ma 2018, Ip 2019, Ku 2020, Vukovich 2020). Their organizing against educational reforms in 2011 was in many ways a profound turning point that gave birth to a movement culture led by students, culminating in the large-scale Umbrella Movement of 2014. Unfortunately, after 79 days of mass street protests, the movement was dispersed by tear gas, forced dismantling of tents, and mass arrests. Internal fracture began to appear, with a cluster of mainly party elites who defended the traditional model of 'peaceful, rational, and non-violent' agitation, in growing distance from a so-called 'radical' wing pushing for direct action and 'leaderless' forms of protest (Pang 2020). Accompanying this split was the rise of various versions of political ideology referred to as 'localism.' An ideology that emphasized not only historical and cultural differences between Hong Kong and the Mainland, localism drew attention to political differences of governmental structures, legal systems, and of course the treatment of those who seek democratic reform and a higher degree of autonomy and political freedom (Ho 2020). The 2019 protests in Hong Kong were thus a bifurcated movement.

Like a disease, political life in Hong Kong has been the case of a chronic battle for hegemony over a people's self-determination (Ibrahim and Lam 2020). In the protests, whether in 2003 over Article 23 or in 2019 over the extradition bill, the streets resemble a hospital, with scenes of protesters being teargassed or struck by police batons replicating the frantic space of the Emergency Room. Remarkably, for many people of Hong Kong, fighting COVID recalls the bonding experience gained from fighting the 'political disease,' as community mobilization in the spirit of 'Hong Kong people saving ourselves!' has been in place as part of our public culture for some time (see Lee 2020, Wan et al. 2020). Meanwhile, with COVID, as with SARS, the government's public health control programme has allowed it to fortify its hegemonic authority, deploying the same police force – now donned in epidemic protective gear

– already well-trained in crowd control, contact tracing, interfering with the media, issuing public fines, and more importantly, squashing any form of public dissent (see Hui 2020). Hong Kong may be the only city in the world where a mask law and an anti-mask law exist compulsorily at the same time. In July 2020, the Hong Kong SAR government promulgated the Prevention and Control of Disease (Wearing of Mask) Regulation, when the colonial-era Emergency Regulations Ordinance to enact a mask ban during protests invoked by the government in October 2019, was still in place. We live within a formal contradiction. Masking/anti-masking appears as an apt political allegory for a city with a history of double afflictions, as well as a people who know how to double down on their resistance (see Pang 2020).

In the United States, meanwhile, there was little to no public health consciousness to speak of, and it showed. In the early days of January 2020, COVID seemed mostly like some distant 'thing' on the news. But as days turned into weeks there emerged a palpable sense that *it* was closing in: a case here, a few more there, and then – by the third week of January, an outbreak in Seattle, Washington, harbinger of the hot-spots that began cropping up all across the nation. By early March, the state of Colorado, home to the other editor of this Special Issue, reported its first major outbreak. Surprising no one, the incidence was linked to one of the state's many international ski resorts, which, like most public accommodations in the United States, had virtually no established protocol for responding to a major public health crisis – even for one everybody could see was coming. In the interregnum between the discovery of COVID in Colorado and the state's first lockdown order (effective March 26, 2020), efforts to prevent the virus's spread amounted mostly to what journalist Derek Thompson (2020) would dub 'hygiene theater': props, scenery, scripts, and stagecraft intended to provide the illusion of exercising some control over this strange and mysterious illness, in the absence of genuine knowledge, widespread testing, and effective prophylaxis. Cafés prohibited reusable mugs out of concern they were potential disease vectors. Bottles of hand sanitizer started appearing on countertops in stores and offices, though often only long enough to be stolen after reports of dwindling supplies. Grocery store shelves, once bursting with merchandise, became eerily sparse as the phrase 'supply chain fragility' crept into public awareness. Here and there people could be spotted wearing face coverings, but more often than not they were dust masks purchased from a hardware store. Almost no one knew they were ineffective at stopping the inhalation of viral droplets, the finer points of particulate filtration having never been a serious topic of public conversation. We had spent our time listening to the heating, ventilation, and air conditioning (HVAC) experts, however, who, for decades, had extolled the virtues of hermetically-sealed, climate-controlled buildings. Slowly it dawned on us that we had become victims of our own recirculated air.

It was like living in a protracted plot twist. Familiar figures, objects, practices, landmarks, infrastructures, institutions, and events had become suddenly, jarringly *other* – no longer as they once were, or had long seemed to be, and now inadequate to maintaining the rhythms and routines that suborned the banality of everyday life (Certeau 1984, Morris 1990, Seigworth 2000). The shutdowns were a way of trying to get a handle on COVID, to be sure, but they were as much a moment of pause to figure out how to retrofit key aspects of life in the United States in such a way as to reflect priorities that should have been in place all along, but were ignored. The move to remote teaching, disruptive though it has been, has nonetheless prompted important conversations about accessibility in education. Similarly, HVAC now seems more a question than a given as ordinary folks debate MERV filter ratings and rediscover the basic function of fresh air. And importantly, mail-in voting, prompted by COVID, has helped enfranchise countless citizens (many belonging to dispossessed populations) who had opted out of electoral politics owing to intimidation, ballot manipulation, calculated suppression, and other nefarious tactics. These revelations have come at the cost of well over a half-million dead and counting.

The pushback has been violent, moreover, with tens of millions of people – emboldened by former President Trump and whipped into a frenzy by conservative media – refusing to accept this moment of reckoning as such, choosing instead to cling to broken ideologies, apparatuses, symbols, and racial and economic hierarchies because they have worked well enough *for them* despite their obvious state of disrepair and injustice. Put differently, the resistance to progressive causes that has manifested since 2020 – causes like Black Lives Matter, the movement to defund the police, the Green New Deal, and more – instances not only the recalcitrance of white supremacy and environmental backlash in the United States, but also the intensity of the effort to prevent the COVID plot twist from ever really twisting. Little wonder so many on the Right have resisted the facticity of COVID, in addition to the need for lockdowns, the use of protective face masks in public settings, the importance of social distancing, prohibitions against mass gatherings, and more. To them, doing so is a way of denying, albeit indirectly, the uncomfortable reality of the need for deep, structural change throughout the United States.

Back in Colorado the ski resorts have reopened for the 2020–2021 season and, as of early February, 13 major COVID outbreaks have already occurred. The worst thus far has been at Winter Park Resort, where 109 employees tested positive. According to county officials, 'these cases have not been traced back to transmission through interaction with visitors but, rather, from social gatherings outside of the workplace and congregate housing' (qtd. in Perrot et al. 2021). The message seems to be that the skiers are safe and, thus, that no one should fear partaking of activities that have earned

Colorado a reputation as the state for outdoor recreation and healthy life-styles. It *should* be a reminder of the degree to which part of the cost of an elite 'healthy lifestyle' is borne, directly or indirectly, by disposable popu-lations with comparatively less access to robust healthcare, adequate housing, and other resources critical for survival during COVID. It is also a reminder that unjust, inequitable, and unhealthy patterns endure, despite whatever plot twist may be occurring.

Readers of this volume, we hope, will provide their own unique, compli-cated, or twisted encounter with COVID, given their unique local histories and accompanying cultural-political configurations of struggle. Many of the essays collected here showcase this kind of mosaic, with different assem-blages that form some kind of outline that helps us to grasp, and remember, the pandemic of our lifetime.

The cultural life of pathogenic diseases

Inasmuch as the COVID-19 pandemic is undeniably a biomedical phenom-enon, the preceding discussion hopefully sheds light on some of the singularities of the crisis, and more importantly, on how the singularities can and do intersect. In some sense this is a familiar line of argument, instanced in countless news reports chronicling the virus' disproportionate impact on historically marginalized communities, as well as in numerous journal issues that have endeavoured to explore COVID from a range of critical standpoints. Collectively, they bear witness to how epidemiological phenomena are rife with all manner of considerations, not least of which are the socioeconomic factors by means of which the virus lands harder on certain bodies.

It is worth reminding that what Cultural Studies brings to the table is a different but related commitment – a commitment to *radically contextualizing* COVID, as well as the broader crucible of issues related to disease, health, and wellbeing, amounting to what Grossberg (2018, pp. 155–157) has called a 'diagrammatic analysis' of an organic crisis. On one hand this represents a call for specificity, or rather, a type of specificity that resists universalizing claims and overarching abstractions. Georges Canguilhem's (1991, p. 200–201) discussion of eye conditions is instructive in this regard. 'In order to discern what is normal or pathological for the body itself,' he writes, 'one must look beyond the body. With a disability like astigmatism or myopia, one would be normal in an agricultural or pastoral society but abnormal for sailing or flying.' This is tantamount to saying that the category 'normal' – or perhaps any medical reality, for that matter – isn't so much ontologically given as situationally dependent, suggesting that any change in the situation (i.e. the context) might in turn provoke a transformation of the norm. Canguil-hem is also suggesting that 'unhealth' isn't strictly a biological state or condition of the body but a relationship of that body to itself, to other bodies, and to the natural and built environments those bodies inhabit.

On the other hand, the process of diagrammatizing COVID means moving beyond discrete specificities to explore how seemingly disparate events, phenomena, figures, and modes of existence link up with one another. On this point we draw inspiration from Roberto Esposito's (2011) *Immunitas,* in which the author traces instances of immunity across medicine, law, religion, society, government, and communication technology. Significantly, Esposito does not treat these as discrete manifestations of immunity but as aspects of an interlocking 'system of systems' that condition, but do not uniquely determine, relations of interiority and exteriority, self and other, commonality and exception, susceptibility and resistance, and more (p. 60). That is to say: one cannot think the category of the biomedical *but* in relationship to all of these other categories – a position reminiscent of E. P. Thompson's (1961, p. 33) argument that one cannot study 'culture' per se but must attend, instead, to 'the dialectical interaction between culture and something that is not culture.'

So what does it mean, then, to explore and chronicle the cultural worlds of COVID-19 – that is, to examine them not within a general framework of culture, but within the specific framework of Cultural Studies? It is worth acknowledging that Cultural Studies' interest in the politics of disease, health, and wellbeing has diminished somewhat in recent years (c.f.: Pezzullo 2007, 2012, 2014, Bennett 2009, 2019), and that the energy surrounding those areas of concern has been absorbed by disability studies, science and technology studies, gender and sexuality studies, environmental studies, and neighbouring fields and disciplines. It is a critical time for *Cultural Studies* – both the field and the journal – to rejoin the conversation.

To approach cultural considerations contextually also means refusing to accept a solid-state definition, or even definitions, of *culture.* Culture, for Cultural Studies, is a variable and not a constant (Williams 1958, Williams 1983, Grossberg 2010, pp. 169–226, Striphas 2016), one that exists and evolves in relationship to specific geo-historical events and, more abstractly, other existential territories (e.g. economy, law, religion, technology, the war machine, etc.). In facing a deadly disease, one should not, in other words, be addressing the 'cultural' aspects without also interrogating how disease, etc. relate to the definitions – indeed, to the very existence – of culture. Once again, as Paula A. Treichler (1999, p. 234) observed with respect to HIV/AIDS:

> culture is typically understood within conventional AIDS discourse in the narrowest and most old-fashioned sense: enrichment, civilization, uplifting art, which fork to use. The sensibility of liberal humanism predominates, while vital contributions of feminist, postmodern, and postcolonial writing and theory are absent.

The lesson is not about theory – far from it – but the interlocking relations between the observable materiality of diseases and the equally hard facticity of culture, understood organically. Once again, by 'theory' in the epidemic, Treichler was arguing for us not to close down prematurely on public political deliberations on those very interlocking relations. As for Cindy Patton, 'theory' was something that helped to reveal how the crisis was 'invented,' understood as a necessary but politically invested process (Patton 1990, 2002).

Timberg and Helperin's (2012) *Tinderbox* may also be instructive here. Like many Western scholars and journalists before them, Timberg and Halperin endeavour to locate the origins of HIV/AIDS in West Africa: specifically, Cameroon and Congo. Importantly, however, the work parts company with most other 'first world chronicles' of so-called 'African AIDS' by subverting the typical narrative formula (Treichler 1999, pp. 99–126, Patton 2002, p. 59). Instead of attributing the growth and spread of HIV/AIDS to traditional sexual practices (e.g. non-monogamy), inadequate sanitation, or perhaps a lack of knowledge of (Western) medical science, Timberg and Halperin situate the AIDS epidemic squarely in the problem space of European colonialism. While they are hardly the first to do so (see Treichler 1999: 115), their work is meticulous in showing how colonial-era projects, including missionary work and resource extraction, led to the development of social and physical infrastructure (e.g. densely populated cities, transportation networks) without which HIV was unlikely to have spread far and wide (Timberg and Halperin 2012, p. 51). Thus, they argue, 'the birth of the AIDS epidemic and colonialism had a more than incidental connection' (p. 35). They reinforce the point, understated here, by referencing the work of Michael Worobey, a molecular biologist whose research on the evolution of HIV has established conclusively that the virus' dominant strain first emerged in the Congo River basin between 1884 and 1924, 'the most rapacious period of German [and Belgian] colonial exploitation in the region' (pp. 49–50).

There are several points here worth emphasizing. The first is to recognize how modern technology and associated infrastructure reterritorialized the Congo basin in such a way as to diminish the prophylaxis otherwise enforced by the physical landscape. 'In the precolonial era, a traveller setting off from the spot that would become Léopoldville [now Kinshasa] eventually would have hit natural obstacles in every direction – jungles, waterfalls, mountains, and the Atlantic Ocean itself – that served as firewalls against the spread of diseases' (Timber's and Halperin 2021, p. 63). While it would be reductive to attribute the global HIV/AIDS epidemic of the 20th and 21st centuries singularly to European colonialism, it seems clear the latter was a decisive element in the epidemic's gradual anthro-medical development as such.

There is, however, a second layer to the colonial story of HIV/AIDS, one that implicates *culture* (i.e. the keyword, the concept) even more directly. '[I]n certain important respects,' observes Nicholas B. Dirks (1992, p. 3), culture was what colonialism was all about … The anthropological concept of culture might never have been invented without a colonial theater that both necessitated the knowledge of culture (for purposes of control and regulation) and provided a colonized constituency that was particularly amenable to 'culture.'

Regrettably, Dirks glosses over the terror and violence that rendered colonial populations 'amenable' to the European cultural conquest (Timberg & Halperin 2012, p. 46, Ismail 2015, pp. 139–140, Mbembe 2019). Yet, the point about *culture's* entanglement with colonialism remains a critical one. If, on some level, the HIV/AIDS epidemic is traceable to European colonialism, and if the story of European colonialism is, as Dirks contends, a story about the emergence, operationalization, and propagation of the modern culture concept, then one can begin to appreciate the degree to which *culture* has been implicated in HIV/AIDS from the very beginning – specifically, as a critical element in the articulation of a new disease complex that would only come to be identified as such a century later. Facing COVID, one wonders about its unique cultural entanglements. For instance, does the Wuhan wet market serve as a stand-in for the tropics (see Alberts 2020)? Does calling COVID a 'Chinese virus' encode not only Sinophobia but also something more troubling in the Western colonial imagination, such as what Žižek has called 'racist paranoia' (see Peters 2020)?

Like the physical landscape, moreover, tropical diseases impeded – but did not completely discourage – the project of culture in Europe's colonies. 'Implicit in the history of tropical medicine,' notes Priscilla Wald (2008, p. 50), 'is the image of tropical places as dangerous and diseased and of disease as resistant to the civilizing project.' Tropical medicine thus emerged in the latter half of the nineteenth century to compensate for the immunological differences and deficiencies endemic to the European body. 'Disease,' Wald (p. 50) puts it, 'was not on the side of the colonizer' (see also Patton 2002). Nor was it exactly on the side of culture, either, a concept whose core logics (racial and ethnic difference; spatial and temporal distance; civilizational hierarchy) would not have made much sense absent the condition in which, through medicine, European bodies might hope to achieve some level of resistance to foreign pathogens. The structure of anticipation reverberates today, as the prospect of receiving a COVID vaccine sets in motion all manner of daydreaming about what may be possible, and 'normal' again, in the near future, and what it may take to get there. Similarly, in the 19th and early 20th centuries, the possibility of medical treatment not only made ethnographic fieldwork (and other types of colonial encounter) more practicable; it was also, on some level, that which enabled would-be colonists to dream in, of, and about culture. 'Even as much of what we now recognize as culture was produced by the colonial encounter, *the concept itself was in part invented because of it* (Dirks 1992, p. 3; emphasis added). And it likely would not have travelled much beyond Europe absent the affordances of tropical medicine which, indeed, deserves to be recognized as a major player in *culture's* own biography.

These examples are meant to reinforce the argument that epidemiological events and viral phenomena don't simply occur *within* culture, as though culture were a container for social and symbolic practices connected, in this particular case, to COVID. They are also offered in the hope of adding depth and dimension to the idea of investigating the cultural aspects of disease, health, and wellbeing. One should resist the temptation to figure culture as though it existed *over here*, the epidemiological *over there,* and somewhere in between, a spot of overlap. It is preferable instead to conceive of the one as a condition or 'grid of intelligibility' for the other (Foucault 1990, p. 93). Within this grid, we offer the following central narratives: one is about a political diagnosis of COVID, while the other grapples with how it has been lived.

Weaponizing COVID

Like previous global pandemics, COVID has had an unfolding political life. Horrific reports have emerged of state manoeuvres in Syria, Uganda, Israel, Russia, China, etc. to test and restrict rights and liberties, and to sow distrust between countries, in the guise of epidemic control (Griffiths 2020, Human Rights Watch 2020, Jolicoeur and Seaboyer 2020, Todman 2020). Clearly, manoeuvring suggests tricky operations that blur sound health sciences with biopolitical contrivances. Between reaffirmation of basic public health necessities (such as masking, social distancing, sanitation, and provision of medical care) and belligerent assertion of the power to instrumentalize suffering (such as differential provision of medical care, including vaccination, between the loyalist and opposition areas of a country, closing down opposition media, closing down the border to restrict immigrant movement, etc.), some states have exploited the grey line of pandemic management for political gains. Of late, vaccine distribution has gone nationalistic, as was predicted by the World Health Organization (WHO). A case in point is the mysterious failure in mid-February 2021 'at the final step' of negotiations between the Taiwanese government and BioNTech (who has struck a deal with the Shanghai-based Fosun Pharmaceutical Group to bring their vaccine to China). 'I was worried about interference from external forces all along and there were many possibilities. I was worried about political pressure. We believed there was political pressure,' said the Health Minister of Taiwan (AFP 2021).

Visions of Orwellian life abound, but they tend to oversimplify things. The warnings about totalizing control can hardly elucidate the profound power struggle taking place between Big Brother and all the Little Ones, for

COVID has only reconfirmed the importance of the dematerialized economy held by the telecommunication and digital giants, many of whom hardly share data with the government in a harmonious way (Hogue 2020). Meanwhile, the wireless technology of Apple and Google, with its geo-locating capacity, is not only exacerbating privacy concerns, it is repeating the nightmare of the digital divide whereby infection control among the less or unconnected population (especially the elderly and the disadvantaged) is sorely needed but hardly made easier.

But no insult and victimization have been more direct than in the racialized attacks on specific citizens and migrants. Blatant Sinophobia aside, the spread of hate speech and physical assault of Asians in general attests to the way a virus is weaponized to compound harm (Kaur 2021). Further, in many places, the macabre map of mortality drawn by COVID mirrors the map of structural inequities, where minorities account for a significantly greater share of deaths from contracting the virus compared to the rest of the population. Routinely, physicians have confirmed that COVID fatality is often the result of 'co-morbidities,' which point to the way many underlying health conditions – associated with poverty and systemic racialized disparities – are the culprit for what would be labelled, simplistically, COVID deaths (see Ejaz et al. 2020, Sanyaolu et al. 2020). Prevalence of the co-morbidities, such as hypertension, obesity, chronic lung disease, diabetes, and cardiovascular disease point to chances of bodily survivability as much as to the warped vectors of society and economy. In many ways, then, COVID is just the latest realization of the processes and practices relating to what Pezzullo and Depoe (2010) have called 'everyday death' (the mirror image of everyday life, in which adverse conditions result in death and dying becoming normalized), or of what Laurent Berlant (2007) has similarly labelled 'slow death.'

Placing 'slow death' within the space of the 'predictable life,' Berlant suggests that the constant, numbing attenuation of life – 'the physical wearing out of a population and the deterioration of people in that population that is very nearly a defining condition of their experience and historical existence' (p. 754) – comes across as extreme and ordinary, simultaneously. She speaks particularly of subordination at the physical level, so that an unhealthy body can only be understood as a produced body (specifically, by 'global/national regimes of capitalist structural subordination and governmentality') (p. 754). The problem is that those who live with it realize the body in distress, if not also in deterioration, has no choice but to continue to struggle to build a life around it. Hence the slowness of death. Hence the predictability of life. This is perhaps why, when COVID racism and countless other discriminatory acts were stirred, no one was seriously shocked. Not even the victims, especially when they were well acquainted with the 'social co-morbidities' that defined their existence. The aftershock of a COVID death, however, often does set sail probing questions about how the ordinary facticity of life has once again ended in tragedy and who is responsible for it, facticity such as the crowdedness of one's living space, whether one has medical insurance for critical events, whether the nature of one's work directly puts one in harm's way, one's religious affiliation, and the colour of one's skin.

Yet in some ways, what Berlant alludes to somehow obscures the apparatus of a 'total continuous war' operated by many governments. In the tactic of using quarantine laws, for instance, which naturalizes a legally-sanctioned separation, classification, and hierarchization of bodies in confronting an 'invisible enemy,' governments are not thinking of, and may even find it impossible to accept, slow death. In a state of exception engineered by the total continuous war against COVID, the exposure to death is often rendered foreseeable (see Dias and Deluchey 2020, see also Assy and Hoffmann 2020, Klingberg 2020). A good number of contributors to this Special Issue speak about the ways in which COVID has been weaponized to escalate existing harms, by states and non-state actors alike. Of these nightmares, racism has been firmly yoked into the history of COVID from the early days.

COVID vulnerabilities

There are many ways to characterize how we have been living through COVID, from enduring social inconveniences, frustrations (and anger) over lockdown orders and travel restrictions, confusion, to separation and boredom. But mourning, we believe, will be remembered as the primary way in which we lived through the crisis. Remembering the horrific figure of 2.6 million-plus who have died from COVID worldwide, we also mourn our existential vulnerability. The ones who live share the same vulnerability as those who have died, because what the coronavirus demonstrates is the profound interdependence of all living species who rely on air to survive. Viruses travel between bodies and across surfaces; their mortal itinerary renders everyone vulnerable in their circulatory path. As Butler (cited in Yancy 2020) puts it:

> Vulnerability is not just the condition of being potentially harmed by another. It names the porous and interdependent character of our bodily and social lives. We are given over from the start to a world of others we never chose in order to become more or less singular beings. That dependency does not precisely end with adulthood. To survive, we take something in. We are impressed upon by the environment, social worlds and intimate contact. That impressionability and porosity define our embodied social lives. What another breathes out, I can breathe in, and something of my breath can find its way into yet another person. The human trace that someone leaves on an object may well be what I touch, pass along on another surface or absorb into my own body. Humans share the air with one another and with animals; they share the surfaces of the world. They touch what others have touched and they touch one

another. These reciprocal and material modes of sharing describe a crucial dimension of our vulnerability, intertwinements and interdependence of our embodied social life.

Given over to a world of others, taking in, and passing along: through these ordinary acts, we weave an existence not unlike the virus itself. And when the virus infects, our bodies' organic armies attack back; what results renders who is the host and who is the guest meaningless, in a zoonotic sense. This is why it is all the more important that in mourning the many who have died, we do not forget the political ineptitude and downright stupidity that have criminally allowed the virus to spread to vulnerable populations, nor do we forget the pervasive structural inequalities under which these vulnerable populations live. Those who perish, whether as host or guest in the zoonotic field, are deaths that are preventable. Their deaths more clearly mark their social and economic vulnerability because of prolonged deprivation from adequate health care, housing, and so on. And for the living – including those who survived the infection episode with lingering health problems – they endure what appears to be permanent disruptions. But for the socially vulnerable, these disruptions are much more than social inconveniences, separation, frustrations with quarantine, boredom, etc. They experience the disruptions in the form of unemployment, homelessness, debt, and abandonment; in short, they experience slow death. Sensing and feeling our existential vulnerability as well as the structural injustices, we mourn COVID, but the predominant way in which we do so has not been through grand public rituals, but more through quiet, lingering sadness. The affective and bodily registers are not lost on many of our contributors to this Special Issue, nor on us.

Indeed, the pandemic has been experienced somatically – sometimes deeply and immediately, as in when the symptoms of COVID manifest (or do not seem to abate); and sometimes more indistinctly, in the way all of us have been compelled to adjust habits, routines, itineraries, clothing choices, modes of self-presentation, and more. These bodily experiences, whether palpable or subtle, are anything but innocent. We mean this not only with respect to particular bodies, but also with regard to the ways in which collective changes in bodily dispositions can, like keywords, possibly instance more fundamental changes to shared conditions of existence. This was the primary argument of Elias' (2000) The Civilizing Process, whose analysis of etiquette books from 16th century Europe explored the connections between the emergence of the purportedly 'civilized' subject of Western modernity and new regimes of affect and bodily comportment. It is not insignificant that he coined the phrase 'structure of feelings' 15 years before its first appearance in Orron and Williams' (1954) Preface to Film, nor that he was a keen observer, like Williams, of cultural 'watchwords' (Elias 2000, pp. 24, 48).

Equally important is the figure whose work, in Elias' view, exemplified this new constellation of sentiments and somatic orientations: Erasmus of Rotterdam (1466–1536). Erasmus' writings are broad-ranging, but central to his repertoire were concerns about disease, public health, and hygiene: 'Turn away when spitting, lest your saliva fall on someone'; 'You should not offer your handkerchief to anyone unless it has been freshly washed' (quoted in Elias 2000, pp. 130, 123). Erasmus also had much to say about the proper places for urinating and defecating (*not* in public), the spread of sexually transmitted diseases, the need for cleanliness and sanitation, and the importance of good ventilation (Cole 1952, p. 530, Elias 2000, pp. 110–111). Notably, Erasmus' mother had died of plague when he was 13, and later, as an adult, he 'frequently moved to escape cholera or the plague – both being frequently observed' in 16th century Europe (Cole 1952, p. 530). Goudsblom (1986, p. 163) contends that 'fear of embarrassment, rather than a concern for health, was the prime reason' behind the brand of advice Erasmus was offering. Still, it is difficult to imagine that repeated outbreaks of plague, cholera, syphilis, and other rampaging diseases had no bearing on Erasmus' views on health and hygiene, nor on public acceptance of the practices he extolled.

Foucault (1977, 2007) makes a similar point. Though it is widely known that he credits Jeremy Bentham for having formulated the panopticon – the prison 'diagram' that emblematized bodily discipline – the plague's contribution to the disciplinary regime is perhaps less well acknowledged. To put it in no uncertain terms: *panopticism was prototyped in the plague*; or, as Foucault (1977, p. 197) puts it, when officials handed down a plague order, they were issuing 'a compact model of the disciplinary mechanism' (see also Foucault 2007, pp. 9–10). Browne (2015, pp. 31–33) further reminds us of how the panopticon was prompted by a voyage Bentham had undertaken in 1785 aboard a ship carrying 18 Black women, all enslaved. While Browne does not address the topic of disease directly, the subject was of paramount concern aboard slave vessels, having much to do with their architecture, their brutal schemes for stowing and managing (terrorizing) human cargo, etc. (see Rediker 2007, pp. 271–276).

The point of this brief historical detour – and, indeed, one of the purposes of this volume – is to conceptualize how pandemics and other disease processes act as contexts, or crucibles, for the emergence of novel structures of feeling and regimes of bodily comportment. This focus should not diminish the aforementioned project of keywords as much as enhance it, by renewing attention to the *gestures* by means of which are embodied specific modes of being, acting, living, dying, and surviving in the world. '[T]he observation of gestures,' Flusser (2014, p. 142) suggests, 'allows us to "decipher" the way we exist in the world. One of the implications of this hypothesis is that modifications we can observe in our gestures allow us to "read" the existential changes we are currently undergoing.' Flusser adds that 'whenever gestures appear that have never been seen before, we have *the key* to decoding a new form of existence' (p. 142; emphasis added). He seems to be proposing a project complementary to keywords, 'key gestures,' in which new techniques of bodily action (or the transformation of established ones) betoken more abstract adaptations to, and of, our shared conditions of existence.

One gesture that figures prominently in Flusser's (2014, pp. 91–97) work is deeply pertinent to the situation today: the gesture of turning a mask around – that is, the act of looking at the interior of a mask before affixing it to one's face. Because Flusser develops the example in relation to Carnival in Rio de Janeiro, the connection to infectious diseases might seem a distant one. The context is telling, however, in reminding us of the complex historical entanglements between disease, masks, and states of exception. Foucault (1977, p. 197–198) observes that, historically, Carnival wasn't strictly a harvest bacchanalia anticipating the long, cold winter ahead. It was also 'a political dream of the plague, which was exactly its reverse: not the collective festival, but strict divisions; not laws transgressed, but the penetration of regulation into even the smallest details of everyday life … ' Agamben (2005, pp. 71–72) goes even further in suggesting that the 'legal anarchy' characteristic of Carnival isn't reducible to the persistence of 'ancient agrarian rites' (c.f.: Bakhtin 1984). Instead, it 'brings to light in a parodic form the anomie within the law, the state of emergency [i.e. exception] as the anomic drive contained in the very heart of the *nomos*' (Agamben 2005, p. 72; emphasis in original).

Understood thus, one might better appreciate why the wearing of masks to help mitigate the spread of COVID-19 has become such a cultural-political flashpoint. The gesture occurs at the nexus of three distinct, if related, states of exception, each of which exists in tension with the other two:

(1) *the legal,* epitomized by the figures of Donald Trump and Jair Bolsonaro, whose opposition to mask mandates and other public health orders was not only widely embraced by their followers, but was also possibly a synecdoche for the hostility each administration has displayed toward to the rule of law;

(2) *the pandemic,* a modality identified as such by Patton (2011) following the SARS outbreak of 2002–2004, which refers to the complex negotiations around 'exceptional laws' and sovereignty that occur when public health crises transcend national borders;

(3) and *the carnivalesque,* which occupies an ambiguous position with respect to the preceding two categories – an apparent other and yet, paradoxically, also evidence of the normalization of a 'world turned upside down' (Stallybrass and White 1986).

The controversies surrounding the gesture of mask wearing also signal how the balance of forces between the three states of exception may be in a process of shifting. How else to explain the seemingly contradictory situation in Hong Kong, noted earlier, in which masks are at once mandated for public health reasons *and* outlawed in cases of political protest? Or similar contradictions in places where face veiling has been banned and criminalized before COVID struck (recall the numerous veil wars in France, etc.)? Or the perverse spectacle of Trump 'triumphantly' removing his mask upon returning to the White House following his emergency hospitalization for COVID? It goes without saying that the facemask-as-gesture is nothing less than a remaking of subjectivity in the shifting everyday anthropology of you/me, bareness/veiling, politeness/incivility, compliance/defiance, affectivity/emotionlessness, and so on. Let us remember that, in some ways, each dyad contains a touch of mourning: with the COVID mask, we grieve our separation, lament the lack of decorum and honesty in our leaders, and regret our sociality diminished through concealed smiles, fogged glasses, muffled voices, frustration, hidden sadness, and numbness.

No normal

There are few certainties where COVID-19 is concerned, but here, at least, is one: we are still very much in the midst of the pandemic. As we write these words, friends and family have taken to social media to mark their one-year COVID 'anniversaries,' mourning loved ones they have lost; posting pictures of precious objects from a year ago (toilet paper, disinfectant, bread …), objects whose status, though once again banal, seems more fragile than before; worrying about the future of employment; recalling the fear and anxiety of the pandemic's early days; reflecting, sometimes bitterly, on the acceptance of new customs and routines; for the lucky few, celebrating inoculations; and observing the whiplash-inducing effects of time passing over the course of an exceptional year. Collectively, these posts strike an ambivalent tone, ranging from 'look how far we've come' to 'look how much we've lost,' and 'maybe now we can return to normal' to 'how much more must we endure?' Meanwhile, nations in the Global North are refusing requests from the Global South to temporarily suspend intellectual property rights for COVID vaccines, thus stymieing efforts to produce cheaper, generic versions of these life-saving products (Reuters Staff 2021). As has often been the case with drugs for HIV/AIDS, the very places in which the 'state of exception' was prototyped (Mbembe 2019, 66–92) are being treated as if they were economically and epidemiologically unexceptional. Furthermore, with reports now surfacing about how COVID-19 is apt to become endemic (Phillips 2021), even in the wake of widespread vaccination in the Global North, the possibility of life 'after COVID' grows evermore faint. At best, it seems, we must learn to negotiate a life, a world, a futurity, *with* COVID.

Meanwhile, as COVID continues to dominate world news, other important life-saving public health work and scientific research has plowed ahead. The challenges of Ebola, HIV, dementia, diabetes, and many other diseases that plague humankind are just as important, but unfortunately, they fell by the wayside of global consciousness. The unprecedented race to develop COVID vaccines has been touted as 'truly historic' by many infectious disease experts and politicians. But how many of us have paid attention to the fact that a vaccine that took scientists years to develop to immunize against Ebola, was finally developed and licensed for use in June 2020, halting the outbreak in the Democratic Republic of Congo and in West Africa that had claimed thousands of lives since 2014 (Branswell 2020)? Major health organizations have also reported important advances in bio-markers for Alzheimer's disease and 'game-changing' developments in the fight against heart and kidney disease associated with diabetes (LaMotte 2020). Going forward with the knowledge of the COVID co-morbidities, as noted earlier, can we afford to neglect the battles in oncology, gene thera-pies, heart health, and so on *in relation to* controlling COVID and its present and future variants?

It would be inappropriate, then, to conclude anything. In closing, we merely wish to signal our hope for this Special Issue: to provide some intellec-tual guidance for the way forward – toward an uncertain future, without guarantees. The essays that follow are grouped into three thematic sections – 'Racializations,' 'Media, Data, and Fragments of the Popular,' and 'Un/knowing the Pandemic' – sections that animate, but do not exhaust, the complex cultural and political life of COVID-19 with respect to identity, technology, and epistem-ology. We fully expect readers to chart their own pathways through the issue, recognizing the realities of unbundled content, the unique ways in which the pandemic has affected us, and the myriad questions that arise when a new pathogen not only touches us all, but refuses to let go.

Acknowledgments

John Erni would like to acknowledge the Fung Hon Chu Foundation for its continued and generous support of his research in the humanities. Ted Striphas wishes to thank Phaedra C. Pezzullo for inspiration for this Special Issue, as well as for important con-versations and research leads that improved the Introduction. The authors also wish to acknowledge Logan Rae Gomez, Managing Editor of *Cultural Studies,* for her editorial assistance on the volume.

Disclosure statement

No potential conflict of interest was reported by the author(s).

Further information

This Special Issue article has been comprehensively reviewed by the Special Issue editors, Associate Professor Ted Striphas and Professor John Nguyet Erni.

References

AFP. 2021. Taiwan says "political pressure" blocking coronavirus vaccine deal [online]. *Hong Kong Free Press*, 18 Feb. Available from: https://hongkongfp.com/2021/02/18/taiwan-says-political-pressure-blocking-coronavirus-vaccine-deal/.

Agamben, G., 2005. *State of exception*. Chicago and London: University of Chicago Press.

Alberts, E.C. 2020. What's in a name? "Wet markets" may hide true culprits for COVID-19 [online]. *Mongabay*, 20 Apr. Available from: https://news.mongabay.com/2020/04/whats-in-a-name-wet-markets-may-hide-true-culprits-for-covid-19/.

Assy, B., and Hoffmann, F.F., 2020. Memento mori: COVID-19 and the political imaginary of death [online]. *Law, culture and the humanities*, Nov. doi:10.1177/1743872120971591.

Bakhtin, M., 1984. *Rabelais and his world*. Bloomington, IN: Indiana University Press.

Bennett, J.A., 2009. *Banning queer blood: Rhetorics of citizenship, contagion, and resistance*. Tuscaloosa, AL: University Alabama Press.

Bennett, J.A., 2019. *Managing diabetes: The cultural politics of disease*. New York: New York University Press.

Berlant, L., 2007. Slow death (sovereignty, obesity, lateral agency). *Critical inquiry*, 33, 754–780.

Branswell, H. 2020. "Against all odds": The inside story of how scientists across three continents produced an Ebola vaccine [online]. *STAT*, 7 January. Available from: https://www.statnews.com/2020/01/07/inside-story-scientists-produced-world-first-ebola-vaccine/.

Browne, S., 2015. *Dark matters: on the surveillance of Blackness*. Durham, NC: Duke University Press.

Canguilhem, G., 1991. *The normal and the pathological*. New York: Zone Books.

Certeau, M.d., 1984. *The practice of everyday life*. Berkeley, CA: University of California Press.

Chen, K.H., and Chua, B.H., eds., 2020. Special issue on the COVID-19 pandemic. *Inter-Asia cultural studies*, 21 (4).

Cheng, J.Y.S. ed. 2005. *The July 1 protest rally: interpreting a historic event*. Hong Kong: City University of Hong Kong Press.

Chung, H., 2020. Changing repertoires of contention in Hong Kong: A case study on the anti-extradition bill movement. *China perspectives* 2020 (3), 57–63.

Cole, H.N., 1952. Erasmus and his diseases. *JAMA: The journal of the American medical association*, 148 (7), 529–531.

Dias, B.L.C.V., and Deluchey, J.-F.Y., 2020. The "total continuous war" and the COVID-19 pandemic: neoliberal governmentality, disposable bodies and protected lives' [online]. *Law, culture and the humanities*, Nov. doi:10.1177/1743872120973157.

Dirks, N.B., 1992. Introduction: colonialism and culture. In: N.B. Dirks, ed. *Colonialism and culture*. Ann Arbor, MI: University of Michigan Press, 1–26.

Ejaz, H., *et al.*, 2020. COVID-19 and comorbidities: deleterious impact on infected patients. *Journal of infection and public health*, 13 (12), 1833–1839.

Elias, N., 2000. *The Civilizing Process: sociogenetic and psychogenetic investigations*. Revised edition. Oxford, UK and Malden, MA: Blackwell Publishing.

Erni, J.N., 2015. A legal realist view on citizen actions in Hong Kong's umbrella movement. *Chinese journal of communication*, 8 (4), 412–419.

Esposito, R., 2011. *Immunitas: The protection and negation of life*. Cambridge, UK: Polity.

Flusser, V., 2014. *Gestures*. Minneapolis: University of Minnesota Press.

Foucault, M., 1977. *Discipline and punish: the birth of the prison*. New York: Vintage Books.

Foucault, M., 1990. *The history of sexuality: an introduction*. New York: Vintage Books.

Foucault, M., 2007. *Security, territory, population: lectures at the Collège de France, 1977–1978*. New York: Picador.

Gates, K., and Leger, M., 2000. On how to have theory in an epidemic: an interview with Paula treichler. *Television & New media*, 1 (3), 383–395.

Goudsblom, J., 1986. Public health and the Civilizing process. *The milbank quarterly*, 64 (2), 160–188.

Griffiths, L. 2020, 3 August. Weaponizing Covid-19 [online]. *Scoop World*. https://www.scoop.co.nz/stories/WO2008/S00015/weaponizing-covid-19.htm.

Grossberg, L., 2010. *Cultural Studies in the future tense*. Durham, NC: Duke University Press.

Grossberg, L., 2018. *Under the cover of chaos: Trump and the battle for the American right*. London: Pluto Press.

Grover, J.Z. 1987. AIDS: keywords. *October*, 43, 17–30.

Ho, L.K.-K., 2020. Rethinking police legitimacy in postcolonial Hong Kong: paramilitary policing in protest management [online]. *Policing*, doi:10.1093/police/paaa064.

Hogue, S., 2020. The power of the "little brothers": surveillance and the future of democracy. In: B. Charbonneau, and C. Lavallée, ed. *COVID-19 and the future of global order* [online]. Centre for Security and Crisis Governance. Available from: https://ras-nsa.ca/publication/covid-19-and-the-future-of-global-order/.

Hui, M. 2020. Hong Kong police are using coronavirus restrictions to clamp down on protesters [online]. *Quartz*, 1 Apr. Available from: https://qz.com/1829892/hong-kong-police-use-coronavirus-rules-to-limit-protests/.

Human Rights Watch. 2020. Uganda: authorities weaponize Covid-19 for repression [online], 20 Nov. Available from: https://www.hrw.org/news/2020/11/20/uganda-authorities-weaponize-covid-19-repression.

Ibrahim, Z., and Lam, J. ed., 2020. *Rebel city: Hong Kong's year of water and fire.* Singapore: World Scientific Publishing.

Ip, I.C., 2019. *Hong Kong's new identity politics: longing for the local in the shadow of China.* New York: Routledge.

Ismail, Q., 2015. *Culture and eurocentrism.* London: Rowman & Littlefield International.

Jolicoeur, P., and Seaboyer, A. 2020. Comparing the weaponization of COVID-19 by China and Russia [online]. *Inside Policy*, 6 Sep. Available from: https://www.macdonaldlaurier.ca/comparing-weaponization-covid-19-china-russia/.

Kane, P.L. 2020. "Unresolved grief": Coronavirus presents eerie parallels for many AIDS advocates [online]. *The Guardian*, 22 Mar. Available from: https://www.theguardian.com/world/2020/mar/22/coronavirus-aids-epidemic-san-francisco.

Kaur, H. 2021. As attacks against Asian Americans spike, advocates call for action to protect communities [online]. *CNN*, 13 Feb. Available from: https://edition.cnn.com/2021/02/13/us/asian-american-attacks-covid-19-hate-trnd/index.html.

Klingberg, T., 2020. More than viral: outsiders, others, and the illusions of COVID-19. *Eurasian geography and economics*, 61 (4-5), 362–373. doi:10.1080/15387216.2020.1799833.

Ku, A.S., 2020. New forms of youth activism: Hong Kong's anti- extradition bill movement in the local-national-global nexus. *Space and polity*, 24 (1), 111–117.

Lamotte, S. 2020. Key 2020 health stories you may have missed because of Covid-19 [online]. *CNN*, 28 Dec. Available from: https://edition.cnn.com/2020/12/28/health/top-2020-health-stories-missed-wellness/index.html.

Law, W.S., 2018. Decolonization deferred: Hong Kong identity in historical perspective. In: L. Cooper, and W-M Lam, ed. *Citizenship, Identity and Social Movements in the New Hong Kong*. 1st ed. Milton: Routledge, 13–33.

Lee, F., 2020. Solidarity in the anti-extradition bill movement in Hong Kong. *Critical Asian studies*, 52 (1), 18–32.

Lee, F., *et al.*, 2019. Hong Kong's summer of uprising: from anti-extradition to anti-authoritarian protests. *China review*, 19 (4), 1–32.

Ma, N., 2018. Changing identity politics: The democracy movement in Hong Kong. In: L. Cooper, and W-M Lam, ed. *Citizenship, Identity and Social Movements in the New Hong Kong*. 1st ed. Milton: Routledge, 34–50.

Mbembe, A., 2019. *Necropolitics.* Durham and London: Duke University Press.

Morris, M., 1990. Banality in Cultural Studies. In: P. Mellencamp, ed. *Logics of television: essays in cultural criticism.* Bloomington, IN: Indiana University Press, 14–43.

Orrom, M., and Williams, R., 1954. *Preface to film.* London: Film Drama Ltd.

Pang, L.K., 2020. *The appearing demos: Hong Kong during and after the umbrella movement.* Ann Arbor: University of Michigan Press.

Patton, C., 1990. *Inventing AIDS.* New York: Routledge.

Patton, C., 2002. *Globalizing AIDS.* Minneapolis: University of Minnesota Press.

Patton, C., 2011. Pandemic, empire, and the permanent state of exception. *Economic and political weekly*, 46 (13), 103–110.

Perrot, L., Boyette, C., and Asmelash, L. 2021. At least 109 employees at a colorado ski resort have tested positive for Covid-19 [online]. *CNN*. Available from: https://www.cnn.com/2021/02/12/us/colorado-ski-covid-19-outbreak-trnd/index.html.

Peters, M.A., 2020. Žlžek on China and COVID-19: Wuhan, authoritarian capitalism, and empathetic socialism in NZ [online]. *Educational philosophy and theory*, doi:10.1080/00131857.2020.1801122.

Pezzullo, P.C., 2007. *Toxic tourism: Rhetorics of pollution, travel, and environmental justice*. Tuscaloosa, AL: University of Alabama Press.

Pezzullo, P.C., 2012. What gets buried in a small town: Toxic E-waste and democratic frictions in the crossroads of the United States. In: S. Foote, and E. Mazzolini, ed. *Histories of the dustheap: Waste, material cultures, social justice*. Cambridge, MA: MIT Press, 119–146.

Pezzullo, P.C., 2014. Contaminated children: debating the banality, precarity, and futurity of chemical safety. *Resilience: A journal of the environmental humanities*, 1 (2). doi:10.5250/resilience.1.2.004

Pezzullo, P.C., and Depoe, S.P., 2010. Everyday life and death in a nuclear world: stories from Fernald. In: R. Asen, and D. Brouwer, ed. *Public modalities: rhetoric, culture, and he shape of public life*. Tuscaloosa, AL: University of Alabama Press, 85–108.

Phillips, N., 2021. The coronavirus is here to stay—here's what that means. *Nature*, 590, 382–384.

Purbrick, M., 2020. Hong Kong: the torn city. *Asian affairs*, 51 (3), 463–484.

Rediker, M., 2007. *The slave ship: A human history*. New York: Penguin Books.

Reuters Staff. 2021. Rich, developing nations wrangle over COVID vaccine patents [online]. *Reuters*, 11 Mar. Available from: https://www.reuters.com/article/us-health-coronavirus-wto-idUSKBN2B21V9?taid=6049610eeaf59800011cdad3&utm_campaign=trueanthem&utm_medium=trueanthem&utm_source=twitter [Accessed 12 Mar 2021].

Sanyaolu, A. 2020. Comorbidity and its Impact on Patients with COVID-19 [online]. *SN Comprehensive Clinical Medicine*, 25 Jun. Available from: https://www.ncbi.nlm.nih.gov/pmc/articles/PMC7314621/pdf/42399_2020_Article_363.pdf.

Seigworth, G., 2000. Banality for Cultural Studies. *Cultural studies*, 14 (2), 227–268.

Stallybrass, P., and White, A., 1986. *The politics and poetics of transgression*. Ithaca, NY: Cornell University Press.

Sterne, J., 2017. What is an intervention? *TOPIA: Canadian journal of cultural studies*, 37, 5–14.

Striphas, T., 2016. Culture. In: B. Peters, ed. *Digital keywords: A Vocabulary of Information society and culture*. Princeton, NJ: Princeton University Press, 70–80.

Tai, B., *et al.*, 2019. Pursuing democracy in an authoritarian state: protest and the rule of law in Hong Kong. *Social & legal studies*, 29 (1), 107–145.

Thompson, D. 2020. The Scourge of Hygiene Theater [online]. *The Atlantic*. Available from: https://www.theatlantic.com/ideas/archive/2020/07/scourge-hygiene-theater/614599/ [Accessed 8 Mar 2021].

Thompson, E.P., 1961. The long revolution (review, parts I & II). *New left review* (9–10), 24–39.

Timberg, C., and Halperin, D., 2012. *Tinderbox: how the west sparked the AIDS epidemic and How the world can finally overcome It*. New York: Penguin Press.

Todman, W. 2020. Assad attempts to weaponize COVID-19 in Syria [online]. *The Hill*, 27 May. Available from: https://thehill.com/opinion/international/498943-assad-attempts-to-weaponize-covid-19-in-syria.

Treichler, P.A., 1999. *How to have theory in an epidemic: a cultural chronicle of AIDS.* Durham, NC: Duke University Press.

Vukovich, D., 2020. A city and a SAR on fire: as if everything and nothing changes. *Critical Asian studies*, 52 (1), 1–17. doi:10.1080/14672715.2020.1703296.

Wald, P., 2008. *Contagious: cultures, carriers, and the outbreak narrative.* Durham and London: Duke University Press.

Wan, K.M., *et al.* 2020. Fighting COVID-19 in Hong Kong: The effects of community and social mobilization [online], *World Development*, 134. Available from: https://www.sciencedirect.com/science/article/pii/S0305750X20301819.

Williams, R., 1958. *Culture and society, 1780-1950.* New York: Columbia University Press.

Williams, R., 1983. *Keywords: a vocabulary of culture and society.* Rev. Ed. New York: Oxford University Press.

Yancy, G. 2020. Judith butler: mourning is a political act amid the pandemic and its disparities [online]. *Truthout*, Apr 30. Available from: https://truthout.org/articles/judith-butler-mourning-is-a-political-act-amid-the-pandemic-and-its-disparities/.

Racializations

COVID -19 and the mundane practices of privilege

Kumarini Silva

ABSTRACT

Moving between the 2015 elections, Covid-19 and the sustained social justice protests in the United States in this essay, I question where and how the pursuit of joy, remedies for boredom and practices of self-care relate to the necropolitical social hierarchies in the United States. In spite of popular declarations that the virus is 'the great equalizer', there is considerable evidence that Covid-19 devastates along established systems of power, rights and values that organize the cultural practices of the everyday. This is especially visible in those who seek self-care from the anxieties of the pandemic, and how and why they seek such care. Driven by a combination of guilt and privilege, along with a deliberate misreading of Audre Lorde's notion of self-care as an act of political warfare, these words and their corresponding practices animate a hubristic right to the good life even at the end of capitalism. Given this, I ask how in the midst of mutating pathological social and political conditions and their corresponding discomforts, self-care and the search for joy have become imbricated in narratives of progressive politics.

(In)#the beginning

Since March 2020, when self-isolation and lockdowns were initiated – in response to the Covid-19 pandemic – the words *joy, boredom* and *self-care* have proliferated across social media and in private conversations, their implicature far exceeding their denotations. Certainly, the need for care of oneself, the desire to feel joy and a sense of beleaguered boredom are widespread, and yet I've grappled with a sense of deep discomfort at the way these words are routinely evoked as a loss of something that is *owed* to the utterer. For example, two recent interactions with acquaintances are emblematic of the ways that words manifest classed and raced losses in this particular moment: one lamenting the lack of *joy* in their life because their regular activities – in particular shopping and vacations – have been interrupted; and the other prioritizing *self-care* because all the news *is just too much*. As these words continue to percolate cross social media and in 'socially distanced' gatherings, they also feed my recent preoccupation with the relationship between love and cruelty, where I contend that love is only recognizable by the intensity of the cruelty that is exerted in the name of that love (Silva 2018). So, where and how does the pursuit of joy, the remedies for boredom, and the practices of self-care reproduce a form of cruelty that is so mundane as to be unrecognizable to even the most thoughtful amongst us? In what ways has American liberal politics emerged over time that allows these words to evade scrutiny in the same way that rabid conservative political performances are scrutinized and critiqued? Certainly the populist movement against masks is easily recognizable as a willful desire to ignore the depth and breadth of the crisis. Take, for example, the obviously racist connotation of comparing isolation and masks to slavery, religious freedom objections, or the well-documented and demented proclamations of the 45th president about the virus. Such utterances are open to criticism from scientific and social positions that are straightforward or less opaque and convoluted than considering the (shorter) long history of care words and their implications that I take up here.

For me, the use of words like boredom, joy and self-care are animated by broader social systems that organize our daily lives, and their use (and misuse) as we navigate 'twin pandemics' – Covid-19 and racism, resulting in the most sustained civil rights movement in the USA since the 1960s – shows how inequality flourishes in a faux-democratic capitalist society in the most ordinary of ways. Essentially, habitus (Bourdieu 2002)[1] becomes a *right* – a right to the good life – even when we are in the midst of sustained chaos and that lamenting its loss as affective pathologies that need remediation has become acceptable.

In focusing on these words and their broader context, I want to consider how the good life becomes one that rests firmly within the necropolitical (Mbembé and Meintjes 2003) hierarchies of the United States and, as such, what they can portent; to tell us of things to come. Such observations, while not new, are an invitation to consider the relationship between mundane words, history, and embodied realities at the end of capitalism. And the ways in which that end is imagined or felt by groups of people follow long established systems of power, rights – including the right to live, the right to die, the right to sacrifice life – and values that organize the cultural practices of the everyday.

Culture and care in (extra)ordinary times

'Anxiety' as the problem and 'self-care' as the solution have been staples in popular culture in recent years (Harris 2017).[2] Especially since the presidential elections of 2015 – with the seemingly[3] shocking defeat of Hillary Clinton – addressing anxiety through self-care, while finding joy in the midst of chaos, have become the words and statements that routinely frame public and private conversations, especially amongst middle-to-upper class, white identified populations. Having politically mobilized – for the first time for many voters – in some magical pursuit of the 'first female president of the United States', that loss manifested in a crisis that underscored their already privileged existence.

That many of these calls for care were part of the process of dealing with 'guilt' – based on the oft cited (and questionable[4]) statistic that 52 percent of white women voters voted for candidate Trump, and guilt by association for being white (or white passing), and/or economically and socially privileged (and therefore less vulnerable to the policies that would follow those election results) – went largely unexamined, or perhaps were too complicated and messy to examine. Contradiction is after all, the de-facto state of this American life,[5] and performative self-care as absolutely necessary for *this particular moment* continues to flourish. One can listen to podcasts, read newsletters and share images about lessons learned, lessons given and lessons shared about #livingyourbestlife with #gratitude even as the economy crashes, unemployment numbers continue to rise and rates of infection multiply. Regardless of the continuing deterioration of the socio-political and economic systems in the United States since the start of the pandemic – including an unstable stock market, a snowballing housing crisis,[6] increasing unemployment figures[7] and sustained social justice protests across the country – the notion that one is entitled to the performed joys of a good life has made a seamless transition to pandemic life.

Perhaps the most ubiquitous and egregious manipulation of this entitlement has been the ways the social justice protests have been folded into the affective pathologies of Covid-19. By this, I mean that so much of the self-care language is also based on the appropriation of an anger and corresponding anxiety about the state of race and racism rather than any direct experience with the condition. For example, Robin DiAngelo's *White Fragility* has been shared widely as a 'must read' on social media, and these endorsements of the book are often accompanied by vows to do the 'heavy lifting' of recognizing white privilege, and a commitment to 'do better', even if that 'work is hard'. This proxy anger and anxiety has also become a justification for self-care. It relies heavily on a co-optation (or deliberate misreading) of Audre Lorde's powerful call to care for oneself in the face of trauma as a form of 'political warfare'. That Lorde saw self-care as a necessary tool for survival in the long and bloody battle for the recognition of one's humanity – and not as a salve for joyous-interruptus – seems irrelevant to those who co-opt the ethico-political aspects of it. As a consequence of 'radicalizing' through care, self-care is deployed through a reinvestment in white middle-class performance of home economics. And, as part of this radical care – in addition to meditation, sewing (facemasks), baking (sourdough), vacations near remote waterways – we are also invited to engage in social media and news cleanses as *acts of political resistance*. Such bucolic pastimes, and the resulting and necessary corollary disengagements are in ironic contrast to the ways that social movements, which are necessarily framed by radical care politics[8], engage in their activism. The Black Lives Matter movement, for example, relies on social and news media to organize, to share safety tips, and politics and policy news that affect their activism that are more in-line with Lorde's notion of radical self-care.[9] Ultimately, for one group 'taking a break' and disengaging from political and social knowledge in the midst of civil unrest is a form of (de) politicized self-care, while for another such performative kinds of care lead to arrests, incarceration, and even death. This cognitive dissonance between those most affected and those seeking self-care and joy reflect the ways such the longer history of such care culture has most recently manifest itself in United States, especially since 2015.[10] In fact, that cognitive dissonance facilitates the most mythologized systematic social structure in the United States: it bolsters a hubristic, unjust and deeply violent system that still believes in meritocracy, even while evidence to the contrary, as I document below, continues to multiply in these times.[11]

The (not so) great equalizer

On March 31st, in a widely recirculated tweet, New York Governor Andrew Cuomo declared SARS-CoV-2 the 'great equalizer' as his brother, news personality Chris Cuomo, announced his Covid-19 positive diagnosis. This declaration was among the first of several such claims regarding the 'democratic' nature of the virus by public officials and medical experts (UNICEF 2020). It's ability to kill 'indiscriminately' marked Covid-19 as unusual – and therefore, especially distressing – in a country that is conditioned to carefully and systematically demarcate the value of human life based on numerous categories and hierarchies too long to note here (and perhaps unnecessary, given their conspicuousness).

In a system where politicians blithely declare that slavery was a 'necessary evil' (Cole 2020) at the same time that protests against the routine murders of black lives continue to take place across the country, Covid-19 as the great morbid equalizer has also continued to magnify existing inequities. As such, while the indiscriminate aspects of the virus, *in theory*, upended the fiction of everyday life for an equally fictitious 'average' American, its longer reach into economic and social spaces has also meant that class/caste politics of precarity and privilege reasserts itself in the ubiquitous laments about the loss of joy through restricted travel, working from home, and in the ways that boredom emerges as a melancholic malaise, ala Freud (1917). Covid-19 then is perceived as an interruption of an imagined copacetic life, and this imagined 'loss' results in a melancholia that animates the need for self-care, and a search for joy. In this search risk/reward falls neatly within the aforementioned precarious/privileged structures of the (extra)ordinary lives of Americans.

For example, even as Covid-19 cases continued to rise in the southern part of the country, where I live, a recent email thread amongst a neighborhood listserv asked for a 'playdate' for their bored pre-teen. The parent also noted that the unsupervised children would be responsible for maintaining social distance, and that while they hope for a playdate in the immediate neighbor-hood they were also open to driving further out. All this, the parent claimed, would give everyone a 'few hours of reprieve'. This parent's request, while more direct, is no different than other comments about the pleasure in the neighborhood coffee shop 'choosing' to stay open because it provides them with somewhere to go and something to do, the capitalist exchange of money and goods providing a 'some sense of normalcy' and an interrup-tion in the monotony and boredom of isolation.

In these declarations of boredom in the face of a deadly virus is a malaise that needs to be 'fixed' through activities that aggressively counter the advice of medical professionals regarding the spread and longevity of the virus itself. But in these interactions the myth of Covid-19 as the great equalizer is upended, since the normalcy and entertainment of one population relies on the labour of another, more hyper-vulnerable population.

For example, *The Guardian* noted on April 8th, that 'While New York's Gov-ernor Andrew Cuomo once called the coronavirus a "great equalizer", data shows the virus has been anything but indiscriminate'. The data the newspa-per referenced was reports from the Economic Policy Institute that show that 'African Americans face a higher risk of exposure to the virus, mostly on account of concentrating in urban areas and **working in essential industries** [my emphasis]'. Only 20 percent of black workers reported being eligible to work from home compared with about 30 percent of their white counterparts (Evelyn 2020). Similar news stories that indicate that African Americans are dying of the virus at greater rates than any other community in the country (Erdman 2020), and that the virus is spreading rapidly in prisons, where social distancing is not possible, and where the inmate population is also likely to be disproportionately African American have also been made public (Williams *et al.* 2020). Such broadly generalized statistical information of the impact of the virus on marginalized communities is juxtaposed against the humanized, and human-interest focused cases (like that of Chris Cuomo) that have become popular on both social media and the press. In fact, as Cuomo was recovering, his wife, Cristina Cuomo and their son also contracted the virus. Their condition, in intimate detail, appeared daily in the press, and Cuomo provided minute details of the impact of the virus on his body, both on twitter and through his news program that he continued to telecast from home. Following their recovery (success story!), Cristina Cuomo has chronicled their 'approach' to recovery in her lifestyle blog under an entry titled 'Cristina Cuomo Corona Protocol Week 3'. In the lengthy post she details their use of, amongst other remedies,[12] 8–10 h of restful sleep each night, a spirometer to oxygenate the lungs, Ayurvedic food from a local restaurant, at-home vitamin C drips and yoga and meditation, directly quoting her yogi who says that 'these conscious, deep breathing exercises activate a life force within us to help us attain a higher state of vibratory energy. They create space in the body and a feeling of joy and ease in the mind and heart' (thepuristonline.com). She ends the entry with quotes from Martin Luther King, Jr. and her brother-in-law, both which reference love.[13]

If my engagement with the Cuomo's treatment plan seems lengthy here, it is for a reason: Cuomo's expensive, and medically unsubstantiated claims to wellness *are wielded with the same normalcy that the melancholic malaise of boredom, and the search for joy in these times deployed by the differently privileged examples I bring up earlier*. And in turn, they are no different than the kinds of care that were popularized and the demographic they were dispensed to, following the elections of 2015.

While individual economic and corresponding social conditions of each of these examples – from politically disappointed progressives in 2015 to Trump-loathing Cuomos in 2020 – may be different, what they share is the belief in a right to the good life that I started this commentary with. One that balances the right amount of activity and nourishment (both consumable and material) that signifies an imagined permanence in their social positions and a stability in their way of live. This stable mirage relies on the labour of entire cross sections of population that have little-to-no access to the kind of leisured boredom that Covid-19 produced for the middle and upper-middle classes, seems of little consequence. It is a form of thoughtless, mundane cruelty, that emerges from a much longer history, which includes settler colonialism and slavery, that established contemporary systems of value for human life. This history, which created systems of racialized hierarchies along economic desires and developments, manifest and mutate even more in the midst of the pandemic. For example, in the addition to the aforementioned Covid-19 impact on African American communities, its devastation on long neglected Native American communities is equally brutal (Friedler 2020). But because practices of systemic genocide are commonplace and even legally and structurally instituted and rationalized over generations (Wagner and Grantham-Phillips 2020), they are hardly noteworthy for those who lament boredom.

End (Times)

The sustained search for a remedy for the malaise of anxiety and disruption Covid-19 brings is not unique to the virus. As with most such events –

whether it is an event like the 9/11bombing or the November 2015 elections more recently – the aforementioned interruption to the good life, as imagined or lived (in most cases the former) certainly brings on a sense of discombobulation. But perhaps the 'difference' we see in the Covid-19 pandemic is that it cast a wider net to bring a previously, relatively shielded cross-sections of the population into the existing necropolitical social fold of this country. That money could not buy medical help (though it did and continues to provide access to different levels of care as I've documented here), nor provide a respite from enforced isolation or even loss, and that it's specific violence is felt intimately, which no amount to cathartic meditation could remedy, certainly produces, in the face of things, Covid-19 as 'different'. And this difference has also meant that broader political shifts and conditions are more intimately felt by populations that been long shielded from the underbelly of American exceptionalism. While political scandals – like Watergate – and civil unrest – whether they are the movements of the 1960s, the LA riots of the 90s, or the more recent protests – have always existed they have also had a different material and temporal insistence in the lives of those not connected to these embodied politics in their daily lives. After all, while Baltimore protested the murder of Freddie Gray, people outside that immediate context and even the neighborhood continued to live their lives, shopping, cooking, raising families, going to work, and socializing.

But now the convergence of a despotic presidency, the continuing fight for civil rights, and a deadly virus forces a reckoning with reality that is deeply unsettling for even those of us who claim a progressive politic. In the midst of all these mutant forces and their corresponding discomfort, self-care and the search for joy then become master terms for reasserting class and economic privilege in the most casually cruel of ways. Such determination is not without precedence, certainly history tells us that. But that determination for an imagined stability, as well as the active participation in that fiction, has also led us to this moment.

This was made even clearer when Covid-19 and the US presidential elections converged under the umbrella of self-care. In the months leading up to the elections on 3 November 2020, entreaties on behalf of the Democratic party, especially on social media, repeatedly invoked better times and a 'return' to 'normalcy' under a Biden/Harris administration.

Certainly, from perspective of anyone with a modicum of intelligence or empathy, 4 more years of the current administration would have been excruciating, and even deadly for a large cross-section of the population; but the notion that we would 'return' to some briefly misplaced past that was universally stable is what is relevant here. Such nostalgic waxing carried with it the same trace of privileged longing that framed the more direct calls for self-care and the right to joy.[14] If we juxtapose the imagined stability that was supposedly 'regained' with the presidential elections against the growing number of Covid-19 cases and fatalities, the increasing numbers of unemployed, the snails-pace distribution of the vaccines, and the meager $600 check approved by the latest stimulus bill, which will increase the savings of the middle and upper middle-class, while providing almost no support for the working classes, a picture emerges of what we can expect in the future: a 'settling' of sorts, along established class, race, and economic lines in the United States, where the gap between those who have resources and the ability to save and increase those resources – and through that, practice self-care in emotional and material forms – and those who either straddled the line between managing and plunging, or those who were already struggling, will be far greater than it has been in recent history. As such, interrogating the interlocking and far-reaching consequences of care – of self and other – as it has emerged over the last several months, and putting it in conversation with broader political and economic systems and their longer histories is especially important as we contemplate the emerging and precarious future where disease, poverty, and environmental and social crises converge. The mundane life practices of Covid-19 are neither outside nor independent of these conditions. Indeed, if we are to learning anything from the 'twin pandemics' and a deranged world leader, it is that without a more critical interrogation of our most mundane practices – with particular attention to the ways we justify and manipulate our own individual needs, dressing it up as forms of radical care – we will likely see far more dire consequences than an immediate loss of joy.

Notes

1. Bourdieu (2002) defines habitus as 'a system of *dispositions*, that is of permanent manners of being, seeing, acting and thinking, or a system of *long-lasting* (rather than permanent) schemes or schemata or structures of perception, conception and action'. While habitus has gone out of fashion in academia, I find Bourdieu's work useful here because of the way he is attentive to the temporality of practices and schemata in both physical and social spaces.
2. Harris (2017) notes that 'The week after the election, Americans Googled the term almost twice as often as they ever had in years past'.
3. I say 'seemingly' here because to assume that her election was predetermined also speaks directly to the unspoken privileges that even the more progressive amongst us engage in. Essentially, to not be prepared for the eventual outcome of that election in 2016 indicates a level of faith in the existing system that the more vulnerable amongst us, from experience, do not have.
4. https://time.com/5422644/trump-white-women-2016/
5. Political and social life in the United States consistently focuses on single issues rather than addressing them as intersecting concerns. For example, we can focus on race or sexism, but not both.
6. https://www.theatlantic.com/ideas/archive/2020/07/americas-health-crisis-is-becoming-a-housing-crisis/614149/

7. As I write this, in mid-2020, the unemployment rate is at 11.1% (https://www.bls.gov/news.release/pdf/empsit.pdf).
8. While there is no space here to go into its longer history, self-care as healthcare was popularized starting in 1950s by the Black Panther movement. In Beyond Berets: The Black Panthers as Health Activist (2016). Mary T. Bassett writes that the Black Panther's ' … vision hewed closely to the fundamentally radical idea that achieving health for all demands a more just and equitable world' (1741).
9. BLM uses the hashtag #blacklivesmatter as a geotag of sorts to communicate with activists on the ground, and to share information about vital care in the spaces they are protesting in.
10. Prior to, and since his election, the 45th president's policies have most negatively impacted the most vulnerable populations in this country, including women, people of colour, and the poor.
11. In my college level classrooms, 'hard work' is always a response I get when I ask how one becomes wealthy in the United States. The correct answer, which is that one must inherit wealth in order to be rich, always seems to surprise students.
12. She also recommends Hydrochlorine baths that have been widely refuted as ineffective by medical practitioners.
13. She writes: Not all of the treatments I talk about here are for everyone, but we can all benefit from eating well and keeping our immunity up. 'Returning hate for hate multiplies hate, adding deeper darkness to a night already devoid of stars. Darkness cannot drive out darkness; only light can do that. Hate cannot drive out hate, only love can do that', said Martin Luther King Jr. And, as our trusted New York governor said, 'Love wins'. https://thepuristonline.com/2020/04/cristina-cuomo-corona-protocol-week-3/
14. Certainly to imagine that this election – framed by white middle and upper-middle class notions of 'electability' and trickle-down policies – is anything more than middle-class self-care, is hubris.

Disclosure statement

No potential conflict of interest was reported by the author(s).

Further information

This Special Issue article has been comprehensively reviewed by the Special Issue editors, Associate Professor Ted Striphas and Professor John Nguyet Erni.

References

Bassett, M.T., 2016. Beyond berets: The Black Panthers as health activists. *American journal of public health*, 106 (10), 1741–1743.

Bourdieu, P., 2002. Habitus. In: J Hillier, and E Rooksby, ed. *Habitus: A sense of place*. Burlington, VT: Ashgate, 27–34.

Cole, D., 2020. Tom Cotton describes slavery as a 'necessary evil' in bid to keep schools from teaching 1619 Project. *CNN.org*. Available from: https://www.cnn.com/2020/07/27/politics/tom-cotton-slavery-necessary-evil-1619-project/index.html [Accessed 28 July 2020].

Cuomo, A., 2020a. Twitter post. March 31. 1213 hrs.

Cuomo, C., 2020b. Cristina cuomo corona protocol, Week 3. *The Purist*. Available from: https://thepuristonline.com/2020/04/cristinacuomo-corona-protocol-week-3/ [Accessed 24 April 2020].

Erdman, S. L., 2020. Black communities account for disproportionate number of Covid-19 deaths in the US, study Finds. *CNN.com*. Available from: https://www.cnn.com/2020/05/05/health/coronavirus-african-americans-study/index.html [Accessed 6 May 2020].

Evelyn, K., 2020. 'It's a racial justice issue': Black Americans are dying in greater numbers from Covid-19. *The Guardian*. Available from: https://www.theguardian.com/world/2020/apr/08/its-a-racial-justice-issue-black americans-are-dying-in-greater-numbers-from-covid-19 [Accessed 9 April 2020].

Friedler, D., 2020. Indian country has entered a devastating new phase of the pandemic. *Mother Jones*, December 4, 2020. Available from: https://www.motherjones.com/coronavirus-updates/2020/12/indian-country-has entered-a-devastating-new-phase-of-the-pandemic/ [Accessed 5 December 2020].

Freud, S., 1917. Mourning and melancholia. The standard edition of the complete psychological works of Sigmund Freud, Volume XIV (1914–1916): On the history of the psycho-analytic movement, papers on metapsychology and other works, 237–258.

Harris, A., 2017. A history of self-care in slate. Available from: http://www.slate.com/articles/arts/culturebox/2017/04/the_history_of_self_care.html [Accessed 8 April 2017].

Mbembé, A., and Meintjes, L., 2003. Necropolitics. *Public culture*, 15 (1), 11–40.

Silva, K., 2018. Having the time of our lives: love-cruelty as patriotic impulse. *Communication and critical/cultural studies*, 15, 79–84.

UNICEF Statement, 2020. COVID-19 does not discriminate; nor should our response. Available from: https://www.unicef.org/press-releases/covid-19-does-not-discriminate-nor-should-our-response [Accessed 16 July 2020].

Wagner, D., and Grantham-Philips, W., 2020. 'Still killing us': The federal government underfunded health care for Indigenous people for centuries. Now they're dying of COVID-19. *USAToday*, October 26. Available from: https://www.usatoday.com/in-depth/news/nation/2020/10/20/native-american-navajo-nation-coronavirus-deaths-underfunded-health-care/5883514002/ [Accessed 5 December 2020].

Williams, T., *et al.*, 2020. Coronavirus cases rise sharply in prisons even as they plateau nationwide. *The New York Times*. Available from: https://www.nytimes.com/2020/06/16/us/coronavirus-inmates prisons-jails.html [Accessed 16 June 2020].

Following the science? COVID-19, 'race' and the politics of knowing

John Clarke ⓛ

ABSTRACT
The UK government has consistently claimed to be 'following the science' in its approach to the pandemic but this claim conceals complex and shifting entanglements of politics and science. The instability of the relationship between politics and science became increasingly visible around the unequal vulnerability of racialized minorities to infection and death from Covid-19. How and when Black and other minoritized deaths matter has become the focus of UK governmental efforts to delay and deflect, in what has been claimed to be the 'best country in the world to be a black person'. Rather than the rule of Science, what the pandemic reveals are the conjunctural contested articulations of science(s) and politics.

This is an unprecedented global pandemic and we have taken the right steps at the right time to combat it, guided at all times by the best scientific advice.

(UK Government spokesperson quoted in the *Guardian*, 22 May 2020, p. 15)

Covid-19 has been both universal and particular: it has connected places around the world in new configurations, breaking established flows and installing new ones. Responses to it have taken distinct national and local forms as governments attempt to manage, control or even ignore the threats to their populations. Here I concentrate on some of the particular political-cultural dynamics of the United Kingdom (while recognizing that its different constituent nations have taken some diverging routes). In particular, I focus on the relationship between science and politics in the response to the pandemic, the racialized inequalities of vulnerability and their interweaving with the insistent claim that 'Black Lives Matter'.

The pandemic – and governmental reactions to it – have evoked many critical responses. Perhaps one of the most far-reaching is Giorgio Agamben's claim that 'the threshold that separates humanity from barbarism has been crossed'. He argued that this transition results from the drive of science to 'split the unity of our vital experience, which is always inseparably bodily and spiritual, into a purely biological entity on one hand and an affective and cultural life on the other.' This spilt has been enabled by 'The Church above all, which, in making itself the handmaid of science, which has now become the true religion of our time, has radically repudiated its most essential principles.' (2020, p. 4). In the UK, as the opening quotation shows, the claim to be 'following the science' has been a recurring theme of the government's approach. This would appear to confirm Agamben's view of the pandemic as enabling the rule of the 'religion of science'.

And yet, I am troubled by two things. First, my experience of the coronavirus lockdown feels strangely different to Agamben's: mine has featured contestation, controversy, outrage and diverse social and political responses. Second, it is not long since attention was being focused on the rise of an anti-intellectual populism in Europe and parts of the Americas. This odd conjunction makes me wonder – and worry – about excessively abstracted conceptions of both science and politics in the face of their currently shifting articulations. Four years ago, many people (including me) were exploring the crystallization of contemporary populist politics around 'anti-expertise' and 'anti-science' arguments in favour of the wisdom of common sense. The position was crisply expressed by the UK Brexit enthusiast and MP Michael Gove in his claim that 'The British People have had enough of experts' (http://www.telegraph.co.uk/news/2016/06/10/michaelgoves-guide-to-britains-greatest-enemy-the-experts; see also Clarke and Newman 2017). In many places, the emergence of what Maskovsky and Bjork-James (2019) have called 'angry politics' was accompanied by a distinctive strain of 'epistemological populism' whose continuing effects remain unevenly visible, in Jair Bolsanoro's Brazil or in the daily psychodrama of Donald Trump's fraught relationship with expertise. Yet in the UK, those politicians who once formed the avant-garde of anti-elitist 'common-sense' have consistently claimed to be 'Following the Science' during this current crisis.

1. Entangling science and politics

This performative deployment of Politics doing the bidding of Science, as if both formations were coherent and singular objects, was recurrently accompanied by a manly rhetoric of 'Having a Plan' (often associated with 'straining every sinew' or 'working day and night' to make it come true). However, this proclaimed unity of science and politics became increasingly unsettled, pulled in different and diverging directions (see Bacevic 2020). Instead, we saw the increasingly fraught entangling of science and politics, with politicians claiming to be merely 'following the science' while scientists complained about being put into a 'political situation'. At one point, Prime Minister Johnson refused to allow government scientists to answer what he defined as 'political questions', specifically about the conduct of his special advisor, Dominic Cummings, in relation to the lockdown rules advocated by the scientists. Among the emerging tangles were:

- The heightened public visibility of science as plural, contestable and incomplete;
- A combative assertion of the 'scientific method' as involving errors, doubts, arguments and probability;
- The sudden disappearance of international comparative mortality data when it became clear that the UK was 'world beating' in its failures (Jones 2020);
- A proliferation of sciences and scientists, and a complex dynamic of inclusion and exclusion of types of science;
- A renewed enthusiasm for those sciences clustered around 'techno-determinism' as the solution to our troubles (for example, in contact tracing) and the relative absence of 'social' sciences;
- And, not least, shifts in which modes of knowledge are valued or excluded. For example, 'experience' based knowledge rarely appears in the policy process but had profoundly disruptive effects in news reports which juxtaposed governmental claims about Protective Personal Equipment (PPE) and accounts from front line workers.

These shifting configurations feel very different from the conception of Science and Politics on offer in a range of critical approaches – in which, to put it crudely, *everything is political* and needs to be revealed as such. Collectively, we have demystified Science, Scientism and the dominant apparatuses of knowledge, justification and calculation – the power-knowledge couplings of our age. But this foundational view of things being political makes it difficult to explore the specific and shifting conjunctural articulations of politics and science.

2. Who gets to die?

Despite governmental claims that 'we are all in this together' (an established Conservative trope), COVID-19 turned out to be anything but an even-handed pandemic. Rather, its impact has been profoundly unequally distributed: in the UK, it has disproportionately affected older people, poor people, people working in low paid but 'essential' occupations (from health and social care to the food chain), and people who are not 'white British' (in census category terms). These are, obviously, not separate categories: racialized minorities in the UK are more likely to live in poverty, to be concentrated in low paid employment and form a disproportionately large part of the health care and social care workforces. Their vulnerability to the virus forms an all too predictable outcome of a pandemic traversing the biopolitics of a racially structured capitalist social formation. This is hardly unique to the UK, but there are distinctively national features of how such biopolitics are translated into policies, practices and, not least, systematic political amnesia.

These unevenly distributed deaths came to public – and eventually political – attention at the intersection of two dynamics: first, the distinctively urban concentrations of the early weeks of the UK pandemic (London and urban centres in the West and East Midlands, all with significant racialized-minoritized populations) and second, the astonishingly visible – literally through the regular publication of their photographs – deaths of 'front line' health and care workers who were disproportionately 'not white British'. As a result, the country became familiar with a distinctive acronym: these were 'BAME [Black, Asian and Minority Ethnic] deaths'. Politicians, health experts, newsreaders and journalists struggled to sound confident in deploying this term which had emerged as a government nomenclature to manage the problem of naming the UK's many Others, offering a broad category, rather than multiple racialized ethnicities. It remains a contested term and has not been adopted as an active identity or form of self-naming (see inter alia, Aspinall 2002, Okolosie et al. 2015). But as an administrative category, it provided a way of naming evident coronavirus-related inequalities.

As news reports and comments by health workers multiplied, a picture of systemically skewed mortality rates emerged. Alongside – and interwoven with – other problems in pandemic governance (e.g. the slow and inadequate supply of PPE to health and social care workers), a story began to take shape about who was dying from COVID-19, centring on its disproportionate concentration among racialized minorities. By the beginning of May 2020, reviews of mortality rates indicated systematic differences (e.g. the Centre for Evidence Based Medicine 2020). The government eventually established an inquiry into BAME death rates. Its report revealed what was already known – and indeed had precipitated the call for an inquiry in the first place: BAME people were dying disproportionately from Covid-19. The report (PHE 2020a) showed that BAME people were twice as likely as white people to die after contracting Covid-19 but was greeted with an angry response for its failure to address the causes of the disparities or propose solutions.

After many critical reactions – ranging from the Muslim Council of Great Britain to the British Medical Association – the government agreed to publish a range of responses and suggestions collected during the consultations undertaken to produce the original report (PHE 2020b). This report was published to relatively greater approval, not least for acknowledging the possibility that 'historic racism' and 'social inequality' might be contributing factors to BAME mortality rates, and the government faced demands that its recommendations be implemented immediately. In a strange side-step, the government called the report 'a descriptive summary of stakeholder insights into the factors that may be influencing the impact of COVID-19 on BAME communities and strategies for addressing inequalities' and announced that it would be taken forward via a further review to be led by Equalities Minister, Kemi Badenoch. To many, this looked like yet another postponement, a strategy wholly in keeping with established governmental responses to questions about systemic or institutional racism.

3. When do Black lives matter?

By this point, the killing of George Floyd by Minneapolis police officers on May 25th had triggered new Black Lives Matter protests in the US, UK and well beyond. In the process, the issue of BAME coronavirus deaths became folded into a wider politics of 'race' and death. As many recognized, George Floyd's last words struck uncanny echoes in the moment of corona-virus: 'I can't breathe' conjoined different forms of systemically racialized oppression and vulnerability (see, for example, Okri 2020). In the UK, it con-nected health inequalities with mobilizations around symbols of colonial history, the continuing effects of the UK's 'hostile environment' policies directed at migrants (Gentleman 2019) and the contemporary policing of black and other racialized communities (involving, for example, the use of stop and search powers or Tasers). However, in a parliamentary debate, Kemi Badenoch (the Minister for Equality) insisted that:

> [L]et us not in this House use statements like 'being black is a death sentence', which young people out there hear, don't understand the context and then continue to believe that they live in a society that is against them. When actually this is one of the best countries in the world to be a black person. (Brewis 2020)

This response was greeted with some scepticism, and suspicions about the government's framing of BAME deaths intensified when the Prime Minister announced a new wider investigation: a Commission on Race and Ethnic Dis-parities. The announcement provoked outrage for several reasons. One was its effective postponement of any immediate action in the current crisis. A second was the catalogue of previous investigations, studies and reports in which racialized inequalities had been reviewed, but with little or no effect on policy or practice (see, *inter alia*, Lammy 2020). A third was that the gov-ernment advisor made responsible for establishing the new Commission (Munira Mirza) had previously insisted that claims of 'institutional racism' were 'a perception more than a reality' and that anti-racist lobby groups and diversity policies encouraged people to 'see everything through the prism of racial difference' (Stone 2020).

The evidence about unequal infection and death rates for Black and other racialized-minoritized groups has been firmly – and, indeed, multiply –

established. What remains contested is how to account for these inequalities, with diverse explanatory frameworks swirling around. Some of these cluster in the realm of the biological: BAME groups have higher levels of 'co-morbidities' (diabetes, cardiovascular disease) and may also have lower levels of Vitamin D which may increase vulnerability to infection. And, not surprisingly, a search continues for the mysterious and elusive 'genetic factor' that may account for differences (as scientific racism makes another comeback: Saini 2019). A second cluster forms around what might be called the socio-cultural sphere, noting that BAME groups tend to live in overcrowded households in more densely populated areas; many live in multi-generational households and practise communal behaviours (from eating to worship) that may contribute to virus transmission. Some also have purported cultural 'flaws' (such as poor English language skills) that allegedly make them immune to public health messages rather than the virus.

This cluster slides into a third which offers a more structural sense of inequality, though often couched in administrative terminology: deprivation, poverty, unequal access to public goods such as housing, health, education and what might be called 'situational racisms' (in workplaces, on the streets, etc.) and the effects of what PHE carefully called 'historic [i.e. as opposed to contemporary] racism'. Finally, individuals and organizations have increasingly demanded attention to the place of institutional, systemic or structural racism in organizing the lives and deaths of these groups. However, it seems likely that prolonged governmental processes of quantifying, acknowledging and denying will bracket the question of whether Black lives matter for the foreseeable future.

4. Which racism is this?

The first report from the government's Race Disparity Unit in October 2020 reasoned its way delicately around the question of racism and its effects, arguing that

> After taking into account the COVID-19 mortality rate in each local authority, controlling for population density, and adjusting for deprivation and socioeconomic position, household composition and occupational exposure, health and disability at the time of the 2011 Census – the *excess risk of mortality* from COVID-19 compared with that of the White ethnic group was reduced for all ethnic minority groups, especially for Black and the combined Pakistani and Bangladeshi ethnic groups. (RDU 2020: 54 – pages unnumbered in original; my emphasis)

This idiosyncratic view of an 'excess' that might be associated with racism after all manner of other socio-economic dynamics have been taken into account both deflects and defers the question of what racism is and how it works. By contrast, arguments about structural racism view 'population density, deprivation, and socioeconomic position, household composition and occupational exposure, health and disability' as intimately and intrinsically connected to the racialised dynamics of the society. A rather different report, commissioned by the Labour Party from Baroness Doreen Lawrence, argued that:

> Covid-19 has thrived on structural inequalities that have long scarred British society. Black and minority ethnic people are more likely to work in frontline or shutdown sectors, more likely to live in poor quality or overcrowded housing and more likely to face barriers to accessing healthcare. Biological factors do not explain the disparity in deaths and infections; Black, Asian and minority ethnic people have been overexposed to this virus.
>
> … Throughout this review, we heard a real sense of frustration that despite the causes of racial inequality being well known, and report after report making recommendations on how to tackle it, little action has been taken. Over the last three years, there have been numerous Government-led reviews, which have cumulatively made over 200 recommendations which could significantly change the experiences of Black, Asian and minority ethnic people in the UK. Yet few of these recommendations have been taken forward effectively. (Lawrence 2020, pp. 24–25)

Forms of knowledge, in this context as in others, have both political affiliations and effects: they are consequential. But these are rarely simple alignments: they shift and they require political work to establish and stabilize their articulations. In the end, I think attention to the conjunctural entanglements of science and politics are more productive than epochal statements about our condition, such as Agamben's. Better to think about the shifting alignments of what counts as political and non-political (including 'Science'), following Rancière's suggestive observation that 'politics is a way of re-partitioning the political from the non-political' (2011, p. 4). This boundary is a necessarily mobile and contested one, where we encounter the articulations of knowledge, power and politics in shifting – and contested – formations. A Foucauldian conception of power/knowledge in which forms of power are constructed, legitimized, and enacted in specific assemblages of agents, practices and technologies offers a productive framing, especially when different forms are viewed as overlaid and articulated (e.g. Isin and Ruppert 2020). However, this needs to be supplemented by a conjunctural view of such shifting formations which explores the ways in which articulations of knowledge, power and politics are always particular to specific moments of time–space – as are the challenges and contestations that they encounter (Newman and Clarke 2018).

Both Covid-19 and the responses to George Floyd's killing have reminded everyone (with some notable exceptions) about the entangled character of the world and where we live and die. But they have also reminded us about the continuing salience of national spaces – including the contradictory roles occupied by national governments and their involvement in political mobilization and de-mobilization. For me, that means giving attention to the overlapping and accumulating crises, contradictions, constructions and con-testations that create what Gramsci – in a compelling image – called 'a series of unstable equilibria'. In those unsettling dynamics, established formations of knowledge, power and politics are also at stake. At such moments, 'race' and the politics of (not) knowing form vital points of connection and disjuncture among the different social forces that are being mobilized (or immobilized).

Acknowledgements

This paper started life as a contribution to a seminar on 'Policy Ontologies' at Birkbeck College. I am grateful to Rachael Dobson for the invitation, to Janet Newman and Paul Stubbs for comments on earlier drafts, and to the editors for suggestions about how to improve it.

Disclosure statement

No potential conflict of interest was reported by the author(s).

Further information

This Special Issue article has been comprehensively reviewed by the Special Issue editors, Associate Professor Ted Striphas and Professor John Nguyet Erni.

ORCID

John Clarke ⓘ http://orcid.org/0000-0003-3968-4713

References

Agamben, G. 2020. "A Question" and "Clarifications" (translated by A. Kotsko). *Inscriptions*, 3 (2), 3–5. https://www.tankebanen.no/inscriptions/index.php/inscriptions/article/view/72.

Aspinall, P., 2002. Collective terminology to describe the minority ethnic population: The persistence of confusion and ambiguity in usage. *Sociology*, 36 (4), 803–816.

Bacevic, J. 2020. There's no such thing as 'following the science' – coronavirus advice is political. *The Guardian*. Available from: https://www.theguardian.com/commentisfree/2020/apr/28/theres-no-such-thing-just-following-the-science-coronavirus-advice-political.

Brewis, H. 2020. UK is 'one of the best countries in the world to be a black person,' says Tory MP. *Evening Standard*. Available from: https://www.standard.co.uk/news/uk/uk-best-countries-black-person-kemi-badenoch-a4459751.html.

Centre for Evidence Based Medicine. 2020. Bame COVID-19 deaths – What do we know? *Rapid Data & Evidence Review*. Available from: https://www.cebm.net/covid-19/bame-covid-19-deaths-what-do-we-know-rapid-data-evidence-review/.

Clarke, J., and Newman, J., 2017. "People in this country have had enough of experts": Brexit and the paradoxes of populism. *Critical policy studies*, 11 (1), 101–116.

Gentleman, A., 2019. *The Windrush betrayal: exposing the hostile environment*. London: Guardian Faber Publishing.

Isin, E., and Ruppert, E. 2020. The birth of sensory power: How a pandemic made it visible? *Big Data & Society*, July–December, 1–15.

Jones, H. 2020. Government 'shamelessly abandons' global comparison of coronavirus deaths. *Metro*. Available from: https://metro.co.uk/2020/05/12/government-shamelessly-abandons-global-comparison-coronavirus-deaths-12692983/.

Lammy, D. 2020. Britain needs leadership on race inequality. Not just another review. *The Guardian*. Available from: https://www.theguardian.com/commentisfree/2020/jun/16/race-inequality-review-boris-johnson-black-lives-matter-david-lammy.

Lawrence, B., 2020. *An avoidable crisis: The disproportionate impact of covid-19 on Black, Asian and minority ethnic communities. A review by Baroness Doreen Lawrence*. London: The Labour Party. Available from: https://www.lawrencereview.co.uk.

Maskovsky, J., and Bjork-James, S., 2019. *Beyond populism: angry politics and the twilight of neoliberalism*. Morgantown, West Virginia: University of West Virginia Press.

Newman, J., and Clarke, J., 2018. The instabilities of expertise: remaking knowledge, power and politics in unsettled times. *Innovation: The European journal of social science research*, 31 (1), 40–54.

Okolosie, L., et al. 2015. Is it time to ditch the term 'Black, Asian and minority ethnic (BAME)? *The Guardian*. Available from: https://www.theguardian.com/commentisfree/2015/may/22/black-asian-minority-ethnic-bame-bme-trevor-phillips-racial-minorities.

Okri, B. 2020. 'I can't breathe': why George Floyd's words reverberate around the world. *The Guardian*. Available from: https://www.theguardian.com/commentisfree/2020/jun/08/i-cant-breathe-george-floyds-words-reverberate-oppression.

Public Health England. 2020a. *Disparities in the risk and outcomes of COVID-19*. London: UK Government. Available from: www.ukgov/phe.

Public Health England. 2020b. *Beyond the data: understanding the impact of COVID-19 on BAME groups*. London: UK Government. Available from: www.ukgov/phe.

Race Disparity Unit. 2020. *Quarterly report on progress to address COVID-19 health inequalities*. London: HM Government. Available from: https://www.gov.uk/government/publications/quarterly-report-on-progress-to-address-covid-19-health-inequalities.

Rancière, J., 2011. The thinking of dissensus: politics and aesthetics. In: Paul Bowman and Richard Stamp, eds. *Reading Rancière: critical dissensus*. London and New York: Continuum, 1–17.

Saini, A., 2019. *Superior: The return of race science*. London: HarperCollins.

Stone, J. 2020. Boris Johnson appoints aide who said institutional racism was a myth and railed against multiculturalism. *The Independent*. https://www.independent.co.uk/news/uk/politics/boris-johnson-westminster-insider-institutional-racism-munira-mirza-a9568456.html.

UK Government. 2020. *COVID-19: understanding the impact on BAME communities*. London: UK Government. Available from: https://www.gov.uk/government/publications/covid-19-understanding-the-impact-on-bame-communities.

'Give me liberty or give me COVID': Anti-lockdown protests as necropopulist downsurgency

Jack Bratich

ABSTRACT
This paper examines the 'anti-lockdown' protests in the US beginning in April 2020 through the concepts of necropolitics (Mbembe) and microfascism (Deleuze and Guattari). The paper argues that these protests are examples of what it coins, *necropopulism*. What if the libertarian, hyper-individualistic, and reactionary populism we witness in these and other manifestations (e.g. mass shooters, alt-right street fights) are both fixated on their identity as a 'people,' yet simultaneously indifferent to their own persistence? Examining the anti-lockdown and anti-masking protests and their precursors, the paper argues that microfascism is infused with homi-suicidal aesthetics. The essay seeks to refine our analysis when it comes to the cultural (necro)politics of this 'downsurgency,' in which decline accelerates rapidly and might even be detached, ultimately, from its own demise. This analysis matters if we are to antagonize this necrotic force, not simply through a battle of ideas but by preventing a fascist social body from being fully activated and mobilized.

The 2020 COVID-19 pandemic has laid bare the unsustainable governance, norms, and social relationships defining racial capitalism. The crisis has illuminated Coronavirus 'disaster capitalism' (Solis and Klein 2020) as well as a mutual aid-based 'pandemic solidarity' (Sitrin and Colectiva Sembrar 2020). Might this rupture open up a terrain of struggle that does not end in a typical post-crisis re-legitimation or restabilization? Indeed, we might be witnessing efforts at a more *belligerent* restoration. As Gramsci (1996, p. 33) put it (and as plenty of commentators have recently re-invoked), this is a moment in which 'the old is dying and the new cannot yet be born: in this interregnum, morbid phenomena of the most varied kind come to pass.' In this brief note I look squarely into one of these morbid phenomena, specifically into individuals and groups who are politically preoccupied with morbidity as such. Beginning with the 2020 anti-lockdown and anti-masking protests in the United States, I sketch out a broad reactionary sensibility characterized by a downward political movement, or downsurgency, that unsettles notions of 'the popular' and populism.

In mid-to late-April 2020, anti-lockdown rallies proliferated across US state capitals, with 'pro-freedom' demonstrators apparently casting paralyzing spells on cops with their displays of armed resistance and weaponized spittle. The rallies, partially sponsored and funded by right-wing organiz-ations, directed their anger at state governors for requiring citizens to wear masks and shutter their businesses, both of which were measures designed to mitigate the pandemic. Somewhat dormant after a series of defeats starting with Charlottesville in 2017, the radical right found its way back into the streets as part of the protests (including the Proud Boys, conservative armed militia groups, and religious fundamentalists). After months of keeping connected through fashwave apocalyptic imagery and armed pepe memes, civil war preppers known as the 'boogaloo bois' also joined the rallies.

How to characterize these anti-lockdown protests? While a range of people showed up in different places, some of the themes were consistent across contexts. Individual mobility and economic jump-starting were prior-itized over public health. Masks were coded not as public-minded pandemic reducers, but as speech mufflers. In an acute expression of longstanding libertarian paradoxes, the anti-masking sentiments called for individual freedom while connecting and expressing them as *collective* hostilities. The protests articulated what Filippo Del Lucchese calls, in describing the popu-lation that seeks tyrants, a 'collection of disconnected, isolated individuals able to act together' (2009, p. 350).

At core, these libertarian notions of freedom emanated from hyper-indivi-dualism. But selfishness is not a sufficient explanation. The ideology of indi-vidualism as the seat of sovereignty extends to the most *familiar*. What appears as selfishness is not anti-social, but a narrowly-defined sociality. It is what Michael Hardt and Antonio Negri (2009) call an identitarian 'love of the same' – a corrupted 'mandate to love thy neighbor, understanding it as a call to love those most proximate, those most like you … .Family, race, and nation, then, which are corrupt forms of the common, are unsurprisingly the bases of corrupt forms of love' (p. 182). This sentiment was found in the Texas lieutenant governor's infamous line, 'There are more important things than living, and that's saving this country for my children and my grandchil-dren and saving this country for all of us.' The 'us' here is an extension of 'my,' invoking blood (family) and soil (nation), while predicated on 'the exclusion or subordination of those outside' (Hardt and Negri 2009, p. 182).

The racial dimension of this homogeneity becomes clear in a pandemic that disproportionately affects communities of colour. Sara Ahmed (2004) argues that racialized affects do not always present themselves as hate of others but as love of one's own (exclusionary and exclusive) identity. The anti-masker cries of 'individual freedom' are in fact passionate protections of the homogenous – of a whiteness that articulates itself through a *disregard* for the lives of Others, an *indifference* to those who are different. The eugenicist tones of the Tennessee anti-lockdown protest sign that said 'Sacrifice the Weak' thus announced a whiteness that determines who is unworthy of care and security.

When US cities erupted in May and June with protests in the wake of the police killing of George Floyd, anti-lockdown demonstrations largely moved off the streets, but the actions amped up. The rallies transformed into distributed direct action, primarily in stores that required masks. Video recordings of shoppers' outbursts went viral, while harassment, threats and violent assaults on employees increased (including at least one killing) (Brown 2020, Castrodale 2020, Miller and Brueck 2020).

Anti-lockdown and anti-masking protests continue a long American tradition of death-driven liberty. The mottos so beloved by libertarians now find COVID clarity. The canonical rallying cry 'Live Free or Die' always seemed to be directed to other citizens as a call to arms, inspiring even martyrdom. In the hands of mini-sovereigns, the phrase now gets a biopolitical makeover, à la Foucault and Mbembe. A demand directed at the government for freedom from it, at the expense of others' lives: *To Let Live Free, and To Make Die*. A similar false binary was found on one sign's new twist on another old motto: 'Give me Liberty or Give me COVID.' Translation: *Give me Liberty AND Give me Death (and throw in some Death to Others as well)*.

None of this should be surprising. Take the gun-worshipping death cult of 2nders, the militant devotees of the US Constitution's Second Amendment, authorizing a right to bear arms. They have declared for years that their totem-weapon could only be 'pried from my cold dead hands.' No wonder that gun stores in different parts of the US were deemed essential, even 'life-sustaining!' To put it succinctly, the accelerated and acute circumstances resulting from COVID-19 are drawing out the *necropolitical* orientations of the US radical and libertarian right.

State necropolitics

Achille Mbembe's (2003) canonical piece defines *necropolitics* as the sovereign power for homicide, 'to dictate who may live and who must die' (p. 11). Mbembe opens his article by noting that Nazism 'became the archetype of a power formation that combined the characteristics of the racist state, the murderous state, and the suicidal state,' and he goes on to trace necropolitical apparatuses back to colonialism's brutal control mechanisms (something analysed earlier by Aimé Cesaire 1972).

Gilles Deleuze and Felix Guattari's (1987) characterization of Nazism resonates with Mbembe's, with an extra emphasis on the self-destructive aspects:

[I]n fascism, the State is far less totalitarian than it is *suicidal*. There is in fascism a realized nihilism. Unlike the totalitarian State, which does its utmost to seal all possible lines of flight, fascism is constructed on an intense line of flight, which it transforms into a line of pure destruction and abolition. It is curious that from the very beginning the Nazis announced to Germany what they were bringing: at once wedding bells and death, including their own death, and the death of the Germans. (p. 230)

Applying these insights to the current conjuncture, we can first turn to the US's former head of state. As Judith Butler (2019) wrote about Donald Trump's response to Congressional attempts at impeachment (the first time), it is increasingly difficult to determine whether his reactions are 'suicidal or a means of triumphant survival.' The essay, succinctly titled 'Genius or suicide?' asks us to consider both simultaneously: 'How are suicide and survival linked in the psychic field we call "Trump"?' I suggest we expand this dynamic ('a death drive left unchecked') to include his fans and followers.

Emboldened by his victory against impeachment in February 2020, Trump began rousing his base during the lockdown protests with tweet-commands such as, 'Liberate Virginia!' (then Michigan, then Minnesota). As Olivier Jutel (2017) notes, Trump is less a strict leader than a permission-giver, a liberator of impulses to allow and encourage enjoyment all the way down. Thus, we need to ask if this tweet-activation also unleashes the 'genius or suicide' impulse in his followers. Add to that the predominantly white constitution of the anti-lockdown protests and we get a lethal cocktails, as succinctly stated by Britney Cooper (2020): 'when whiteness has a death wish, we are all in for a serious problem.'

As President, and even perhaps since his term has ended, Trump is the CEO of the homi-suicide state. Indeed, his public denials about COVID's severity became a defining mark of the final months of his term. He retweeted widely dismissed claims for cures, engaged in misinformation wars against his critics and incited his base to confidently continue their despot-friendly protests and preparations for conflict. For him, the BlackLivesMatter uprisings in May and June 2020 presented an opportunity to deflect criticisms of his COVID response by aggrandizing himself as the law-and-order president. He no longer needed to be interested in surges of COVID cases, only in surges of federal armed agents into cities against despot-unfriendly protestors. Trump's ongoing gutting of the biopolitical infrastructure in favour of militarized repression seems to fulfil former political advisor Steve Bannon's grand objective of 'the deconstruction of the administrative state' (Prupis 2017). Such a despotic and martial version of security exemplifies Deleuze and Guattari's (1987) claim that fascism produces 'a flow of absolute war whose only possible outcome is the suicide of the State itself. ... [one that] would rather annihilate its own servants than stop the destruction' (230–231).

Cultural necropolitics

Mbembe primarily focused on the necropolitical dimensions of *state* institutions. But we need to move beyond the state form, as recent events show that necropolitics are also carried out primarily by non-state actors.[1]

Before the anti-maskers, we saw this collective homi-suicidal display in the alt-right street demonstrations of 2015–2017. The pro-Trump assemblies often looked like a costumed re-enactment of dead regimes. Roman gladiators, Spartan fighters, medieval knights, and Nazi troopers were all re-mixed into a cosplay gathering for fans of lost empires. In addition to being MAGA[2] youth troops, their carnivalesque attachment to mythic ruins gave first glimpses into this interregnum's morbid direction – less an uprising than an accelerated and violent downsinking. We could call this *cultural necropolitics*.

Cultural necropolitics have roots in fascist culture, encapsulated in the famous insight by Walter Benjamin (1969/2007, p. 242) that fascism seeks to 'experience its own destruction as an aesthetic enjoyment of the first order.' While cinema (and its subject, the spectator) was the media form for this aesthetic (see also Buck-Morss 1992), today's digital culture is, on the whole, more participatory and networked.

Cultural necropolitics are also part of what Deleuze and Guattari called *microfascism* – the subjective domain that exists prior to a fascist state apparatus. Microfascist culture is not reducible to practices and artifacts expressing an authoritarian identity, nor to the recruiting ground for organized movements (e.g. the 'alt-right'); it is a sphere of the development of capacities, or subjectivation. The interregnum's morbid aesthetic is manifest in this digital culture as irony (disavowal), resentment, rage, shitposting (a will to freedom as transgressive and 'fun'), and strategic abjection (claims to victimhood). A range of ordinary affects (armored cruelty, depression, shock, numbness) infuse the senses and activate sensibilities. Culture not as lifestyle, but as *deathstyle*: a subjectivity that gives to itself a mode of non-existence. Such a deathstyle is not inert – its participatory, peer-to-peer goading and incitements unleash lethal phenomena. As a result, microfascist culture develops a networked body (individualized and collectivized) capable of killing and of being killed.

The contemporary cultural production of microfascist subjectivity includes the anti-lockdown protestors (who also form a network of COVID spreaders) as well as the racially motivated mass shooters who have leapt from online 'chan' culture into streets, big box stores, mosques, and clubs. In addition, manosphere-fueled 'lone wolves' attack women (partners, exes, strangers), birth control centres, yoga classes, college campuses and other spaces where women tend to congregate. Patriarchal revenge and control killings, some spectacular while most are ordinary, synthesize popular misogyny (Banet-Weiser 2018), gendertrolling (Mantilla 2015), and everyday sexism (Bates 2014) into the United States' own version of femicide. All told, cultural necropolitics forms subjects who embrace 'new technologies of destruction … represented by the massacre' (Mbembe 2003, p. 34).

Necropolitical microfascism is a nihilism formed in the spirit of defeat, disillusionment, and deflation. This networked minority acts desperately to guard a patriarchy and white supremacy increasingly losing legitimacy in the interregnum. These passionate defenders of servitude to ruins seek unwilling participants during their collapse, particularly women and people of colour. Reactionary and resentful, this downward vortex takes populism along with it because it is indifferent, ultimately, to its own demise. It fights by accelerating its decline – less an insurgency than a *downsurgency*.

Our conventional political terminology needs to capture this process better in order to understand the logics that undergird the anti-lockdown protests. The homi-suicidal tendency disorients contemporary discourses (e.g. populism or democracy) that continue to invoke a persistent 'people' even when the enemy is not ultimately attached to its own survival. This 'populism' is lacking a *bios*, much less a *demos*. With its self-immolating death networks and techno-subjective ruination, at best we are confronted with a *necropopulism*: a populism that, under the banner of specific types of people (white, masculinized, Christian), seeks to extinguish the life that allows any people to persist.

Necropopulism traffics in performative memories of the never-existing and of the dead, invoking ghosts of the Southern 'Lost Cause,'[3] medieval and ancient warrior masculinity, and lost empires. Necropopulism is cheered by some in their costumes and public-health indifference, while others operate on the more violent end of the homi-suicidal spectrum, creating a stochastic supply of killers (by gun, car, spit, and other weapons).

One can turn to an odd etymological twist of the word 'popular' to distill the operations. While the origins of its meaning are murky, the Latin *populor* meant to destroy, pillage, and lay to waste (Populor 2020). It refers to an invasion that despoils, a raid that plunders. *Populor* thus combines population and depopulation. Today's necropopulism returns us to the *populor*, generating a *populorism* that just might be the line of flight-becoming-line of abolition that Deleuze and Guattari find at the core of fascism.

One or many abolitions?

During the Michigan anti-lockdown protests of April 2020, one barely-teen white male protestor carried a sign declaring, 'Even Pharaoh freed slaves during the Plague.' This artifact prompts a query: did the demonstrators hold similar placards during the Black Lives Matter (BLM) protests a month later in support of the closest approximations to slaves today – the incarcerated, and those killed by police? The answer is, of course, no, for that would mean they are interested in an expansive freedom for others. Instead, they clamor for a license to exert despotic power, even a libertine taste for cruelty.

In some ways, we could say we live in a moment where competing and hostile abolitionist movements are confronting each other: on the one hand, the nihilistic and eliminationist version enacted in microfascist cultural necropolitics – the freedom entwined with walls, borders, and chants of 'lock them all up!'; on the other, the life-affirming abolitions that seek decarceration, the defunding of police, and to 'free them all!'

Surging to prominence during the George Floyd and BLM uprisings, the prison and police abolition movements seek to dismantle the repressive state as a project of race- and class-based social justice. Moreover, gender-based abolitions of patriarchy and against femicide are on the rise. With the Ni Una Menos movement starting in 2015 and the Un Violador en tu Camino project of late 2019/2020, Latin American feminists have strengthened and advanced memetic transmission and street performance as solidarity and antagonism. Key here is their recognition that everyday interpersonal violence resonates with macro-violence (extractivism, structural repression). In addition, these are explicitly counter-necropolitical projects, forming as 'Women Rising in Defense of Life' (Gago and Aguilar 2018). These projects understand the future neither as ruined nor through the deathmaking styles of settler capitalist patriarchy but through the life-making work of social reproduction (as the linking of daily struggles around care).

Community defense, collective security, communal modes of existence: all that is life-affirming can oppose the death-machines in their final act of necro-populist sovereignty. This means creating worlds, shaping relations, and making forms-of-life against fascist lines of abolition and deconstructive states. During COVID collapse, we have seen emergency commons formed through mutual aid, recovery efforts through self-organized networks of support and repair, uprisings for social reproduction (e.g. #CareNotCops), and the reconfiguration of the most intimate gendered relationships as examples of antifascist compositions of subjectivity.

The emergent field of collapsology (Gadeau 2019) could use an analysis of the popular (and *populor*) mutations that will slouch from cascading ruins. In an interregnum marked by the confrontation of abolitions, an anti-fascist cultural studies can assess the terrain of uprisings, even their most morbid phenomena. This matters if we are to antagonize this force, align with the life-affirming abolitions, and defeat an enemy on its cultural and subjective territory.

Notes

1. Others have extended Mbembe's concept to contemporary practices of femicide (Wright 2011, Threadcraft 2017) or offered similar ones: *necroculture* (Thorpe 2016), political *necrophilism* (Fromm 1973, Daly 1978, Castronovo 2001), *necro-capitalism* (Banerjee 2008) and the *necrocene* (McBrien 2016). Together, this

cluster highlights how the homi-suicide dynamic has been synthesized across multiple levels (interpersonal, cultural, planetary, and economic).
2. 'Make America Great Again,' the slogan from Trump's first presidential campaign.
3. Let's not forget that the rise of the Confederacy myth originated in a graveyard ritual. The remaining statues and monuments act as reminders but also as marble zombies (the standing dead) while the neo-confederates of today ride with ghosts.

Disclosure statement

No potential conflict of interest was reported by the author(s).

Further information

This Special Issue article has been comprehensively reviewed by the Special Issue editors, Associate Professor Ted Striphas and Professor John Nguyet Erni.

References

Ahmed, S., 2004. Affective economies. *Social text*, 22 (2), 117–139.
Banerjee, S.B., 2008. Necrocapitalism. *Organization studies*, 29 (12), 1541–1563.
Banet-Weiser, S., 2018. *Empowered: popular feminism and popular misogyny*. Durham, NC: Duke University Press.
Bates, L., 2014. *Everyday sexism*. London: Simon & Schuster.
Benjamin, W., 1969/2007. *Illuminations*, trans. H. Zohn. New York, NY: Schocken Books.
Brown, D. 2020. "I feel threatened!": Viral video shows shopper throwing tantrum, but who protects workers? *USA TODAY* [online], 8 July, Available from: https://www.usatoday.com/story/money/2020/07/08/i-feel-threatened-who-protects-shoppers-angry-anti-maskers/5389199002/ [Accessed 5 August 2020].
Buck-Morss, S. 1992. Aesthetics and anaesthetics: Walter Benjamin's artwork essay reconsidered, October 62, 3–4.
Butler, J. 2019. Genius or Suicide. *London Review of Books* [online], 24 October, Available from: https://www.lrb.co.uk/the-paper/v41/n20/judith-butler/genius-or-suicide [Accessed 2020].
Castrodale, J. 2020. Teenage ice cream shop employees are getting harassed by anti-maskers. *Vice* [online], Available from: https://www.vice.com/en_us/article/m7j5ka/teen-ice-cream-shop-employees-are-getting-harassed-by-anti-maskers [Accessed 5 August 2020].
Castronovo, R., 2001. *Necro citizenship: death, eroticism, and the public sphere in nine-teenth-century United States*. Durham, NC: Duke University Press.

Césaire, A., 1972. *Discourse on colonialism*, trans. J. Pinkham. New York: Monthly Review Press.

Cooper, B. 2020. *Twitter* [online], 28 April, Available from: https://twitter.com/ProfessorCrunk/status/1255117671273824257 [Accessed 10 August 2020].

Daly, M., 1978/1990. *Gyn/ecology: the metaethics of radical feminism*. Boston, MA: Beacon Press.

Deleuze, G., and Guattari, F., 1987. *A thousand plateaus*, trans. B. Massumi. Minneapolis: University of Minnesota Press.

Del Lucchese, F., 2009. Democracy, multitudo and the third kind of knowledge in the works of spinoza. *European journal of political theory*, 8 (3), 339–363.

Fromm, E., 1973. *The anatomy of human destructiveness*. New York: Holt, Rinehart and Winston.

Gadeau, O., 2019. A brief chronology of the media coverage of collapsology in France (2015–2019). *Multitudes*, 76 (3), 121–123.

Gago, V., and Aguilar, R.G., 2018. Women rising in defense of life. *NACLA report on the Americas*, 50 (4), 364–368.

Gramsci, A., 1996. *Prison notebooks volume 2*, ed. and trans. J.A. Buttigieg. New York, NY: Columbia University Press.

Hardt, M. and Negri, A., 2009. *Commonwealth*. Cambridge: Harvard University Press.

Jutel, O. 2017. Donald Trump's Libidinal Entanglement with Liberalism and Affective Media Power. *Boundary2* [online], 23 October, Available from: http://www.boundary2.org/2017/10/olivier-jutel-donald-trumps-libidinal-entanglement-with-liberalism-and-affective-media-power/ [Accessed 8 January 2020].

Mantilla, K., 2015. *Gendertrolling: how misogyny went viral*. Santa Barbara: Praeger.

Mbembe, A. 2003. Necropolitics, trans. Libby Meintjes. *Public Culture*, 15(1), 11–40.

McBrien, J., 2016. Accumulating extinction: planetary catastrophism in the necrocene. In: J.W. Moore, ed. *Anthropocene or capitalocene? Nature, history, and the crisis of capitalism*. Oakland: PM Press, 116–137.

Miller, M., and Brueck, H. 2020. Anti-maskers are the new anti-vaxxers. *Business Insider* [online], Available from: https://www.businessinsider.com/anti-maskers-are-new-anti-vaxxers-threatening-public-health-coronavirus-2020-7 [Accessed 5 August 2020].

Populor. 2020. https://www.latin-is-simple.com/en/vocabulary/verb/5537/ [Accessed 2020].

Prupis, N. 2017. Bannon Heralds "Deconstruction of Administrative State" and Trump's "New Political Order" *Common Dreams* [online], Available from: https://www.commondreams.org/news/2017/02/23/bannon-heralds-deconstruction-administrative-state-and-trumps-new-political-order [Accessed 14 July 2020].

Sitrin, M. and Colectiva Sembrar, ed. 2020. *Pandemic solidarity: mutual aid during the covid-19 crisis*. London: Pluto Press.

Solis, M., and Klein, N. 2020. Coronavirus is the perfect disaster for "disaster capitalism". *Vice* [online], Available from: https://www.vice.com/en_us/article/5dmqyk/naomi-klein-interview-on-coronavirus-and-disaster-capitalism-shock-doctrine [Accessed 2 August 2020].

Threadcraft, S., 2017. North American necropolitics and gender: On #BlackLivesMatter and Black femicide. *The South Atlantic quarterly*, 116 (3), 553–579.

Thorpe, C., 2016. *Necroculture*. New York: Palgrave Macmillan.

Wright, M.W., 2011. Necropolitics, narcopolitics, and femicide: gendered violence on the Mexico-U.S. border. *Signs: journal of women in culture and society*, 36 (3), 707–731.

Racism is a public health crisis! Black Power in the COVID-19 pandemic

Lisa B. Y. Calvente

ABSTRACT
The article argues the covid-19 pandemic – including its laws and representations – has produced a context in which normalized crisis has become both abnormal and unacceptable. By examining a series of circulated images, this article highlights how the ordinances of the pandemic brought about a break in the racialized and racist normalcy of Black death and response. In doing so, it argues that racism and colonial violence are essential to white sovereignty and underscores the role of cultural studies in theorizing Black Power and decolonization. It calls for a critical (re)turn to these concepts to solidify a popular praxis for social justice and equity.

It is a fact that most black countries live under a colonial regime. Even an independent country such as Haiti is in fact in many respects a semicolonial country. And our American brothers themselves are, by force of racial discrimination, artificially placed at the heart of a great modern nation in a situation [that] is comprehensible only in reference to a colonialism, abolished to be sure, but one whose aftereffects still reverberate in the present.

– Aimé Césaire 2010, p. 127

The COVID-19 pandemic has disrupted the contemporary stage of neoliberal capitalism. Through images appearing in national and local news media, the United States, along with observers in many nations across the globe, viewed a series of murders and brutalities exacted against predominantly Black residents. Television watchers and avid social media users were compelled to stop, watch and listen through the shelter-in-place mandates that were pushed across many nations. In this, the normalization of crisis was suddenly disrupted by repeated instances of chaos tied closely to racism and white privilege.[1] This article examines a series of circulated images in an effort to highlight how laws and policies associated with the pandemic brought about a break in the flow of racial performativities.[2]

Circulated, storied images illustrate how informal channels of communi-cation shape the ways in which normalized knowledges circulate.[3] Networks of talk quite often accompany the brutalities of white supremacy and anti-black and – brown racism, serving as alternative, resistant channels for knowl-edge and information that undermine normative proclamations of whiteness – and perhaps save many Black and Brown lives in the process.[4] But circulated images do more than just serve as windows into parallel networks of talk; they also possess the potential to influence popular formations for change. Building on these ideas, this article argues that the disruption of the ordinary acceptance of crisis brought forth by circulated, storied images lies within the history of Black Power and decolonization, and that a critical (re)turn to these concepts can help solidify a popular praxis for social justice and equity in the now.

Masking (in) Black & White

Approximately three weeks from the first confirmed case of COVID in New York City (NYC) on March 1, 2020, the city, with a population of over 8 million people, became the epicentre of the coronavirus pandemic, at the time accounting for approximately 5% of the globally infected (Chakrabarti and Kotsonis 2020, McKinley 2020). Contrary to the slow initial response, Gov-ernor Andrew M. Cuomo, like many other government officials, swiftly enacted a strict social distancing and stay-at-home strategy, one that included the shutting down of city businesses and public transportation, as well as the mandatory use of facemasks in public. Within weeks, many people came to understand and witness firsthand how racial disparities con-nected to the pandemic. A video posted on Twitter on April 11, for instance, showed the New York Police Department (NYPD) detaining a little Brown boy for violating social distancing laws by selling chips on the train to help support his homeless family (Cheney-Rice 2020). The child, who was accompanied by his parents and a sibling, was distraught and crying as officers pulled him off the train, threw his jacket on the floor, and kicked and threw his chips on the platform. Witnesses voiced their disdain for the treatment of the child and many donated to the family's Cashapp in response to the police abuse; as of July 9, 2020, the viral video had garnered 1.6 million views.

On May 2, 2020 three days before the video of Ahmaud Arbery's murder in South Georgia was released to the public, another video was circulated on Twitter showing the brutal confrontation with, and arrest of, Donni Wright, a bystander who had witnessed two non-white youths abused and arrested in New York City (NYC) for having allegedly violated social distancing laws (Cheney-Rice 2020). The NYC video shows four police officers forcing a young male onto the ground with witnesses yelling in protest; one of the officers has his knee on the youth's neck. The same officer, Francisco Garcia, without a mask, points his taser at Wright. He repeatedly tells Wright to 'move the fuck back, right now' as he approaches Wright and then states, 'Don't flex. Don't flex.' The use of slang from Garcia, coupled with his stance, depicts the officer's approach less as one of protection and service and more as that of a rival ready to attack the opposition. Garcia then grabs Wright – who up until this point is outside of the camera frame – swings him down, and repeatedly smacks him in the face and head as Wright remains on the floor. Wright did not resist.

The two-minute and four-second video of Wright and Officer Garcia shows an accumulation of neighbours screaming in protest as additional officers arrived on the scene. When local news covered the confrontation between Officer Garcia and Donni Wright, the police violence against residents was said to have been in the East Village section of New York City; however, the more accurate location of the incident was in the Lower East Side, at a bodega across the street from Jacob Riis Public Housing. Riis, which encompasses 13 buildings of between 6 and 14 stories and over 1700 housing units, is one of the city's numerous public housing projects that have been under scrutiny for its poor conditions, retaliatory actions for tenant complaints, and crime, in addition to police abuse and hyper-surveillance (Mai and Annesse 2016, Chiel 2017, Ramirez 2018). National coverage of this incident limited the video to Garcia approaching and smacking Wright and juxtaposed it with another, shorter clip of a park ranger who was pushed into a lake in Austin, Texas, as he attempted to enforce a six-foot social distancing mandate with a party of white youths who were 'unlawfully drinking and smoking' (Elliott 2020, p. 2).[5] It was also reported that the young man who had pushed the ranger was charged with attempted assault of a public servant. A witness commented that the park ranger was 'being really sweet and understanding' before he was pushed (Elliott 2020, p. 3).

The viral video of Wright's assault received more than 400,000 views and 400 responses as of July 9, 2020, many of which focused on the differences between white life and Black life. A number of posts pointed specifically to the armed protesters, unmasked, yelling and shoving their way into the legislative floor in Michigan's State Capitol just days before. Of the protestors who had made their way into the house chamber, Lieutenant Brian Oleksyk of the Michigan State Police stated, 'people were just venting their frustrations in a loud manner,' and 'once they were able to do that … people were pleasant and polite' (Egan 2020, p. 1). On April 30, 2020, coverage of the same Michigan protest displayed white men, women, and children with swastikas, U.S. Civil War-era Confederate battle flags, and similar signs, some of which stated, 'Tyrants get the rope,' 'Give me liberty or death,' 'Freedom,' and 'Tyrant Bitch' (Beckett 2020, Egan 2020, p. 1, p. 2. The slogan, 'Tyrant Bitch,' was intended specifically for Gretchen Whitmer, democratic governor of Michigan, who in other images was likened to Adolph Hitler and was later depicted by another protestor with a naked doll on a noose in one hand and an ax in the other (Beckett 2020, Vallejo 2020).

The naked doll on a noose was condemned by one female protestor, who attempted to rip it from the hands of the sixty-year-old man who was holding it, rightfully stating that the man's act was a hate crime that would not be tolerated (Vallejo 2020). Nevertheless, its symbolic presence and the depiction of the man as a victim demonstrated the rising tone of the scene, which was supported by President Trump's tweets to 'Liberate Michigan' (Mauger and LeBlanc 2020, p. 1, Vallejo 2020). These same tweets from the President were later underscored to have been influential in an anti-government militia group's foiled plot to abduct Governor Whitmer, storm Michigan's State Capitol (again), and incite a civil war. Thirteen men were charged with conspiracy, terrorism and weapons violations, and, in response, Governor Whitmer stated that such militia group extremists 'heard the president's words not as a rebuke but as a rallying cry – as a call to action' (Bogel-Burroughs, Dewan, and Gray 2020, p. 1).

More videos began surfacing and circulating after the appearance of two videos showing Ahmaud Arbery's stalking and murder by three white men. On May 6, 2020, 21-year-old Dreasjon 'Sean' Reed was shot multiple times, to death, by Indianapolis police, after two unmarked police cars claimed to have seen Reed 'nearly hit several cars' (Bogel-Burroughs 2020, p. 1). Reed streamed the chase on Facebook Live (the video was later posted on YouTube), and thousands watched while he pleaded for someone to come and help him. He parked his car and a foot chase ensued; shots were then fired, and they continued to be fired as Reed lay on the ground. Indianapolis Police Chief Randal Taylor confirmed that a total of 15 shots were fired, 13 from an officer's gun and 2 from a gun that was found near Reed's body, though Taylor also stated that it could not be determined 'which shots were fired when' (Bogel-Burroughs 2020, p. 1). There were no body or dash cameras, and, since Reed was literally running for his life, his phone did not capture the shooting. However, witnesses can hear a detective state, 'Think it's going to be a closed casket, homie' after Reed and his phone chillingly cease to move (Bogel-Burroughs 2020, p. 1).

On May 13, 2020, the same day Michigan police and armed protestors had their 'peaceful' encounter, and less than two weeks before the recorded murder of George Floyd, five NYPD officers accosted a 22-year-old mother, Kallemah Rozier, for not wearing her mask properly. The video shows Rozier escorted by officers as she ascends the stairs of the Barclays Center station in Brooklyn. She is heard saying, 'Don't touch me' and slaps one of the officer's hands away, as the officer seemingly reaches for her neck (Verde 2020). Officers then pin Rozier to the ground as she struggles and yells, while another officer holds back her five-year-old child. Again, witnesses are heard yelling to the officers that their behaviour was excessive; they can also be heard pleading with them to stop, if only because her baby is with her and she is wearing her mask (Verde 2020).

Collectively, these incidents are not just about the deaths of George Floyd, Breonna Taylor, Elijah McClain, and Dreasjon Reed; they are about the accumulation of state-sanctioned and state-inflicted racial violence that has been experienced, witnessed, and circulated on a vast scale through social media.

Un-Masking racism, White sovereignty, and Black Power

Videos of police brutality and murder and their circulation, however, have done little to shift the tide toward structural change for social justice and racial equity. The victims of state-sanctioned racial violence are often re-cast as criminals and threats while officers, in the rare instances they are held accountable, are generally depicted as 'bad apples' (Calvente and Smicker 2019, p. 145). Accountability also does not equate to conviction or even criminal charges as in the death of Breonna Taylor, the shooting of Jacob Blake, and in the aforementioned Wright assault. The viral video of Officer Francisco Garcia's physical assault of Mr. Wright on the Lower East Side garnered swift action from the NYPD, causing them to drop the charge against Wright for assaulting a police officer and to shift the criminal investigation toward Officer Garcia and two additional officers – a process that typically takes years (Southall 2020). Officer Garcia, however, retired prior to his scheduled departmental hearing on the Wright assault, which enabled the officer to avoid providing testimony that could be used against him and the two other officers in a criminal investigation; Garcia's retirement also enabled him to receive his pension for his eight years as an NYPD officer, a luxury he would not be afforded if he were found guilty and terminated (Southall 2020).

Yet, if we listen to the voices and organizations made audible in and through these instances of state-sanctioned racial violence – and perhaps more importantly, manifested in the virtual and actual protests in recent months for Black and Brown lives for defunding the police, and for an end to structural racism – we are again reminded that a racist within a culture of racism is the norm, not the outlier (Fanon 1967). Utilizing the works of Frantz Fanon and of the Black Panther Party, cultural studies has made this distinction in its foundational work on mugging in Britain, *Policing the Crisis* (Hall *et al*. 1978). Here, the authors underscore the centralization of racial oppression and the articulation of Fanonian decolonization into popular Black Power politics in urban spaces throughout the United States and Britain (Hall *et al*. 1978). The centralization of racial oppression pushed forth racism as *the* primary defining factor of Black life in the (post)modern world.

Along these lines, Ture (formerly Carmichael) and Hamilton's definition of racism proves significant: 'the predication of decisions and policies on considerations of race for the purpose of subordinating and maintaining control over that group' (1992, p. 3). Additionally racism, 'as a system assembling race in the world,' not only produces race and racial difference but continues to reassemble race and racist strategies (Gilroy *et al.* 2019, p. 188). Such assemblages obscure how racism affects us all simultaneously and for the maintenance of white supremacy and sovereignty. Nevertheless, the reliance on particular goods and services (e.g. packed meat and other mass-produced household items, cleaning and maintenance, and at-home delivery) on the one hand, and the disposability of the exploited, often invisible 'non-worker' on the other, have contributed to the fact that Covid-19 death, both socio-economic and physical, is predicated deeply and profoundly on racism.[6]

For Malcolm X, colonialism was white supremacy, and white supremacy was deeply embedded in the fabric of both the Constitution of the United States and the broader tapestry of the western world (X 2020). Achille Mbembe develops a similar claim in his interpretation of the writings of Frantz Fanon, arguing that colonial violence has three dimensions that work simultaneously to ensure colonial sovereignty (2012). Colonial violence was 'institutional insofar as it oversaw the entrenchment of subjugation by force, the origin of which was dependent on force and the maintenance of which was dependent on force' (2012, p. 22). Colonial violence was embedded in the daily lives of the colonized and manifested itself in varied strategies of control in physical, 'spatial and topological terms, extended both horizontally and vertically. Moreover, searches, unlawful assassinations, expulsion and mutilation targeted the individual subject who had to be monitored down to his every breath. This violence was imposed even on language' (Mbembe 2012, p. 22). Finally, colonial violence simultaneously targeted and attacked both the subject's psyche and their body physically as it 'intended to do nothing less than decerebrate' (Mbembe 2012, p. 22).

In the United States, colonial-racial violence was made inseparable from so-called democracy, materialized through Jim Crow and lynching and solidifying 'the permanent authority of whiteness' (Hesse 2017, p. 592). For Barnor Hesse, 'white sovereignty is the historical assemblage of repeated colonial-racial violence' (2017, p. 592); it legitimizes and even demands the exclusion and expendability of indigenous and subordinate populations – including and especially those marked as belonging to Blackness – while ensuring that only white bodies possess a legitimate claim to violence as in the 'pleasant' gun-toting protestors in Michigan. For Ture and Hamilton (1992, p. 5), as for Césaire in the epigraph opening this article:

To put it another way, there is no 'American dilemma' because Black people in this country form a colony and it is not in the interest of the colonial power to liberate them. Black people are legal citizens of the United States with, for the most part, the same *legal* rights as other citizens. Yet they stand as colonial subjects in relation to the white society. Thus, institutional racism has another name: colonialism.

The Covid-19 pandemic has rearticulated the point that many of us are marked as secondary by virtue of our 'secondariness' (Hall *et al*. 1978, p. 390). It is in this context that Black politics has again 'been obliged to adopt a more populist approach to its constituency and to work from a *community* base' that has propagated 'the ghetto and the politicization of the unemployed' as 'key political factors' (Hall *et al*. 1978, p. 387). The pandemic has inadvertently provided a context for Black empowerment.

Conclusion: and then we had to vote for Joe Biden?

When superstar Cardi B discovered that U.S. Bernie Sanders had ended his bid for the presidency of the United States, she got on Instagram and scolded her followers for not voting. She then stated that she would now have to vote for former Vice-President Joe Biden. Biden, in his effort to secure the young urban Black and Brown vote – one that Sanders was thought to possess – appeared on NYC's The Breakfast Club with radio host Charlamagne tha God. When Biden wanted to leave before the interview had concluded, Charlamagne informed him that they had more questions and Biden replied, 'You've got more questions? Well, I tell you what, if you have a problem figuring out whether you are for me or for Trump, then you ain't Black' (Bradner, Mucha, Saenz 2020). When Charlamagne said it had nothing to do with Trump but his community, Biden responded, 'Take a look at my record, man!' (Bradner, Mucha, Saenz 2020)

While Joe Biden has acknowledged that his role in helping to pass stringent policing laws as a United States Senator was a mistake, he has also stated that he would not defund the police. Biden later made his way onto the Breakfast Club for a second time, but this time as Charlamagne tha God's 'Donkey of the Day' for having called Donald Trump the first racist president. Charlamagne stated, "Racism is the American way, ok? Donald Trump is not the first, and sadly, he won't be the last, alright? Saying Donald Trump is the first racist president is a lie, ok? It's a lie that relinquishes America of all responsibility of its bigotry … How the hell can Donald J. Trump be the first racist president in a country where 12 presidents before him owned slaves? Whatcha going to tell me, slavery wasn't racist? It was just business?' (Caralle 2020). Charlamagne *does* know Biden's record – and that of the United States as well.

In the midst of the global pandemic and widespread political unrest, U.S. Congressman John Lewis passed away. During his speech at the Civil Rights leader's funeral, Former U.S. President Bill Clinton stated, 'There were two or three years there where the movement went a little too far toward Stokely but in the end, John Lewis prevailed' (Jeffries 2020, p. 1). As indicated by Clinton's comment, white sovereignty not only asserts its power through repeated colonial violence but also through a continued renunciation of Black Power. This pattern is also evident in the various representations of Black Lives Matter (BLM) protestors as both violent and inciting of violence even though, according to The Armed Conflict and Event Data Location Project (ACLED), of '7,750 Black Lives Matter demonstrations in all 50 states and Washington D.C. that took place in the wake of George Floyd's death between May 26 and August 22,' 93% of BLM protests were peaceful (Mansoor 2020, p. 2). ACLED's study also found that state authorities 'disproportionately used force while intervening in demonstrations associated with the BLM movement, relative to other types of demonstrations,' and BLM protesters were also victimized through 'dozens of car-ramming attacks,' some of which were exacted by members of right-wing extremist groups (as cited in Mansoor 2020, p. 3). Black Power *is* the antithesis of white sovereignty.

Former U.S. President Barack Obama also spoke at Lewis's funeral, evoking details of Lewis' life to push for the John Lewis Voting Rights Act: legislation that would combat the calculated and systemic weakening of the United States' Voting Rights Act of 1965, a landmark piece of legislation that prohibited racial discrimination. President Obama added that we must continue to march to strengthen the JLVR Act and incorporate former inmates, in addition to citizens in Washington D.C. and Puerto Rico.[7] These efforts, for President Obama, would provide voters with the 'power to choose their politicians, not the other way around' (Cineas 2020, p. 10). As Fanon (1967) forewarned in his appeal to Africans for decolonization, however, the reliance of voter participation can bind us tighter to the racial colonial violence of white supremacy. In contrast, Black Power is the fundamental understanding that 'there can be no social order without social justice' (Ture and Hamilton 1992, p. 53).

Black Power does not rely on the very structure that aims to oppose and even annihilate it. As John Lewis' mentor Dr. Martin Luther King, Jr. described it, Black Power is 'a call to black people to amass the political and economic strength to achieve their legitimate goals' (2015, p. 192). For King, Black Power is a love and affirmation of Blackness that is both economic and psychological – and also necessary (King 2015). For us, as cultural studies scholars, Black Power as revealed during the Covid-19 pandemic prompts a return to the study of the popular with racism and colonial violence as the primary mode of white sovereignty – to borrow from Hall (Hay, Hall, Grossberg 2013), a conjunctural moment within a larger conjuncture spurred by colonization and enslavement. Black Power is a practice with the collective 'people' at its core, a people that has been and can be 'constituted as a force against the power-bloc' (Hall 1980, p. 239); it is community-based with the ultimate goal of an 'effective share in the total power of the society' (Ture and Hamilton 1992, p. 47). What we do with this moment is open to interpretation and possibilities, and cultural studies is in a unique position, through its methods and objectives, not only to interpret the world in various ways but also to change it.[8]

Notes

1. For a discussion on the normalization of crises, see Calvente and Smicker (2019) and Grossberg (2018).
2. For a discussion of colonial and racial performativity, see Bhabha (1994).
3. For a discussion on informal channels of communication, see Hall et al. (1978).
4. For historical examples of parallel communicative networks, see Scott (1990); see also Mills (2007) and Delgado (2009). For examples of contemporary black politics that parallel politics proper, see Iton (2008) and Spence (2013); see also Brock (2020).
5. For national news coverage of both the Wright assault and the Texas park ranger assault, see World News Tonight with David Muir, May 4, 2020, Season 11, Episode 123. Last accessed: July 13, 2020. Available from: https://abc.com/shows/world-news-tonight/episode-guide/2020-05/04-monday-may-4-2020
6. Black and Brown bodies who are exposed more to pollution than their white counterparts in part because of redlining strategies and additional informal and formal segregation laws of the not too distant past are also dying at a faster rate (Villarosa 2020). Black Americans and Latinx/os/as make up a majority of the front-line workers in part because they have been streamlined into particular occupations. Majority minority is the case across healthcare, public transportation, and janitorial services in addition to even policing in cities like New York. Additionally, over '60% of warehouse and delivery workers in most cities are people of color' (NBC Associated Press 2020, p. 1) Simultaneously, Black and Brown workers are also facing higher unemployment rates than their white counterparts with Black and Latinx women facing the greatest risk of unemployment (Gould and Wilson 2020, Kochhar 2020). Indigenous peoples have also faced an exponential death toll and, while tribes received relief, they had to sue to get it (Ackee 2020, Goden 2020).
7. In the 2016 Presidential election, approximately 6.1 million voters were ineligible to vote due to felony disenfranchisement and Black Americans are disenfranchised at a rate four times greater than non-Blacks (Uggen, Larson, and Shannon 2016). Latinas/os are also disproportionately impacted by felony disenfranchisement though generally not greater than Black Americans; however, the proportion varies throughout the states and there is an undercounting of incarcerated Latinos due to the continued reliance of racial categories in prisons rather than ethnicity (Demeo and Ochoa 2003). Additionally, millions of Americans cannot vote for the president because they live in Guam, the Virgin Islands, Northern Mariana Islands, American Samoa, and Puerto Rico unless they move to the mainland (Murriel 2016).
8. In the 11th Theses on Feuerbach, Karl Marx argues, 'The philosophers have only interpreted the world, in various ways; the point is to change it' (Marx 1888);

Barnor Hesse uses this same text to critique Afropessimism in his twitter account, *Blues and Abstract Truth*; he writes: 'Lessons from 2020: A footnote to Marx's 11th thesis on Feuerbach: Afropessimists have hitherto only interpreted the anti-Black world in one way; their point is not to change it' (Hesse 2020).

Disclosure statement

No potential conflict of interest was reported by the author(s).

Further information

This Special Issue article has been comprehensively reviewed by the Special Issue editors, Associate Professor Ted Striphas and Professor John Nguyet Erni.

References

Ackee, R., 2020. How covid-19 is impacting indigenous people in the U.S. *PBS Newshour*, 13 May. Available from: https://www.pbs.org/newshour/nation/how-covid-19-is-impacting-indigenous-peoples-in-the-u-s [Last accessed 25 Jul 2020].

Associated Press, 2020. People of color, women shoulder front-line work during pandemic. *NBC News*, 4 May. Available from: https://www.nbcnews.com/news/nbcblk/people-color-women-shoulder-front-line-work-during-pandemic-n1199291 [Last accessed: 7 March 2021].

Beckett, L., 2020. Armed protestors demonstrate against Covid-19 lockdown at Michigan capitol. *The Guardian*, 30 April. Available from: https://www.theguardian.com/us-news/2020/apr/30/michigan-protests-coronavirus-lockdown-armed-capitol [Last accessed 13 Jul 2020].

Bhabha, H.K., 1994. *The location of culture*. London: Routledge.

Bogel-Burroughs, N., 2020. Indianapolis police face growing questions after killing 3 people in 8 h. *The New York Times*, 7 May. Available from: https://www.nytimes.com/2020/05/07/us/sean-reed-indianapolis-shooting.html [Last accessed 25 Jul]..

Bogel-Burroughs, N., Dewan, S., and Gray, K., 2020. F.B.I. says Michigan anti-government group plotted to kidnap Gov. Gretchen Whitmer. *The New York Times*, 8 October (updated November 3, 2020). Available from: https://www.nytimes.com/2020/10/08/us/gretchen-whitmer-michigan-militia.html [Last accessed December 30, 2020].

Bradner, E., Mucha, S., Saenz, A., 2020. Biden: 'If you have a problem figuring out whether you're for me or Trump, then you ain't black.' *CNN*, 22 May. Available from: https://www.cnn.com/2020/05/22/politics/biden-charlamagne-tha-god-you-aint-black/index.html [Last Accessed: 7 March 2021].

Brock, A., 2020. *Distributed blackness: African American cybercultures*. New York, NY: New York University Press.

Calvente, L., and Smicker, J., 2019. Crisis subjectivities: resilient, recuperable, and abject representations in the new hard times. *Social identities*, 25 (2), 141–155.

Caralle, K., 2020. Charlamagne Tha God calls Joe Biden 'Donkey of the Day' for saying Donald Trump is the 'first racist president' and blames him for making Kanye 'a viable option.' *DailyMail*, 24 July. Available from: https://www.dailymail.co.uk/news/article-8557549/Charlamagne-Tha-God-calls-Biden-donkey-day-saying-Trump-racist-president.html [Last Accessed 7 March 2021].

Césaire, A., 2010. Culture and colonization. *Social text*, 28 (2(103)), 127–144.

Chakrabarti, M., and Kotsonis, S. 2020. How New York city became the epicenter of the coronavirus pandemic. *On Point*, 13 April. Available from: https://www.wbur.org/onpoint/2020/04/13/new-york-city-epicenter-pandemic [Last accessed 9 Jul 2020].

Cheney-Rice, Z. 2020. Even during a pandemic, the NYPD is still the NYPD. *Intelligencer*, 5 May. Available from: https://nymag.com/intelligencer/2020/05/nypd-social-distancing-enforcement-run-amok.html#comments [Last accessed 9 Jul 2020].

Chiel, E. 2017. Police floodlights are unlikely to reduce crime, but could harm your health. *Vice*, 25 February. Available from: https://www.vice.com/en_us/article/z48j83/police-floodlights-are-unlikely-to-reduce-crime-but-could-harm-your-health [Last accessed 17 Jul 2020].

Cineas, F. 2020. "The March is Not Over:" Read Barack Obama's Eulogy for John Lewis. *Vox*, 30 July. Available from: https://www.vox.com/2020/7/30/21348062/john-lewis-funeral-barack-obama-eulogy [Last accessed 31 Jul 2020].

Delgado, R., 2009. The law of the noose: A history of Latino lynching. *Harvard civil rights – civil liberties law review*, 44, 297–312.

Demeo, M.J., and Ochoa, S.A. 2003. Diminished voting power in the Latino community: The impact of Felony disenfranchisement laws in ten targeted states. *MALDEF*, December. Available from: https://static.prisonpolicy.org/scans/diminishedpower.pdf [Last Accessed 31 Jul 2020].

Egan, P. 2020. Capitol protestors urge an end to Michigan's state of emergency. *Detroit Free Press*, April 30. Available from: https://www.freep.com/story/news/local/michigan/2020/04/30/capitol-protesters-urge-end-michigan-state-of-emergency/3055294001/ [Accessed 10 Jul 2020].

Elliott, J.K. 2020. Park ranger pushed into lake while telling crowd about coronavirus rules. *Global News*, May 5. Available from: https://globalnews.ca/news/6906158/coronavirus-park-ranger-pushed/ [Last accessed 13 Jul 2020].

Fanon, F., 1967. *Toward the African revolution: political essays*. Haakon Chevalier, trans. New York, NY: Grove Press.

Gilroy, P., et al., 2019. A diagnosis of contemporary forms of racism, race and nationalism: a conversation with Professor Paul Gilroy, *Cultural studies*, 33 (2), 173-197.

Goden, M., 2020. 'We know what is best for us.' Indigenous groups around the world are taking COVID-19 responses into their own hands. *Time*, 29 May. Available from: https://time.com/5808257/indigenous-communities-coronavirus-impact/ [Last accessed 7 March 2021].

Gould, E. and Wilson, V., 2020. Black workers face two of the most lethal conditions for coronavirus-racism and economic inequality. *Economic Policy Institute*, 1 June. Available from: https://www.epi.org/publication/black-workers-covid/ [Last accessed 7 March 2021].

Grossberg, L., 2018. *Under the cover of chaos: Trump and the battle for the American right*. London: Pluto Press.

Hall, S., 1980. Notes on deconstructing 'the popular'. In: R. Samuel, ed. *People's history and socialist theory*. London: Routledge, 227–240.

Hall, S., et al., 1978. *Policing the Crisis: mugging, the state, and law and order*. London: MacMillan Press, LTD.

Hay, J., Hall, S., and Grossberg, L., 2013. Interview with Stuart hall. *Communication and critical/cultural studies*, 10 (1), 10–33.

Hesse, B., 2017. White sovereignty (…), Black life politics: "The N****r they couldn't kill.". *The South atlantic quarterly*, 116 (3), 581–604.

Hesse, B., 2020. Lessons from 2020. *Twitter*, 26 December. Available from: https://twitter.com/barnor_hesse?ref_src=twsrc%5Egoogle%7Ctwcamp%5Eserp%7Ctwgr%5Eauthor [Last accessed 4 Jan 2021].

Iton, R., 2008. *In search of the Black fantastic: politics and popular culture in the post civil rights era*. New York, NY: Oxford University Press.

Jeffries, H. K., 2020. Opinion: Stokely Carmichael didn't deserve Bill Clinton's during John Lewis's funeral. *The Washington Post*, 1 August. Available from: https://www.washingtonpost.com/opinions/2020/08/01/stokely-carmichael-didnt-deserve-bill-clintons-swipe-during-john-lewiss-funeral/ [Last accessed 7 March 2021].

King, M.L., 2015. *The radical king*. Cornel West, ed. Boston, MA: Beacon Press.

Kochhar, R., 2020. Hispanic women, immigrants, young adults, those with less education hit hardest by COVID-19 job losses. *Pew Research Center*, 9 June. Available from: https://www.pewresearch.org/fact-tank/2020/06/09/hispanic-women-immigrants-young-adults-those-with-less-education-hit-hardest-by-covid-19-job-losses/ [Last accessed 7 March 2021].

Mai, A., and Annesse, J. 2016. NYPD officer shoots emotionally disturbed man in Lower East Side housing complex. *New York Daily News*, 26 January. Available from: https://www.nydailynews.com/new-york/man-shot-nypd-east-side-housing-complex-article-1.2509504 [Last accessed 21 Jul 2020].

Mansoor, S. 2020. 93% of Black lives matter protests have been peaceful, new report finds. *Time*, 5 September. Available from: https://time.com/5886348/report-peaceful-protests/ [Last accessed 29 Dec 2020].

Marx, K. 1888. Theses on Feuerbach. *Marx/Engels Internet Archive*, 1995. Available from: https://www.marxists.org/archive/marx/works/1845/theses/theses.htm [Last accessed 4 Jan 2021].

Mauger, C., and LeBlanc, B. 2020. Trump tweets 'liberate Michigan,' two other states with Dem Governors. *The Detroit News*, 17 April. Available from: https://www.detroitnews.com/story/news/politics/2020/04/17/trump-tweets-liberate-michigan-other-states-democratic-governors/5152037002/ [Last accessed 15 Jul 2020].

Mbembe, A., 2012. Metamorphic thought: The works of Frantz fanon. *African studies*, 71 (1), 19–28.

McKinley, J. 2020. New York City region is now an epicenter for the coronavirus pandemic. *The New York Times*, 22 March. Available from: https://www.nytimes.com/2020/03/22/nyregion/Coronavirus-new-York-epicenter.html [Last accessed 9 Jul 2020].

Mills, C.W., 2007. White ignorance. In: S. Sullivan and N. Tuana, eds. *Race and epistemologies of ignorance*. Albany, NY: State University of New York Press, 13–38.

Murriel, M. 2016. Millions of Americans can't vote for President because of where they live. *The World*, 1 November. Available from: https://www.pri.org/stories/2016-11-

01/millions-americans-cant-vote-president-because-where-they-live [Last accessed 31 Jul 2020].

Ramirez, J. 2018. Tenant says NYCHA tried to evict her for complaints on conditions. *Spectrum News*, 30 April. Available from: https://spectrumlocalnews.com/nys/hudson-valley/news/2018/05/01/jacob-riis-houses-tenant-says-nycha-tried-evict-her-for-complaints-about-conditions [Last accessed 20 Jul 2020].

Scott, J.C., 1990. *Domination and the Art of resistance: hidden transcripts*. New Haven, CT: Yale University Press.

Southall, A. 2020. Officer who pressed a knee into Bystander's Neck Leaves N.Y.P.D. *The New York Times*, 28 October (Updated 5 November 2020). Available from: https://www.nytimes.com/2020/10/28/nyregion/nypd-officer-francisco-garcia.html?referringSource=articleShare [Last accessed 30 Dec 2020].

Spence, L.K., 2013. *Stare in the darkness: The limits of Hip Hop and Black politics*. Minneapolis, MN: University of Minnesota Press.

Ture, K., and Hamilton, C.V., 1992. *Black Power: the politics of liberation*. New York, NY: Vintage Books.

Uggen, C., Larson, R., and Shannon, S. 2016. 6 Million lost voters: state level estimates of Felony disenfranchisement, 2016. *The Sentencing Project*, 6 October. Available from: https://www.sentencingproject.org/publications/6-million-lost-voters-state-level-estimates-felony-disenfranchisement-2016/ [Last accessed 31 Jul 2020].

Vallejo, J., 2020. Naked doll hanging by a noose prompts fight at armed anti-lockdown protest in Michigan. *Independent*, May 14. Available from: https://www.independent.co.uk/news/world/americas/lockdown-protest-michigan-fight-doll-noose-gretchen-whitmer-a9515381.html [Last accessed 15 Jul 2020].

Verde, B., 2020. See it: Cops aggressively arrest mom who improperly wore face mask in Brooklyn Subway Station. *Brooklyn Paper*, 13 May. Available from: https://www.brooklynpaper.com/video-cops-arrest-mom-social-distancing/ [Last accessed 10 Jul 2020].

Villarosa, L., 2020. 'A terrible price': The deadly racial disparities of Covid-19 in America. *The New York Times Magazine*, 29 April. Available from: https://www.nytimes.com/2020/04/29/magazine/racial-disparities-covid-19.html [Last accessed: 7 March 2021].

X, M. 2020. *The end of white world supremacy: four speeches*. Imam Benjamin Karim, ed. New York, NY: Arcade Publishing.

Asian Americans as racial contagion

Madhavi Mallapragada

ABSTRACT
The convergence of racism against Asian Americans and the tightening of borders to prohibit and control the entry of Asian immigrants during the COVID-19 pandemic, though distressing, is not unprecedented. It is in fact a repetition of a historical pattern where exclusion or restriction of Asian immigration and racist scapegoating of Asian Americans converge and surge during periods of public health crises in the United States. Yellow Peril narratives, Orientalist tropes of 'filthy, backward and morally depraved' Asians, and racialized discourses about disease, migration, and belonging, which have historically played a crucial role in the cultural production of Asians as a racial contagion, have reemerged in the context of COVID-19, although the specific discursive conditions and impact are not always identical. Nonetheless, reduced to their bodies, which in turn are ethno-stigmatized (by their presumed connection with China), Chinese Americans and Asian Americans are being invested with the epidemiological properties associated with COVID-19 – infectious, contaminating the air around them, and contagious. While Asian Americans are being viewed as an embodied form of the contagion that needs to be expelled, Asian immigrants are being projected as a potential risk and as a future threat that needs to be contained. The anti-Asian racism during COVID-19 illuminates the through lines of white supremacism and virulent nativism that are integral to the foundation of the United States and its past and present imaginaries of 'American' national identity, culture, and security. Asian Americans are being reminded, yet again, of the precarity of their belonging within the white American nation, and their vexed condition redirects our attention to the need for a more contextualized analysis of the complicated entanglement of ideologies of liberal multiculturalism and racial capitalism with those of settler colonialism and white supremacy in the current socio-political moment.

Across the United States, the COVID-19 pandemic has fuelled a spike in every-day racism and hate crimes against Asian Americans. Between March and December 2020, the STOP AAPI HATE reporting centre documented more than 2,800 self-reported incidents that include being set on fire, stabbed, spit on, verbally bullied with racial slurs, and vandalized[1] (STOP AAPI HATE Reports 2020). Asian Americans in the medical and health care professions have reported dealing with racist patients who refuse to be treated by 'Asian' doctors over fears of contracting the 'China virus' (Jan 2020). Across the country, in streets, neighbourhoods, public transit, and workplaces, Asian Americans are being re-traumatized as the familiar racist insults of 'go back home,' and 'go back to whatever Asian country you came from' are hurled at them (Sanchez 2020).[2]

The pandemic has also resulted in the suspension and restriction of immigration, mostly from Asian countries, into the United States. The United States Citizenship and Immigration Services, following the orders in Presidential Proclamations (issued in April and June 2020), stopped issuing immigrant visas/green cards, non-immigrant employment visas like the H-1B, and dependent family visas like the L-2.[3] Immigration was further tightened by the addition of new guidelines and requirements to the legal process of transitioning from nonimmigrant to immigrant status (US Department of State-Bureau of Consular Affairs 2020). A short-lived proposal by the U.S. Immigration and Customs Enforcement would have required international students enrolled in online learning for Fall 2020 to voluntarily leave the United States or face deportation (Treisman 2020). Although none of the pandemic-spurred immigration regulations are country-specific, they disproportionately affect applicants from Asia, notably, from China, India, Korea, and the Philippines (and black and brown populations, globally).[4]

The convergence of racism against Asian Americans and the tightening of borders to prohibit and control the entry of Asian immigrants during the COVID-19 pandemic, though distressing, is not unprecedented. It is in fact a repetition of a historical pattern where exclusion or restriction of Asian immigration and racist scapegoating of Asian Americans converge and surge during periods of public health crises in the United States (Trauner 1978, Shah 2001). Yellow and Brown peril narratives (Lee 2015), Orientalist tropes of 'filthy, backward and morally depraved' Asians (Said 1978), and racialized discourses about disease, migration, and belonging (Molina 2006), which have historically played a crucial role in the cultural production of Asians as a racial contagion, have reemerged in the context of COVID-19, although the specific discursive conditions and impact are not always identical. In this essay, my aim is to foreground the value of a historical perspective to better understand the COVID-19 pandemic-related construction of Asian Americans as diseased, contagious and as a threat. In the concluding section, I reflect on the precariousness experienced by Asian Americans (due to hate crimes) in the context of neoliberal discourses of multiculturalism in US media industries where the presence, the participation and the 'success stories' of Asian Americans is crucial to the representation of the industries as being racially diverse and inclusive. While contagion narratives produce Asian Americans as threats, and diversity narratives imagine Asian Americans as desirable, their simultaneous presence in contemporary public culture opens up a productive line of enquiry into the making, unmaking, and remaking of race, generally, and more specifically of Asian Americans as 'raced' subjects in COVID and so-called post-COVID times.

'China virus' and 'alien' risks: racist tropes and white supremacy

The Trump administration's racial scapegoating of China by using the terms 'China/Chinese virus,' 'Wuhan Flu', 'Kung Flu,' and 'China ban,' and by advancing an unsubstantiated claim that the virus is a Chinese state-engineered bioweapon, has politicized the pandemic (Brumfiel 2020, Chiu 2020). Despite community outrage, appeals from health officials, the FBI warning of a spike in hate crimes, and a rebuke from the World Health Organization for violating the organization's guidelines relating to the naming of diseases (WHO 2015), President Trump and his allies continued using racist terminology while discussing the pandemic. There is a long history of naming epidemics after people, places, animals and racist stereotypes (Kaur 2020). Examples include naming the Zika virus after a Ugandan forest, Ebola after a Congolese river, MERS after the Middle East region and the nineteenth and twentieth centuries cholera epidemics and bubonic plagues after 'Asiatics' and 'Orientals,' respectively. The World Health Organization recently acknowledged that such practices stigmatize and endanger the communities 'named' in the disease and announced their decision to end them (WHO 2015). For the Trump administration, however, reframing a pathogen as 'China virus' is part of a broader attempt to steer attention away from their disastrous response to the pandemic (Epimonitor 2020) and towards the incendiary idea that COVID-19 is a threat from abroad and a manifestation of a Chinese contagion that has infiltrated the nation's borders.

Political relations between the United States and China, while historically complex, were particularly tense under the Trump administration. Sinophobia has an important role in the American national imaginary, and American media and popular culture play a key role in shaping its ideological power and impact at a systemic and interpersonal level. Orientalist and racist tropes such as the 'Yellow Peril' and 'dirty' Chinese (Xing 1998), narratives of unassimilable Asian immigrants (marking them as perpetual foreigners within the nation) (Lowe 1996), and stereotypes about Chinese and Asian cultural identities, practices and communities persist to this day. Within the racial and cultural regimes of America, people of Asian descent, regardless of their legal citizenship, continue to experience sustained racism. Utterances such as – 'Look, it's a Chinese – he's got Corona!'; or ' … bringing that Chinese virus over *here*' (emphasis mine); and 'Take your disease that's ruining our country and go home' (California Report 2020) and related physical attacks, which have been documented during the COVID-19 pandemic, indicate that the use of the racist rhetoric by politicians has sanctioned its wider usage among everyday Americans. More importantly, it conveys the emotive register of the term 'China virus' for nativists and white supremacists, who feel called upon to (re)invest and act upon the 'foreign' threat to the American nation – not of the virological kind, but of the immigrant-as-'alien' kind.

When racists view Asian Americans, especially Chinese Americans, as embodiments of the COVID-19 disease, they are reproducing entrenched ideologies, attitudes and practices about Asian immigrants, illness, and epidemics in the United States (and globally). Chinese American bodies, the spaces they inhabit and the neighbourhoods associated with them, such as Chinatowns, are being recast as a racial contagion – that in turn, must be shunned, contained and expelled.

The antecedent to the 2020 'racial contagion' discourse can be traced back to the 'medical scapegoating' (Trauner 1978) of Chinese immigrants in California (and the West Coast) during the late 1800s and early 1900s. When San Francisco – a hub for Chinese immigration during this period and home to the oldest Chinatown district in the country – experienced a smallpox outbreak in 1875–76, it was blamed on the 'lying and treacherous aliens' who lived in Chinatown, the latter described as a 'laboratory of infection,' with its 'foul and disgusting vapors.' (Trauner 73) (the miasma theory of disease popular at the time influenced public belief that diseases were caused by malodor). Xenophobic attitudes towards Chinese immigrants engendered narratives that presented them as economic threats, culturally inferior, uncivilized, incapable of assimilating, and morally perverse. As sanitary reform measures of the city's health officials failed to contain the spread of disease, the 'vile and disease-breeding' (Shah 2001, 4) Chinatown's immigrants were blamed. Regulating the bodies, the morality and the mobility of immigrants was hence linked to the containment and expulsion of disease. Feeding on white economic and racial anxieties, in the 1880s, a rat poison brand advertisement with the slogan, 'they must go,' linked the theme of Chinese expulsion to pest eradication while also exploiting prevailing ideas about the 'exotic' (rat) food cultures of the immigrants (Daniel K. E. Ching Collection Archive). During the 1870s and 1880s, racist cartoons with the slogan, 'Chinese must go' depicted immigrant labourers in traditional attire and pigtails being chased or kicked by white society. Such representations upheld anti-Chinese sentiments and helped shape the passage of the nation's first race and immigration-based legislation: the Chinese Exclusion Act of 1882, which banned the entry of Chinese immigrant labour into the United States (National Archives 2004). Popular media images and constructions of the time articulated the themes of epidemic outbreaks and immigration influx to imaginations of a nation under threat to justify a support for anti-immigration legislation. In a magazine cover illustration titled, 'San Francisco's three graces' published shortly after the Chinese

Exclusion Act of 1882, the diseases of malaria, smallpox and leprosy appear as ghost-like apparitions floating over San Francisco's Chinatown (The Wasp 1882). The racialized and racist logic – that epidemics are an outcome of immigration – undergird the strategies of monitoring, quarantining and possible expulsion that were adopted by the Quarantine station that was opened in 1891 and later by the Angel Island Immigration Station, the leading port of entry into the United States from Asia, as a response to the fears over parasitic and infectious diseases (Angel Island Conservancy).

Over the course of the twentieth century, popular imaginations and media representations continued to construct Asian Americans and Asian immigrants as a menace and infestation. For example, early Hollywood depictions of fictional Chinese villains (notably Fu Manchu and Ming the Merciless) and of the Japanese as foreign invaders shaped Yellow peril narratives while South Asian immigrants were described as 'hindu hordes' and a 'dusky peril.' (Puget South American 1906) Even as so-called positive representations emerged – such as the fictional character of Chinese detective Charlie Chan (1920s–1950s) and Asian Americans as non-threatening, hard-working, high-achieving, culturally traditional, economically successful and politically apathetic 'model minorities' (1960s onwards) – the associations of 'Asians' with threats and risks have persisted (Xing 1998). Stereotypical discussions of the 'Asian' advantage and Asian Americans as overachievers, for example, captures an undercurrent of racial panic, while anti-immigrant labour lobbying and legislation (notably over the H-1B visa for high-skilled labour) explicitly links 'Asian' threats to American workers and their economic security. In the context of disease outbreaks, the discrimination, stigmatization and fear experienced by Asian Americans during the 2003 SARS outbreak offers another example of the fear of contagious 'Asian' bodies (Fang 2020).

During the 2020 pandemic, the narrative threads of 'infected Chinese,' 'Asian' threats and border problems have come into play. Reduced to their bodies, which in turn are ethno-stigmatized (by their presumed connection with China), Chinese Americans and Asian Americans are being invested with the epidemiological properties associated with COVID-19 – infectious, contaminating the air around them, and contagious. Despite wearing masks and practicing social distancing in public spaces, they are being called 'diseased,' and accused of 'having coronavirus' (Siegal 2020). Physical attacks and 'go back to your country' utterances close out the racist logic that since Asian Americans are *the* virus, they pose an immediate threat and hence need to be removed as a de-contamination and safety measure. Relatedly, Chinatowns have been vandalized, and Asian restaurants have been special targets (Fernando and Mumphrey 2020). Given the apparent zoonotic origins of COVID-19 and the spotlight on bats, racist and Orientalizing views about Chinese/Asian foods and meat markets are being aired, especially on social media (Brandon 2020).

While Asian Americans are being viewed as an embodied form of the contagion that needs to be expelled, Asian immigrants (inclusive of non-immigrant 'aliens') are projected as a potential risk and as a future threat that needs to be contained. Since prospective immigrants are physically outside the boundaries of the United States – and therefore their bodies are not readily available to materialize into an immediate threat – it is instead their intent to enter the U.S. for work, study or family reunification purposes that is reframed within the contexts of risks and security. Using the language of loss – the loss of jobs and income for American workers because of layoffs during the pandemic and the loss of potential re-employment opportunities because of the 'threat of competition' from immigrant labour (Trump 2020a, 2020b) – which resonates in the context of the lethal and devastating trajectory of the pandemic in the United States, the border-related measures put in place by the Trump administration's immigration ban articulate a lockdown on (Asian) immigration to the protection and recovery of the American nation symbolized through the figures of American workers and their economic futures.

Confronting racism in neoliberal multicultural times

The tragic resonance between anti-Chinese sentiment in the historical past and in the unfolding present reiterates the value of viewing the racial crisis during COVID-19 through a historical lens. The American Medical Association's recent declaration that racism is a structural barrier to equity and a public health threat, while not a revelation to racially minoritized communities, is significant especially for the visibility it might bring to efforts to dismantle systemic racism (O'Reilly 2020). Relatedly, numerous public conversations and focus stories about race during COVID-19 have been on the structural disparities in healthcare access that are responsible for the disproportionate levels of infections and death in communities of colour. A USA Today story (Cava 2020) connects the alarming rates of illness and death in San Francisco's Asian American communities to lack of funds, necessary information, and cultural stereotypes about Asian Americans as 'model minorities' and being economically well-off, which in turn made it harder for struggling Asian Americans to admit they needed help and resources, and easier for the city to render them invisible. When evaluating the damaging effects of the Yellow peril myth, or its stereotypical counterpart, the 'model minority' myth, the liberal strains of white supremacism in contemporary mainstream media must be foregrounded. To understand the relationship between racism and public health during this pandemic, it is necessary to rope in sites of analyses like media and popular culture, but also to let our analysis be informed by an intersectional frame where the impact of historical supremacist tropes can be viewed in the context of prevailing neoliberal multicultural ones.

A crucial frame relating to race in contemporary America, and one that has been strategically adopted by U.S. media and communication industries, is one where the 'multicultural is new mainstream,' and 'diversity is good for business' (Nielson 2013). This manifests itself in the form of images, representation, rhetoric and some institutional changes to seemingly reflect America's multiracial demographics. Diversity narratives and inclusivity practices are upheld as a sign that both American media and its culture at large have shed historic tendencies shaping the racist past and have undergone a racial reckoning necessary to embrace the multicultural present. Within liberal discourses of media multiculturalism, the rhetoric of racial diversity and inclusivity is often performative and does not extend to a fundamental rethinking of the racial structures and hierarchies that shape mainstream media institutions. Therefore, although Asian Americans have made meaningful gains in recent decades towards greater and diverse representation and participation within American public and popular culture, they continue to experience the material effects of structural racism, white privilege, and cultural stereotypes. In this context, it is significant that the mainstream media outlets that carry multiple stories relating to anti-Asian hate and discrimination have been called out for their gratuitous use of images of East Asian people and Chinatowns in their coverage of the pandemic, thereby reinforcing the racialization of the disease as Chinese (Burton, 2020). The anti-Asian racism during COVID-19 illuminates the through-lines of white supremacism and virulent nativism that are integral to the foundation of the United States and its past and present imaginaries of 'American' national identity, culture, and security. The ideologies of white nationalism, of people of colour as a threat to the 'American' body politic, and of xenophobia directed towards people of Asian descent, which have historically been instrumental in constructing the American nation, are at work in the present context; relatedly, white entitlement and white grievance is on display yet again in the rhetoric and actions implicating racially minoritized Asian Americans as a threat to public safety.

While hate crimes against Asian Americans are being widely denounced and there has been pushback in the form of public outcry, community advocacy, and media awareness and information campaigns, it is important to interrogate what kinds of ideologies are being weakened or strengthened through the different explanations and strategies that are being advanced in discussions of hate crimes, anti-racist measures, and community responsibility. For example, some denouncements of anti-Asian racism revert to the cultural mythology of America as a land of immigrants (as if to say we are all immigrants, so don't target Asian Americans). However well-intentioned, the invoking of the myth strengthens and preserves an origin story of the founding of America that erases the genocide of Native Americans and indigenous communities and the enslavement of Black people. It also flattens the diverse and distinct histories of migration, racialization and community formation within the communities that are invoked within the category of 'Asian American.' Another strategy, exemplified through the op-ed of Asian American politician Andrew Yang, published in *The Washington Post*, puts a substantial onus of ending anti-Asian racism on Asian Americans themselves. In a twenty-first century recasting of the model minority frame, Yang urges Asian Americans to 'embrace and show our American-ness in ways we never have before. We need to step up … wear red white and blue, volunteer, fund aid organizations, and do everything in our power to accelerate the end of this crisis. We should show without a shadow of a doubt that we are Americans who will do our part for our country in this time of need' (Yang 2020). Such contentions, while problematic for setting up an ideal of the patriotic Asian American, do not fundamentally interrogate the issues of whiteness as well as systemic and interpersonal racism that engender hate crimes against Asian Americans. Lastly, since March 2020, civic engagement through data collection of hate crimes (such as the STOPAPPIHATE's reporting centre), as well as public advocacy through interactive and social media campaigns (#WashtheHate, #Iamnotavirus, #STOPAAPIHATE and #MakeNoisetoday on Twitter and YouTube for example), have been two key ways in which Asian Americans are speaking up against hate, pushing back against stereotypes, and engendering a shared sense of belonging for fellow Asian Americans. While these measures are crucial in letting Asian Americans shape public conversations around racism and anti-racism, the upsurge in hate crimes and violence against Asian Americans – especially senior citizens between January-March 2021 – is a sobering reminder of the dangers inherent in racially minoritized voices claiming space and attention, dangers that don't necessarily disappear even in the face of legislation such as the COVID-19 Hate Crimes Act being proposed as of March 2021 by Asian American lawmakers, Representative Meng and Senator Hirono (Yam 2021).

In this moment of rupture, when fresh imaginings of 'community' are possible (and potentially emergent), it is tragic and enraging that racism and xenophobia – especially their latent forms – towards Asian Americans have intensified under the guise of contagion metaphors and erupted in the form of racist speech acts, vicious hate crimes, and inhumane anti-immigration regulations. Asian Americans are being reminded, yet again, of the precarity of their belonging within the white American nation, and their vexed condition redirects our attention to the need for a more contextualized analysis of the complicated entanglement of ideologies of liberal multiculturalism and racial capitalism with those of settler colonialism and white supremacy in the current socio-political moment.

Notes

1. Actual numbers are estimated to be much higher, given the historical trend of underreporting hate crimes.
2. In a White House memorandum dated 26 January 2021, President Biden acknowledged the 'significant harm' caused to AAPI communities by hate crimes during the pandemic and issued guidance to the Department of Justice to collect hate crime data and assist with the reporting of anti-AAPI hate incidents (see Biden Jr. 2021 in references).
3. On 24 February 2021, President Biden issued a proclamation revoking the Trump administration's ban on the issuance of immigrant visas wherein he noted that immigration bans do not advance the interests of the United States. However, the prior administration's ban on employment visas like the H-1B remains in effect and are set to expire on 31 March 2021.
4. Chinese and Indian citizens routinely account for two of the five largest national groups that receive immigrant visas, making them lawful permanent residents of the United States (see Baugh 2019 in references). A majority of the H-1B visas are annually allotted to Filipino, South Korean, Chinese and Indian professionals (see Characteristics of H-1B Specialty Occupation Workers 2020 in references). Students from Asia make up the majority of international students in the United States with Chinese and Indian students accounting for almost half of them (see Announcements 2019 in references).

Disclosure statement

No potential conflict of interest was reported by the author(s).

Further information

This Special Issue article has been comprehensively reviewed by the Special Issue editors, Associate Professor Ted Striphas and Professor John Nguyet Erni.

References

Angel Island Conservancy, Quarantine Station. Available from: https://angelisland.org/history/quarantine-station/ [Accessed 5 January 2021].
Announcements, 2019. Number of international students in the United States hits all-time high. The Power of International Education, 18 November. Available from:

https://www.iie.org/Why-IIE/Announcements/2019/11/Number-of-International-Students-in-the-United-States-Hits-All-Time-High [Accessed 5 August 2020].

Baugh, R., 2019. U.S. lawful permanent residents: 2018. Department of Homeland Security, 1 October. Available from: https://www.dhs.gov/sites/default/files/publications/immigration-statistics/yearbook/2018/lawful_permanent_residents_2018.pdf [Accessed 5 August 2020].

Biden Jr., R.J., 2021. Memorandum condemning and combating racism, xenophobia, and intolerance against Asian Americans and Pacific Islanders in the United States. The White House, 26 January. Available from: https://www.whitehouse.gov/briefing-room/presidential-actions/2021/01/26/memorandum-condemning-and-combating-racism-xenophobia-and-intolerance-against-asian-americans-and-pacific-islanders-in-the-united-states/ [Accessed 1 March 2021].

Brandon, J., 2020. Coronavirus misinformation is spreading on social media. Will Facebook and Twitter react? 26 February. Forbes. Available from: https://www.forbes.com/sites/johnbbrandon/2020/02/26/coronavirus-misinformation-is-spreading-on-social-media-will-facebook-and-twitter-react/?sh=447e9530785e [Accessed 5 January 2021].

Brumfiel, G., 2020. As Trump pushes theory of virus origins, some see parallels in lead-up to Iraq war. NPR, 6 May. Available from: https://www.npr.org/2020/05/06/851043242/as-trump-pushes-theory-of-virus-origins-some-see-parallels-to-iraq [Accessed 3 January 2021].

Burton, N., 2020. Why Asians in masks should not be the "face" of the coronavirus. Vox. 6 March. Available from: https://www.vox.com/identities/2020/3/6/21166625/coronavirus-photos-racism [Accessed 5 January 2021].

California Report, 2020. Over 800 COVID-19-related hate incidents against Asian Americans take place in California in three months. STOP AAPI HATE Reports, 30 June. Available from: http://www.asianpacificpolicyandplanningcouncil.org/wp-content/uploads/CA_Report_6_30_20.pdf [Accessed 6 July 2020].

Cava, D. M., 2020. Asian Americans in San Francisco are dying at alarming rates from COVID-19: Racism is to blame. USA Today News. 18 October. Available from: https://www.usatoday.com/in-depth/news/nation/2020/10/18/coronavirus-asian-americans-racism-death-rates-san-francisco/5799617002/ [Accessed 5 January 2021].

Characteristics of H-1B Specialty Occupation Workers, 2020. Fiscal year 2019 annual report to congress. Department of Homeland Security. 5 March. Available from; https://www.uscis.gov/sites/default/files/document/reports/Characteristics_of_Specialty_Occupation_Workers_H-1B_Fiscal_Year_2019.pdf [Accessed 5 August 2020].

Chiu, A., 2020. Trump has no qualms about calling coronavirus the 'Chinese Virus.' That's a dangerous attitude, experts say. The Washington Post, 20 March. Available from: https://www.washingtonpost.com/nation/2020/03/20/coronavirus-trump-chinese-virus/ [Accessed 22 March 2020].

Daniel K.E. Ching Collection, Archive. Rough on Rats. Chinese Historical Society of America. Entry/Object ID CHSA-01056. Available from: https://chsa.org/exhibits/collections/chsa-collections-database/ [Accessed 3 January2020].

Epimonitor, 2020. Epimonitor: the voice of epidemiology. Available from: https://www.epimonitor.net/EIS-Officers-Letter-In-Support-Of-CDC.htm [Accessed 3 January 2021].

Fang, J., 2020. The 2003 SARS outbreak fueled Anti-Asian racism. Coronavirus doesn't have to. The Washington Post, 4 March. Available from: https://www.washingtonpost.com/outlook/2020/02/04/2003-sars-outbreak-fueled-anti-asian-racism-this-pandemic-doesnt-have/. [Accessed 5 January 2021].

Fernando, C. and Mumphrey, C., 2020. Racism targets Asian food, business during Covid-19 Pandemic, *AP News*. 20 December. Available from: https://apnews.com/article/donald-trump-race-and-ethnicity-pandemics-wuhan-animals4d25738ab49597d0de1517383a9108d2 [Accessed 5 January 2021].

Jan, T., 2020. Asian American doctors and nurses are fighting racism and the coronavirus. *The Washington Post*, 19 May. Available from: https://www.washingtonpost.com/business/2020/05/19/asian-american-discrimination/ [Accessed 1 June 2020].

Kaur, H., 2020. Yes, we long have referred to disease outbreaks by geographic places. Here's why we shouldn't anymore. *CNN*, 28 March. Available from: https://www.cnn.com/2020/03/28/us/disease-outbreaks-coronavirus-namingtrnd/index.html [Accessed 3 January 2021].

Lee, E., 2015. *The making of Asian America*. New York: Simon and Schuster.

Lowe, L., 1996. *Immigrant acts: on Asian American cultural politics*. Durham: Duke University Press.

Molina, N., 2006. *Fit to be citizens? Public health and race in Los Angeles, 1879–1939*. Berkeley: Univ. of California Press.

National Archives, 2004. National archives presents databases for "Chinese Exclusion Act" (RG 85) Records. 28 July. Available from: https://www.archives.gov/press/press-releases/2004/nr04-75.html [Accessed 5 January 2021].

Nielson Consumer Report, 2013. Significant, sophisticated and savvy: the Asian American consumer. Nielson, 3 December. Available from: https://www.nielsen.com/us/en/insights/report/2013/significant-sophisticated-and-savvy-the-asian-american-consumer-report-2013/. [Accessed 5 January 2021].

O'Reilly, B.K., 2020. Racism is a threat to Public Health. 16 November. *AMA*. Available from: https://www.ama-assn.org/delivering-care/health-equity/ama-racism-threat-public-health [Accessed 5 January 2021].

Puget South American, 1906. Have we a Dusky Peril? Hindu Hordes Invading the State 16 September. South Asian American Digital Archive. Available from: https://www.saada.org/item/20111215-549. [Accessed 1 March 2021].

Said, E., 1978. *Orientalism*. New York: Pantheon Books.

Sanchez, H., 2020. Fear, avoidance, being told to go back to their country: what it's like to be Asian in Colorado in the time of coronavirus. *Colorado Public Radio*, 31 March. Available from: https://www.cpr.org/2020/03/31/fear-avoidance-being-told-to-go-back-to-their-country-what-its-like-to-be-asian-in-colorado-with-coronavirus/ [Accessed 1 August 2020].

Shah, N., 2001. *Contagious divides: epidemics and race in San Francisco's Chinatown*. Oakland: University of California Press.

Siegal, I., 2020. Woman called 'diseased' in possible coronavirus-based Manhattan subway station attack. 6 February. NBC New York. Available from: https://www.nbcnewyork.com/news/local/crime-and-courts/woman-called-diseased-in-possible-coronvirus-based-manhattan-subway-station-attack/2280090/ [Accessed 5 January 2021].

STOP AAPI HATE Reports, 2020. STOP AAPI HATE Reporting Center. Available from: http://www.asianpacificpolicyandplanningcouncil.org/stop-aapi-hate-reports/ [Accessed 3 January 2021].

The Wasp, 1882. San Francisco's three graces. Chinese in California collection. Identifier No. 304. Calisphere: University of California. Available from: http://content.cdlib.org/ark:/13030/hb8x0nb2zm/?layout=metadata&brand=calisphere [Accessed 5 January 2021].

Trauner, J., 1978. The Chinese as medical scapegoats in San Francisco, 1870–1905. *California history*, 57 (1), The Chinese in California (Spring), 70–87. Univ. of California Press in association with the California Historical Society.

Treisman, R., 2020. ICE agrees to rescind policy barring foreign students from online study in the U.S. *National Public Radio*, 14 July. Available from: https://www.npr. org/sections/coronavirus-live-updates/2020/07/14/891125619/ice-agrees-to-rescind-policy-barring-foreign-students-from-online-study-in-the-u [Accessed 18 July 2020].

Trump, J.D., 2020a. Proclamation suspending entry of immigrants who present risk to the U.S. labor market during the economic recovery following the COVID-19 Outbreak. The White House, 22 April. Available from: https://www.whitehouse. gov/presidential-actions/proclamation-suspending-entry-immigrants-present-risk-u-s-labor-market-economic-recovery-following-covid-19-outbreak/ [Accessed 30 April 2020].

Trump, J.D., 2020b. Proclamation suspending entry of aliens who present a risk to the U.S. labor market following the coronavirus outbreak. The White House, 22 June. Available from: https://www.whitehouse.gov/presidential-actions/proclamation-suspending-entry-aliens-present-risk-u-s-labor-market-following-coronavirus-out break/ [Accessed 24 June 2020].

US Department of State-Bureau of Consular Affairs, 2020. US Visa news. Available from: https://travel.state.gov/content/travel/en/News/visas-news.html [Accessed 10 August 2020].

WHO, 2015. WHO issues best practices for naming new human infectious diseases. World Health Organization, 8 May. Available from: https://www.who.int/mediacentre/news/notes/2015/naming-new-diseases/en/ [Accessed 5 April 2020].

Xing, J., 1998. *Asian America through the lens: history, representations, and identities.* Lanham: Altamira Press.

Yam, K., 2021. Asian American lawmakers reintroduce legislation to combat Covid-related hate Crimes. *NBC News*. 11 March. Available from: https://www.nbcnews. com/news/asian-america/asian-american-lawmakers-reintroduce-legislation-comb at-covid-related-hate-crimes-n1260749 [Accessed 11 March 2021].

Yang, A., 2020. We Asian Americans are not the virus, but we can be part of the cure. *The Washington Post*. 1 April. Available from: https://www.washingtonpost.com/opinions/2020/04/01/andrew-yang-coronavirus-discrimination/. [Accessed 5 January 2021].

COVID-19 and 'crisis as ordinary': pathological whiteness, popular pessimism, and pre-apocalyptic cultural studies

Josh Smicker

ABSTRACT

In this essay I elaborate the concept of 'pathological whiteness' as a way to articulate and understand the ways in which openness to infection, transmission and death by COVID-19 has become a central element of US white conservative subjectivities, discourses and embodied practices during the pandemic. Of particular importance are the ways in which potential or actual infection is understood and enacted as a biological threat to racialized others through the weaponization of one's own body, with infection and transmission of COVID serving as a form of racist necropolitical violence mobilized to defend and maintain white supremacist policies and futures. I analyse some of the key logics and examples of this pathological whiteness, and situate it within a broader cultural conjuncture defined by what [Calvente, L. and Smicker, J., 2019. Crisis subjectivities: resilient, recuperable, and abject representations in the new hard times. *Social Identities*, 25 (2), 141–155] have discussed as 'crisis as ordinary.' I briefly explore some of the main relationships of pathological whiteness to crisis as ordinary, and conclude by gesturing to some possible considerations for contemporary cultural studies work when trying to analyse and intervene into this cultural formation.

Almost everywhere the law of blood, the law of the talion, and duty to one's race – the two supplements of atavistic nationalism – are resurfacing. The hitherto more or less hidden violence of democracies is rising to the surface, producing a lethal circle that is increasingly difficult to escape. *Nearly everywhere the political order is reconstituting itself as a form of organization for death.*
                                                              – Achille Mbembe, *Necropolitics*

Another end of the world is possible.
 – Graffiti seen at multiple sites during the US anti-racist protests of July 2020

On 30 April 2020, as the number of COVID-19 cases across the United States were beginning to rapidly rise, a group of armed, white, right-wing protesters participating in what they called 'The American Patriot Rally' (Figure 1) forced their way into the Michigan state Capitol to protest the extension of mandatory stay-at-home orders meant to help 'flatten the curve' of the pandemic in the state that was part of the public health response designed by Gretchen Whitmer, its Democratic governor. Organized by a private Facebook group called 'Michigan United for Liberty,' members of the protest were variously wearing pro-Trump gear, swastikas, confederate flags, and the Hawaiian shirts that have become the standard uniform of the race war-baiting 'Boogaloo bois', and participants also included members of other white nationalist paramilitary organizations like the Three Percenters and the Oathkeepers.[1] A large contingent of the group armed with AR-15 assault rifles (the firearm brand of choice employed in recent terrorist massacres like the Las Vegas shootings and the Pulse nightclub shootings, among many others) took up a position in the balcony of the statehouse that directly overlooks the members of the state Senate, which was read by its members as such a substantive threat that several Michigan senators wore bulletproof vests (BBC 2020). Beyond their firearms the lack of any personal protective gear, the sheer size of the crowd, and its physical proximity to capitol security and legislators also meant that the bodies of the protestors themselves were weaponized through their potential transmission of the COVID virus. Donald Trump's response to this violent disruption of the process of a state's democratic governance was to send the participants an encouraging tweet instructing them to 'LIBERATE MICHIGAN.'

The combination of the severity of the threat of violence and/as infection and the explicit encouragement of these tactics from the president, the national Republican party, and conservative media more generally ended

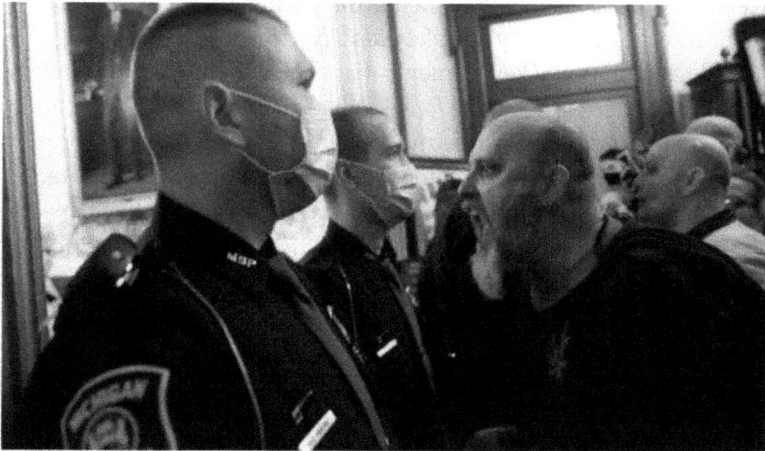

Figure 1. Protestors at the 'American Patriot Rally' at the Michigan Statehouse.

up making this a successful assault on the democratic process and a proof of concept for other assaults on state capitols (as in Oregon) and the 1/6 insurrection. Two weeks later another Michigan state legislative session was cancelled when planning for the follow-up protest (dubbed 'Judgment Day') began featuring even more direct calls for physical violence, sexual assault, and/or the assassination of Gov. Whitmer on private Facebook groups including 'Michigan Unite for Liberty' (Welch 2020). The simultaneous allusion to religious apocalypse and the spectacular violence of the *Terminator* franchise seems appropriate enough, as the online discussion began to increasingly include posts making arguments such as 'plain and simple she needs to eat lead and send a statement to the rest of democrats that they are next' and that the participants 'gotta go in, grab her by the hair and drag her down the street for everyone to see. Get the gallos [*sic*] ready' (Neavling 2021). After Michigan newspapers shared this information with Facebook, the 'Michigan Unites for Liberty' group was shut down for violating the company's policies on hate speech and incitement of violence.

I would suggest that the 'American Patriot Rally' has largely served as the prototype for the white conservative reaction to the pandemic in the United States, and has only intensified in the wake of the anti-racist movements that have emerged during the pandemic as a response to both the disproportionate impact of COVID on communities of colour and the highly visible and currently unpunished murders of Ahmad Arbury, George Floyd, and Breonna Taylor (among others) during quarantine, suggesting that the one thing that could remain 'normal' during COVID was officially sanctioned anti-Black violence. The 'American Patriot Rally' and similar conservative organized protests and quotidian performances during COVID-19 – most obviously the 1/6 assault on the U.S. Capitol in a final violent attempt to overturn the democratic election of Joe Biden–s erve as points of articulation between a number of elements composing what can best be thought of together as a conjuncturally specific *pathological whiteness*.

There are a number of key elements that compose this specific modality of pathological whiteness. First, *the foregrounding of white grievance politics* and the presumption of unfair treatment, persecution, and disproportionate suffering because of one's whiteness (a weaponized 'reverse racism').[2] Second, the *literalization of this weaponized whiteness* via the paramilitarization of 'mainstream' white conservative politics and the increasing acceptance, centrality, and normalization of threatened or actual political violence by overlapping networks of state and non-state actors, including the necropolitical violence of spreading the virus to others . Third, *an increasing popular extremism*, as law enforcement and 'mainstream' conservative politicians actively encourage, support, and even participate in what were previously understood as 'fringe' or 'extremist' elements of these formations.[3] Fourth, the *prominent role of viral conspiracy theories and other forms of online misinformation* as the primary sources for 'news' and meaning-making, serving as the main lenses for understanding the broader cultural context in general and COVID-19 and its proper responses in particular (e.g. QAnon, the medical 'conspiracy' to deny the efficacy of hydroxychloroquine as a treatment option,'Plandemic', etc.).[4] Fifth, and most importantly in this context, *an openness by participants to exposure, infection, transmission, illness, and death by COVID-19* for themselves but more importantly racialized others, i n the service of white supremacist conservative politics.[5] These elements are affectively organized and driven by a structure of feeling composed primarily by moods of fatalism, pessimism, rage, and spite that Lawrence Grossberg (2017) has termed 'passive nihilism' and which might now be better understood as having morphed into an aggressively 'active nihilism,' which of course also has its own sadistic pleasures.

My understanding of this pathological whiteness is based on the extensive critical race theory literature analysing the politics of white racist resentment, white supremacist violence, 'toxic' white masculinities and subjectivities, and anti-black racism.[6] Especially central to the particular conjunctural understanding of pathological whiteness under COVID are Bernadette Calafell's (2015) discussion of the 'monstrosity of whiteness' and Kane Race's (2016) thoughts on 'the pathological' as a descriptor of post-Trump quotidian conservative performance. In her analysis of the cultural construction of James Holmes ('the Aurora shooter') as a type of long-suffering and relatable white victim through news accounts and social media commentary, Calafell elaborates an understanding of white monstrosity as primarily defined by its constant generation of a 'gray area as the nebulous and confusing space where responsibility for inappropriate actions becomes tangled and lost' which in turn serves abet or 'excuse white male violence,' particularly if it is justified as a way to avoid or counteract 'infection by Otherness' (Calafell 2015, 41–42).

This definition of monstrous whiteness as an abdication of both personal and social responsibility which legitimizes, if not actively demands, racist violence can in turn be put in productive conversation with Race's discussion of 'the pathological.' He argues that 'the pathological' can serve as a generative concept for thinking through new forms of hegemonic minoritization – 'when a hegemonic social identity – in this case, white and heteromasculinist – starts to understand itself as an aggrieved and embattled minority' (Race 2016, 1). Referring to the increasing number of 'excessive' performances of white racism occurring under the Trump regime that are often captured on video and shared virally on social media, Race suggests that "losing their shit' is a polite way of putting it: what we have here is a series of highly public, abusive outbursts, precipitated by feeling of entitlement to special treatment that are apparently frustrated' (Race 2016). Taken together, Calafell's 'white monstrosity' and Race's 'pathological' are useful in both linking together and understanding more recent performances of pathological whiteness.

While a few specific examples of pathological whiteness will be discussed in more detail below, it is important to underscore the breadth and intensity of these everyday white conservative performances, which have recently included a wide-ranging set of examples that includes attempts to whitewash Black Lives Matter murals and messages in public spaces, to wearing Nazi flag face masks as a response to mask mandates, to spitting on people to potentially infect them with COVID, to demonstrating police K-9 takedowns on a volunteer dressed as Colin Kaepernick, among many others. Like Trumpist politics more generally, these reactionary and often improvised COVID-19 conservative performances have constellated and fused into a more general social formation of what I understand as a mode of *subjunctive violence*. I use the term subjunctive violence to capture how white male threats of violence, especially online, are increasingly fused with elements of satire, absurdism, humour, denial, and/or gaslighting in a way that is meant to (a) *obfuscate* if they are 'real' threats or not, and to blur the boundaries between their 'online' and 'real' status (b) to provide *plausible deniability* about the seriousness of the threats, often to avoid criminal liability or deplatforming; (c) to enable a *delayed public decisio*n on their reality for as long as possible, usually operating in the register of 'too late'; and (d) *to intensify the confusion and terror experienced by its victims* due to all of the above, an infliction of suffering meant to function as a key component of the threatened violence whether it is 'actualized' or not (Race 2016).[7]

The mission statement of this pathological whiteness is perhaps most clearly articulated in Republican Texas Lt. Governor's Dan Patrick's well-publicized claim that not only should elderly and high-risk populations in the United States be *willing* to suffer infection and death for the sake of 'the economy' (which in all of these discourses is bizarrely abstracted from the obvious economic impacts of an ongoing pandemic through the conservative false dichotomy of the need to prioritize either 'public health' or 'the economy') but that they should be *happy* to do so for the sake of the 'younger' and 'fitter' populations that would somehow presumably benefit from their illness, hospitalization, and demise. Patrick suggests that senior citizens and high-risk populations should gladly 'take a chance on [their] survival in exchange for keeping the America that America loves for its children and grand-children,' since after all 'there are more important things than living' (Knodel 2020, Madani 2020). Expressed this way, pathological whiteness under COVID-19 functions as a particular racist formation that shapes a 'political organization of death' premised on the direct valorization of infection, transmission, illness, and death by COVID of vulnerable others (especially racial others), and if necessary one's self, in the service of broader white conservative goals (Mbembe 2019). While these proximate goals are often pandemic-related (rolling back public health regulations more rapidly, not wearing face masks or engaging in any other individual risk mitigation, not admitting any mistakes have been made by the Trump regime) they are more generally about preserving and expanding white supremacy, preferably through inflicting 'ambient horror,' excess suffering, and death on socio-political Others (Kelly 2017). It is a (patho)logic of self-destruction that is meant to cause harm specifically to non-white communities, an affective attitude and politics where, as Adam Serwer (2018) has concisely noted 'the cruelty is the point,' a cruelty that at this juncture has its own infectious qualities since 'once malice is embraced as a virtue, it is impossible to contain.'

While Patrick's call for an embrace of illness and death in the service of an abstracted economy and a desired white futurity serves as the best representative anecdote of this pathological whiteness, numerous other figures of its operating logics have been rapidly accumulating over the last several months. In terms of popular representations, there have been a proliferation of 'viral' images of unsafe conservative protests against public health measures meant to contain the virus being directly or indirectly compared to media representations and narratives of zombies and zombification, for example, with memes juxtaposing scenes from another mass, non-masked, and non-socially distanced conservative protest at the Ohio capitol with shots from the TV show *The Walking Dead* or the film *Shaun of the Dead* (Figure 2); or, iterating on the genre of recordings of quotidian racist violence perpetrated by white women that have come to be colloquially known as 'Karens', the video of 'Zombie Karen' responding to not being able to enter a New Orleans bar by ramming herself against the door multiple times before giving it a theatrical lick that also carried a very real and embodied epidemiological threat (Figure 3). In these and similar actions captured and circulated online, the simultaneous self-exposure to coronavirus and the deliberate positioning of one's own body as a biological weapon meant to threaten others are central to their presumed efficacy.

Far from being limited to individual or marginal conservative discourses and actions, however, this pathological whiteness is also foundational to the official national response to the pandemic by the Trump regime. This response, such as it is, has been premised on denial, indifference, and scapegoating, particularly when what that regime viewed as the 'right people' (i.e. non-white, non-conservative, 'blue state' residents) were primarily the ones getting sick and dying.[8] This has perhaps been evidenced most clearly in reporting around Jared Kushner's expansive role in the pandemic response, which has been characterized by a typical blend of incompetence (relying on Facebook posts to gather information and intelligence about the virus; giving his old college roommate a leading role on the response team despite lack of qualifications) and active malice (Eban 2020, Lahut 2020). Recent reporting has suggested that even the underdeveloped and piece-meal national plan to respond to the pandemic developed by Kushner's

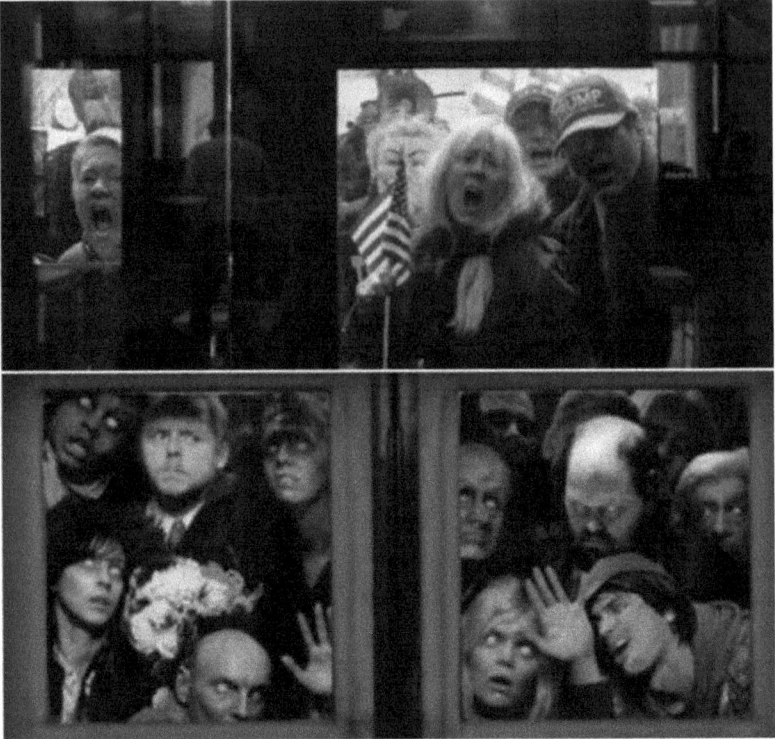

Figure 2. Conservative protestors at the Ohio statehouse juxtaposed with a promotional still for Shaun of the Dead.

team was abandoned in part because of a sentiment in the Trump administration that since at that point 'the virus had hit blue states hardest, a national plan was unnecessary and would not make sense politically. "The political

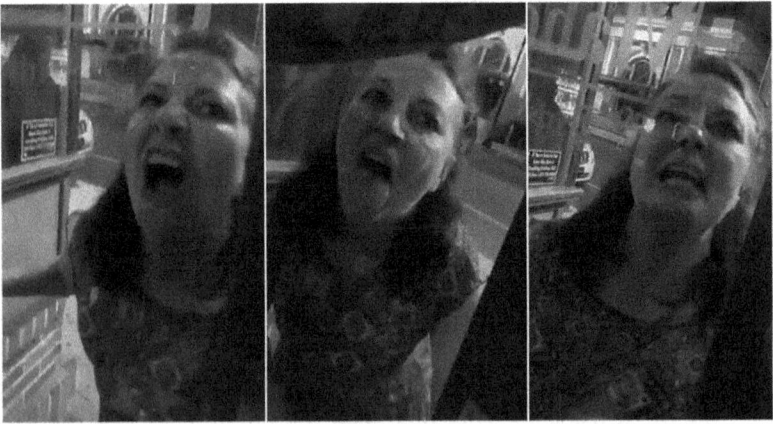

Figure 3. Stills from 'Zombie Karen' viral video.

folks believed that because it was going to be relegated to Democratic states, that they could blame those governors, and that would be an effective political strategy"' (Eban 2020).

Of course, as both a public health and political plan this has been a spectacular failure, leading to the United States having one of the worst pandemic responses in the world (it has recently entered an even more dire 'new phase' according to White House coronavirus task force coordinator Dr. Deborah Birx) and is as of this writing requiring such basic interventions as Dr. Birx giving televised press conferences to remind people in rural areas that they are not in fact magically protected from the virus after its outright denial or association with liberal, urban elites in conservative media (Stracqualarsi 2020). Within the administration, refusing to wear a mask and actively engaging in other risky behaviour has been transformed both into a conservative bona fide and a signal of loyalty to Trump, even if that entails personal infection or death. Indeed, that was the outcome for most of the central members of the Trump administration, as dozens of Trump administration officials, family members, and Trump himself contracted COVID-19, with the nomination party for Amy Coney Barrett identified as a probable super-spreader event for GOP elites. While Trump and many in his inner-circle were able to survive this infection, largely due to access to top-tier health care and experimental and exclusive therapeutic options like Regeneron's monocolonal antibody treatment, others were not so fortunate.

For example, former GOP presidential hopeful Herman Cain is the highest profile conservative politician to die from COVID-19 after presumably contracting it at a non-masked and non-socially distanced Trump rally in Tulsa, OK. This again underscores the ways in which pathological whiteness primarily impacts non-white people even if they are trying to actively support, participate in, and benefit from that pathological whiteness. As Damon Young of *Very Smart Brothas* suggested in a memorial article for Cain entitled 'White People Won't Save You,' Cain 'died how he lived – tragically, stupidly, and clutching onto an anchor of white supremacy, hoping it would save him from drowning, not realizing it had bound his arms too' (Young 2020). Given what might now very well be the irreversible spread of the virus throughout the United States and the pathological embrace of it as a performance of white conservative identity, it is clear that the Trump 'response' was to simply to hope that a defeated and demoralized American populace 'just gets used to dying of coronavirus' and 'learns to live with the virus being a threat,' a calculated futility and exhaustion reminiscent of what Lauren Berlant (2007) has discussed as 'slow death' and what Lisa Calvente and Smicker (2019) have analysed elsewhere as 'crisis as ordinary.'

All of these elements that compose the formation that I have been discussing as pathological whiteness were articulated and mobilized in 1/6 insurrection, when an armed mob of Trump supporters successfully stormed the U.S.

capitol building, leading to the evacuation of members of Congress, the inter-ruption of the certification of the presidential election, the deaths of five people, and a currently unknown number of new COVID-19 infections. As of this writing, the events leading up to the assault, as well as a detailed and accurate account of what actually happened that day, are still being pieced together. All of the broken windows haven't even been replaced. However, it serves as an alarming example of the multilayered and intercon-necting networks that compose pathological whiteness, with the twin assaults on the election – by Republican Senators and Representatives within the capitol and the armed mob outside it – coming together even more directly with politicians like Rep. Boebert publicly sharing movements and locations of Democratic politicians mid-assault on social media. While the members of Congress (as well as former Vice President Pence) narrowly avoided physical harm at the hands of the mob, as they were hiding from them GOP representatives refused to wear face masks in their safe room leading to the at least four confirmed COVID infections amongst their col-leagues. The call is, quite literally coming from inside the House.

Understanding the complexity and stakes of the ongoing COVID-19 pan-demic within a more general context of crisis as ordinary provides a segue into thinking about what specific interventions cultural studies in particular might afford in this moment. I would argue that a meaningful engagement with crisis as ordinary, especially under the intensified conditions of COVID-19, demands a simultaneous reconsideration of some key conceptual and praxical elements of contemporary cultural studies work. Conceptually, it is clear that a context of crisis as ordinary, and especially one of COVID-19, pathological whiteness, and the various economic, political, and cultural responses it has generated, necessitate a rethinking and reimagining of central cultural studies concepts like hegemony, counter-hegemony, the popular, and organic crisis (among others). It is increasingly obvious, for example, that we are in a moment where white conservative politics in the US have largely abandoned any meaningful investment or engagement in what we would typically characterize as hegemonic politics, understood broadly as the attempt to secure power through democratic means via the production and maintenance of popular consent and a shared 'common sense,' as 'teeth-gritting' those popular formations may be. Instead, as the central necropoltical role of normalized violence and death in formations of pathological whiteness sketched above make clear, there has been a marked shift towards an *anti-hegemonic* politics by American white conserva-tives defined by a combination of articulated techniques meant to secure white conservative minoritarian rule (what John Erni, in helpful comments on this manuscript, described as the production of a 'common non-sense'). These range from the *explicitly illegal* (asking for and accepting foreign elec-toral interference; mainstreaming and mobilizing violent paramilitary organizations; stealing absentee ballots, as in NC's 9th congressional district; armed insurrection), to the *extra/quasi-legal* (refusing to consider Supreme Court nominees during election years; using DHS rules meant to respond to terrorist attacks to assemble a quasi-legal executive security force to suppress lawful protests; using technical loopholes to give candidates for government positions who failed to receive Congressional approval de facto versions of those jobs, changing the legal and administrative powers of political positions that they lose to Democrats, most obvious in the stripping away of the powers of the governorships of North Carolina and Wisconsin, etc.), to the *questionably legal* (microtargeted gerrymandering; restrictive voter ID laws; closures of polling sites, etc.). All of these semi-legal tactics are backed by implicit and/or explicit threats of direct white supremacist violence.[9]

In terms of practice, providing both an accurate and thorough account of 'what's going on,' as well as identifying zones and methods of interventions to combat the contagion of pathological whiteness demands the type of work that is broadly understood as definitional for cultural studies' interdisciplinary and political project. C ultural studies is often fundamentally defined in canonical texts by its interdisciplinarity; its focus on conjunctural analysis; its collaborative and collective engagement, research, and writing; and its situation within a broader intellectual community that cuts across academia, government, activist communities and popular culture. This type of cultural studies work, most often typified by referencing the collaborative and cross-disciplinary development and authorship of *Policing the Crisis*, has always been difficult to actually produce and sustain.

The challenge is intensified in an intellectual, and specifically academic, context of generalized precarity, disinvestment, and active governmental (and increasingly public) hostility, producing an academic context that is increasingly unreceptive to the production of knowledge that might be understood or experience as 'critical', 'controversial', 'uncomfortable' or 'unproductive.' It can be even more difficult to translate this type of work (long, arduous, conflictual, exhausting) work into popular forms and modalities beyond the academy or closed intellectual circles. However, the Trump presidency, pandemic, and insurrection, as well as the revitalization of movements for racial and economic justice under these conditions underscore the absolute urgency of this work. We need to take this moment of intensified crisis and uncertainty to re-evaluate our role as cultural studies practitioners and think critically about what types of interventions we want to make, and are in fact capable of making. In a moment of popular pessimism on both the right and left, a moment of what I would argue is an understandable pessimism of the intellect *and* pessimism of the will, we might still haltingly explore together what spaces and practices those feelings and experiences of exhaustion, hopelessness, vulnerability, precarity, just not giving a fuck, and having nothing left to lose might open up, or more accurately, re-open and re-activate.

Notes

1. The Three Percenters are an anti-government militia based on the false histori-cal claim that only 3 percent of the inhabitants of the original U.S. colonies opposed the British monarchy and fought in the American Revolutionary War, and who see themselves as a similar small but elite group of 'real Ameri-cans.' The Oathkeepers are an anti-government militia founded in reaction to the election of Barack Obama and is primarily composed of ex-military and law enforcement, who believe that the democratically elected government of the U.S. has in fact been 'coopted by a shadowy conspiracy that is trying to strip Americans of their rights' (Sparling and Grasha 2021). The Boogaloo Bois are best understood as an 'absurdist internet culture' adjacent to both groups like the Proud Boys and troll sites like 8kun 'defined by ideas and termi-nology that are simultaneously ridiculous and terrifying,' whose core conceit is a nihilistic desire for a second American Civil War (Mooney 2021). These reaction-ary groups form overlapping networks whose connections have intensified throughout the candidacy and presidency of Trump, and along with the Proud Boys are as of this writing broadly seen as likely responsible for the most extreme violence of the 1/6 insurrection at the U.S. Capitol (Savage et al. 2021; Goldman et al. 2021).

2. For more on the updating, consolidation, and mobilization of white grievance politics and narratives of white victimization in the post-Obama era, see especially Skocpol and Williamson's (2012) The Tea Party and the Remaking of Republican Conservatism, Hoschild's (2016) Strangers in Their Own Land: Anger and Mourning on the American Right, Ashley Jardina's (2019) White Iden-tity Politics, Ibram X. Kendi's (2019) How to Be An Antiracist, and Ijeoma Olou's (2020) Mediocre: The Dangerous Legacy of White Male America. The key throughline of these works is the clear production of a white 'Christian' ethno-nationalist identity that is framed as under assault by the basic existence of racialized Others, who are perceived as illegitimate economic and political sub-jects threatening 'real' white Americans.

3. Examples of this convergence range from the successful election of Republican Qandidates (candidates for election who endorse the Qanon conspiracy that Democratic politicians are running a secret network of child sexual slavery and cannibalism that is on the verge of being revealed and shut down by Trump) such as Reps. Marjorie Taylore Greene and Lauren Boebert (who is cur-rently under investigation for her potential role in aiding the 1/6 attacks) to a majority of House Republicans endorsing Trump's false claims and of election fraud their subsequent vote against the certification of the results of the U.S. presidential election after the insurrection.

4. Online disinformation campaigns around COVID-19 have been a key point of articulation between different online communities such as the anti-vaxxer movement, previously mentioned right-wing extremists, conspiracy theories like Qanon, and 'mainstream' Trump supporters and Republicans more gener-ally. There is now a fairly well-defined feedback loop between extremist online content, 'mainstream' conservative media, and conservative politicians, where outlandish claims on messages boards and social media get amplified

by more famous media personalities like Tucker Carlson and Rush Limbaugh, who then are in turn cited by conservative politicians to justify their antidemocratic actions, which is taken as evidence by the conspiracy theorists that they were correct and their claims are legitimate since real politician are citing and responding to them. The Republican vote against certifying the presidential election is the most recent and extreme example of this, with politicians like Ted Cruz justifying their vote by claiming that many people had concerns about the integrity of the election, while of course leaving out the ways in which they helped generate and normalize those very concerns. For a helpful introduction to how these overlapping disinformation networks operate, see Starbird (2017).

5. For works that elaborate relevant discuss the literalization of 'toxic' whiteness and masculinity more generally, see Metzl (2019) and Case and Deaton (2020). For the disproportionate harm that this pathological whiteness still inflicts on communities of colour see Pezzullo (2007) and Clark (2019). For discussions of the production and performances of toxic white masculinity online see Nagle (2017), Salter and Blodgett (2017), and Condis (2018)

6. While a comprehensive summary of the literature is beyond the scope of this essay, my understanding of these broader racial formations is particularly reliant on the bodies of work and conceptual framings of critical race theorists such as Frantz Fanon, Aime Cesiare, C.L.R. J ames, Stuart Hall, Paul Gilroy, Sylvia Winters, Achille Mbembe, Fred Moten, Alexander Wehilye, Sharon Patricia Holland, Patricia Hill Collins, David Scott, and Kara Keeling.

7. This logic of subjunctive violence is present in practices like the Proud Boy initiation rituals, which include rituals such as being 'beat in' by members until the initiate is able to list the name of five different breakfast cereals. Here the absurdity is simultaneously a direct element of the violence, a cover for its 'seriousness', and also a bearer of a 'secret meaning' (in this case about masculine self-control that is also connected to the ban on masturbation). As Gavin McInnes, the founder of the Proud Boys, put it 'you must get the crap beaten out of you by at least five guys until you can name five breakfast cereals' because in addition to being funny, it is also training for 'better adrenaline control. Both physical fighting and arguing require you to maintain your composure and not get petty ... defending the West against the people who want to shut it down is like remembering cereals as you're being bombarded with ten fists' (Nickalls 2017). As we have now seen, this particular blend of absurdity and violence allowed many law enforcement personnel, journalists, academics, and more to be stuck wondering how seriously to view groups like the Proud Boys as an actual threat until they were already roving the halls of the U.S. Capitol looking for politicians to kidnap or kill. Practices like 'doxing' (finding and releasing personal information about individuals online), 'swatting' (used doxed personal information to call in police teams to those locations with the intent of causing property damage, injury and/or death) and 'manifesting' (posting plans and justifications for violence online, which might end with there or might end in actual attacks as in Santa Barbara, Christchurch, and El Paso terror attacks) are also key examples of this concept.

8. While it is too recent to definitively say, preliminary reports from the Biden administration seem to suggest that there was literally no plan at all for COVID-19 vaccinations developed by the Trump administration. According to

one source in the Biden administration there was a 'complete lack of vaccine distribution strategy under former President Trump' and that their team would have to 'start from square one because there simply was no plan' (Lee 2021). If confirmed, this is another example of how actions by the Trump administration that were often described as simply 'unconventional' and 'rude'—in this case not meeting with members of the incoming Biden team—were actually disguising and enabling inaction that will lead to people's deaths.

9. While a more in-depth account of these shifting and interconnected juridical formations within the political strategies of the contemporary U.S. conservative movement are beyond the scope of this paper, a critical cultural studies framework that can help make sense of them is present in recent work by John Erni (2019), particularly in his discussion of the 'juris-cultural' and multiple 'legal modernities'

Disclosure statement

No potential conflict of interest was reported by the author(s).

Further information

This Special Issue article has been comprehensively reviewed by the Special Issue editors, Associate Professor Ted Striphas and Professor John Nguyet Erni.

References

Berlant, L., 2007. Slow death (sovereignty, obesity, lateral agency). *Critical inquiry*, 33 (4), 754–780.

Calafell, B., 2015. *Monstrosity, performance, and race in contemporary culture*. New York: Peter Lang.

Calvente, L. and Smicker, J., 2019. Crisis subjectivities: resilient, recuperable, and abject representations in the new hard times. *Social identities*, 25 (2), 141–155.

Case, A. and Deaton, A., 2020. *Deaths of despair and the future of capitalism*. Princeton: Princeton University Press.

Clark, A., 2019. *The poisoned city: flint's water and the American urban tragedy*. New York: Metropolitan Books.

Condis, M., 2018. *Gaming masculinity: trolls, fake geeks, and the gendered battle for online culture*. Iowa City: University of Iowa Press.

Coronavirus: Armed protestors enter Michigan statehouse, 2020. *BBC* [online]. Available from: https://www.bbc.com/news/world-us-canada-52496514.

Eban, K., 2020. How Jared Kushner's secret testing plan 'went poof into thin air'. *Vanity Fair* [online]. Available from: https://www.vanityfair.com/news/2020/07/how-jared-kushners-secret-testing-plan-went-poof-into-thin-air.

Erni, J., 2019. *Law and cultural studies: a critical rearticulation of human rights*. London: Routledge.

Goldman, A., *et al.*, 2021. Investigators eye right wing militias at capitol riots. *The New York Times* [online]. Available from: https://www.nytimes.com/2021/01/18/us/politics/capitol-riot-militias.html.

Grossberg, L., 2017. *Under the cover of chaos: Trump and the Battle for the American right*. New York: Pluto Press.

Hoschild, A., 2016. *Strangers in their own land: anger and mourning on the American right*. New York: The New Press.

Jardina, A., 2019. *White identity politics*. Cambridge: Cambridge University Press.

Kelly, C., 2017. It follows: precarity, thanatopolitics, and the ambient horror film. *Critical studies in media communication*, 34 (3), 234–239.

Kendi, I.X., 2019. *How to be an antiracist*. New York: One World.

Knodel, J., 2020. Texas Lt. Gov. Dan Patrick suggests he, other seniors willing to die to get economy going. *NBC News* [online]. Available from: https://www.nbcnews.com/news/us-news/texas-lt-gov-dan-patrick-suggests-he-other-seniors-willing-n1167341.

Lahut, J., 2020. Jared Kushner asked his college roommate to create a national coronavirus testing plan, according to a new report. *Business Insider* [online]. Available from: https://www.businessinsider.com/kushner-hired-college-roommate-national-covid-coronavirus-testing-plan-2020-7.

Lee, M., 2021. Biden inheriting nonexistent coronavirus plan and must start 'from scratch,' sources say. *CNN* [online]. Available from: https://www.cnn.com/2021/01/21/politics/biden-covid-vaccination-trump/index.html.

Madani, D., 2020. Dan Patrick on coronavirus: 'more important things than living'. *NBC News* [online]. Available from: https://www.nbcnews.com/news/us-news/texas-lt-gov-dan-patrick-reopening-economy-more-important-things-n1188911.

Mbembe, A., 2019. *Necropolitics*. Durham: Duke University Press.

Metzl, J., 2019. *Dying of whiteness: how the politics of racial resentment is killing America's heartland*. New York: Basic Books.

Mooney, M., 2021. The Boogaloo bois prepare for civil war. *The Atlantic* [online]. Available from: https://www.theatlantic.com/politics/archive/2021/01/boogaloo-prepare-civil-war/617683/.

Nagle, A., 2017. *Kill all normies: online culture wars from 4chan and Tumblr to Trump and the alt-right*. New York: Zero Books.

Neavling, S., 2021. Gov. Whitmer becomes target of dozens of threats on private Facebook groups ahead of armed rally in Lansing. *Detroit Metro Times* [online]. Available from: https://www.metrotimes.com/news-hits/archives/2020/05/11/whitmer-becomes-target-of-dozens-of-threats-on-private-facebook-groups-ahead-of-armed-rally-in-lansing?media=AMP+HTML&utm_source=feature&utm_medium=home&utm_campaign=hpfeatures&utm_content=HomeTopFeature&__twitter_impression=true.

Nickalls, S., 2017. Why The Proud Boys Initiation Ritual Involves Cereal. *Yahoo News* [online]. Available from: https://sports.yahoo.com/why-proud-boys-initiation-ritual-194947464.html.

Pezzullo, P., 2007. *Toxic tourism: rhetorics of pollution, travel and environmental justice.* Tuscaloosa: University of Alabama Press.

Olou, I., 2020. *Mediocre: the dangerous legacy of white male America.* New York: Seal Press.

Race, K., 2016. Pathological. *Crossroads in cultural studies conference*, [online]. Available from: https://www.academia.edu/30685870/Pathological

Salter, A. and Blodgett, B., 2017. *Toxic geek masculinity in media: sexism, trolling, and identity politics.* New York: Palgrave MacMillan.

Savage, C., *et al.*, 2021. 'This Kettle is Set to Boil': New Evidence Points to Riot Conspiracy. *The New York Times* [online]. Available from: https://www.nytimes.com/2021/01/19/us/politics/oath-keepers-capitol-riot.html

Serewer, A., 2018. The cruelty is the point. *The Atlantic* [online]. Available from: https://www.theatlantic.com/ideas/archive/2018/10/the-cruelty-is-the-point/572104/.

Skocpol, T., and Williamson, V., 2012. *The tea party and the remaking of republican conservatism.* London: Oxford University Press.

Sparling, H. and Grasha, K., 2021. Who are the Oath Keepers, Ohio state regular Milita. *Cincinatti Inquirer* [online]. Available from: https://www.cincinnati.com/story/news/2021/01/21/ohio-militias-who-oath-keepers-ohio-state-regular-militia/4231869001/.

Starbird, K., 2017. Information wars: a window into the alternative media ecosystem. *Medium* [online]. Available from: https://medium.com/hci-design-at-uw/information-wars-a-window-into-the-alternative-media-ecosystem-a1347f32fd8f.

Stracqualarsi, V., 2020. Birx warns US is 'in a new phase' of coronavirus with more widespread cases. *CNN* [online]. Available from: https://www.cnn.com/2020/08/02/politics/birx-coronavirus-new-phase-cnntv/index.html.

Welch, D., 2020. Michigan cancels legislative session to avoid armed protestors. *Bloomberg* [online]. Available from: https://www.bloomberg.com/news/articles/2020-05-14/michigan-cancels-legislative-session-to-avoid-armed-protesters?fbclid=IwAR3Jp17kTlbZZBROHZC2JIB14gPx7GT8lOmOuq_XQ1oGmtfnOc8QA3p6-Ec.

Young, D., 2020. White people won't save you. *The Root* [online]. Available from: https://verysmartbrothas.theroot.com/white-people-wont-save-you-1844558680.

COVID-19 and the affective politics of congestion: an exploration of population density debates in Australia

Sukhmani Khorana 🅐

ABSTRACT

This essay considers the post-COVID-19 debates over the level of migration to Australia to understand how the rhetoric of 'affective congestion' which is used for population management has changed. On the one hand, it demonstrates that the concerns of white bodies regarding congestion are taken more seriously by the political and media mainstream than those of new migrants. On the other, it shows that COVID-19 is bringing the injustice of this approach to light, as seen in the case of the harsh lockdown imposed on public housing estates in Melbourne. Finally, it argues for population density planning that uses the 'mobility justice' framework and makes a case for developing affective capacities in addition to building infrastructure.

Introduction: population congestion and mobility justice

At the time of writing this article, the COVID-19 pandemic is in full swing across the globe, giving new meaning to physical distance between unrelated individuals, to public gatherings, mass transit, and congested dwellings. Australia's second largest city of Melbourne is in the midst of a second wave of infections and suburbs with a high density of migrant and working-class residents are being targeted for another lockdown. In fact, nine 'towers' which are public housing estates in these areas are also being surveilled by the police, and their occupants cannot leave even for stocking up on essentials (Wahlquist and Simons 2020). This unprecedented measure has led to several critiques of the Victorian state government's heavy-handed approach, as well as the federal government's reluctance to provide income support to temporary visa-holders, meaning that they were likely at work in high-contact jobs and hence more exposed (Albeck-Ripka 2020). There have also been comparisons with Singapore which was similarly commended for controlling infections early until an outbreak was discovered in neglected (and cramped) quarters of migrant workers. This begs the question – in a post COVID-19 world, what is new about scapegoating working class and migrant populations in these contexts? Relatedly, what can we learn about the politics of congestion and how it is affectively deployed by dominant political and media discourses to effect the above-mentioned scapegoating?

Human geographers have used the 'mobility justice' approach (see Sheller 2018) to understand and advocate for a more equitable distribution of space and related mobility resources, including access to travel and time spent commuting. In the aftermath of COVID-19, the 'Untokening Network' (comprised of mobility justice advocates) released a statement to reflect on this moment and issue a set of recommendations for planners, governments and local communities. In their reflection, they surmise, 'While we are facing unique challenges, what is not unique is that the most marginalized have the least choice to stay safe at home and are more likely to have a precarious safety net in weathering this moment' (Untokening Network 2020). They also note the racialised nature of this precarity and suggest that mobility justice requires that 'we hold the lives and the work of our BIPOC front line workers and communities as sacred, rather than sacrificial' (Untokening Network 2020). This paper attempts to apply these foundational principles on mobility justice in the new context of COVID-19 to the Australian case of population and migration, and the affective politics engulfing these debates.

Population debates in Australia: pre-election and post-COVID-19

Only a year and a half before COVID-19 impacted the population and immigration debates, the Australian government's approach to these issues right before the federal election was making headlines. This was also about the same time as a state election in New South Wales (or NSW, the nation's most populous state). At the height of the election campaign, NSW Premier Gladys Berejiklian declared, 'I would be irresponsible if I did not identify the issues that matter to our communities. People are *concerned about the character of their environments* [emphasis mine], people are concerned about their quality of life moving forward, and so am I' (Saulwick 2018). While there is clear conflation of population control with environmental sustainability in her comment, there is no lucidity in terms of who is voicing this concern, why they are feeling anxious, and what the state and federal governments plan to do about it (other than slowing the migration intake).

As NSW went to the polls a couple of weeks later, and a federal election loomed on the horizon in 2019, politicians (and their mediated discourses) appeared to be selectively listening to and amplifying certain kinds of concerns. Until September of the previous year, Prime Minister Scott Morrison had dismissed any suggestions that the permanent migration numbers needed to be cut to control population in the major cities. The very next month, however, there was a major policy backflip, and the PM suggested there was uneven population growth across the big brown land (Gothe-Snape 2018). By December, the federal treasurer was meeting state and territory treasurers in Canberra to discuss congestion and population growth. This was largely an opportune occasion for the Morrison Government to unveil their new $19 million 'regional visa' plan for potential permanent migrants (No Author 2019). It was presented as a win-win: Sydney, Melbourne and south east Queensland get some room to breathe, and regional areas get to boost their economies and fill job vacancies. In the wake of the COVID-19 pandemic in 2020, there are already calls for radically reducing immigration from both sides of the political spectrum, seemingly due to economic reasons (No Author 2020). At the same time, there are concerns that those on temporary work visas could be further jeopardized – their numbers have gone up as permanent migration numbers have faced the axe, and a significant percentage of frontline workers such as nurses are on such visas (Boucher 2020).

What interests me in the above two sets of narratives (that is, pre-election, and post-COVID-19) is the explicit linking of what is perceived to be over-population to seemingly legitimate concerns about the environment or the economy when the policy directives implicitly scapegoat new and future migrants. It is this group on whose behalf others can make life-changing decisions; it is this group that is deemed too desperate to enter or remain in Australia; it is these bodies, and their presence on our clogged roads, their odours in our crammed trains that are perceived to be excessive to our cities, even as economists highlight how reliant we are on the annual skilled migrant intake for GDP growth (Kehoe 2018). Even in the aftermath of the COVID-19 pandemic, their lives are both more expendable, and blamed for either the origins of the virus (Chinese-Australians), or its continued spread by failing to heed public health advice in the case of the above-mentioned Melbourne suburbs (Albeck-Ripka 2020).

This raises the question of what is really going on when there is a politicized reference to urban congestion. According to Melissa Butcher, population management that ostensibly attempts to curb congestion usually reproduces or magnifies existing power dynamics with respect to racial and other kinds of diversity:

> managing diversity is the key thrust of policies that ostensibly target congestion, as the result of affective responses to the close proximity of difference and what it represents, namely, unpredictability ... infrastructural and intercultural capacities can enable the navigation of diverse, crowded urban space, but are developed and deployed within extant frameworks of pre-existing power

relationships that can also shift the burden of congestion onto others (2014, p. 460).

Butcher also emphasizes the role of affect in the way that urban space is used, developed and navigated. This is significant for the overview of population density debates in Australia in this article because it means that certain affective responses can also be adapted to changing conditions. As it stands, most of these embodied reactions to congestion are rooted in 'cultural frames of reference' that entail 'an accumulation of knowledge that delineates who, what and how many is permissible in which space and when, and that engenders what is civil and uncivil behaviour' (Butcher 2014, p. 461). The challenging of these boundaries inevitably leads to discomfort and falling back on ready-made templates of identity such as ethnicity, class, gender, age and others to both explain the affective reflex, and make a judgement. This means that those meeting normative standards (that is, white, middle-class etc) are more likely to be seen as experiencing congestion. On the basis of this, the rest of this article will unpack the congestion debates in reference to those considered to be its 'most-impacted subjects', that is, white settlers, followed by new migrants who cannot afford to live near the city centre and are seen as causing said congestion. To conclude, I will consider what pre and post-COVID-19 conditions means for affective experiences of population density, and how affect can be mobilized to bring about 'mobility justice'.

Whiteness and affective congestion

Before COVID-19 and the above-mentioned elections, some political commentary and media analysis usefully highlighted the importance of long-term infrastructure planning, and how Sydney and Melbourne lagged on this front in the early 2000s relative to projected growth (Maios 2018). Likewise, the Victorian Labor government raised objections to the regional visa programme, suggesting that the funds being invested in it would short-change infrastructure funding (Packham and Baxendale 2019). The chairperson of the Federation of Ethnic Communities Councils of Australia (FECCA) welcomed the creation of jobs in regional areas, but added 'governments have to be far more visionary in planning for the future'. Given that the last major backflip on population policy – that of former Prime Minister Kevin Rudd almost a decade ago (Gordon 2010) – was triggered by unfavourable opinion polling, one ought to ask whether amplified sentiment or measured evidence was informing the planning agenda.

The amplified sentiment itself was selective and remains so in the sense that it perpetuates the idea of congestion as being generated by a static or mobile gathering of non-white bodies, but that evokes affective discomfort only for white bodies. For instance, an article in the *Australian Financial*

Review just before the NSW election began with a quote from a daily commuter in Parramatta, which is at the heart of Sydney's migrant-dominated western suburbs (Kehoe 2018). She was cited as being married to a Lebanese man, and still thinking the place is over-populated. This was followed by an analysis of a Fairfax poll, which concluded that most Sydneysiders don't want more migrants or further development. What was not clear from this sampled polling was, once again, who are these people that fear congestion? Perhaps the previous anecdote of the harried ordinary commuter in a domestic partnership with a migrant is meant to assuage any readerly concerns about the veiled racism of those attributing congestion to excessive migration. Still, where is the invisible-but-always-too-present non-white migrant here?

Concerns around congestion and its link to migration were also brought to the fore before the election campaign as a result of the use of the term 'white flight' by then NSW Opposition Leader, Luke Foley. Himself representing the western Sydney electorate of Auburn, he expressed concern that Anglos moving out of middle-rung suburbs in the west, and a high proportion of migrants and refugees moving into them was creating undue pressure on services (Davies 2018). However, his comments were taken out of context due to the history of the term 'white flight', which connotes a kind of spatial racism in the US where it is believed to have originated. In his book on the postwar movement of middle class Anglo families from the African-American dominated-inner city to the suburbs (hence termed 'white flight') in cities like Los Angeles, Avila concludes that recent migratory developments mean that whites are now a demographic minority, and this could lead to new urban social relations (2004, p. 208). This means that whiteness is no longer the defining principle of urban culture and identity in LA, and the landscape itself is changing to accommodate more novel forms of spatiality, such as the street-oriented cultures of the newest immigrants (Avila 2004, pp. 208–209). While these developments are also likely afoot in the western suburbs of Sydney, and comparable areas of Melbourne, the dominant media and political discourse about them in Australia continues to centre whiteness and its affects.

The above phenomenon came to light once again during the NSW state election campaign itself when then Opposition Leader Michael Daley (who had replaced Foley) made a reference to 'Asians with PhDs' taking jobs from 'our young children' (Clift 2019). In this instance, he apologized but also defended his comments as being about economics and housing affordability in Sydney rather than linked to race. What was implicit in his remarks was the othering of non-white migrants, whether recent arrivals or long-term Australian citizens as they seem to have not been included in the category of those impacted by said affordability issues.

To make progress in this debate, it is vital for politicians and the media to acknowledge that they are conflating largely white middle class concerns with the anxiety of the 'wider community'. Why is this unsayable? It is likely that recent migrants and ex-refugees matter less in political terms, are seen as less likely to mobilize to save their suburbs from over-development. On the contrary, this has been moderately successful when undertaken by citizen volunteer groups in the suburb of Marrickville in Sydney's inner west, or politicians with a say in councils like Ryde (Saulwick 2019). What is equally vital to point out here is that the government advocating for cutting permanent migration during the election campaigns was also the very same one that has fuelled frenzied building developments (often over-priced or poorly-planned) in parts of Sydney and Melbourne. This means that while ordinary people from a range of backgrounds might be rightly con-cerned about the pace of construction, and too many cranes and road blockages in their neighbourhoods, they are sometimes being wrongly encouraged to point the finger at migration. Gorton ascribes this fear to 'the emotional intrusions of the other', which in turn leads people to retreat-ing and fortifying their own surroundings (2007, p. 338).

In the wake of the second wave of the COVID-19 outbreak in Melbourne in July 2020, the spatial othering of migrants that is taking place is less about a literal white flight, and more akin to setting up whiteness as separate from the practices in migrant-dominated suburbs. According to Sara Ahmed, this kind of fear 'involves relationships of proximity, which are crucial to establish-ing the "apartness" of white bodies' (2004, p. 63). Therefore, social space is aligned along racialised lines, as has been witnessed in the coverage of the above-mentioned suburbs as well as the public housing estates that faced increased policing. For instance, when the clusters in these areas were first identified, the Victorian chief health officer attributed it to misinformation amongst migrants. He alleged that they were likely sourcing information from social media from their countries of origin, or relying solely on their net-works of friends as opposed to credible government sources (Davey and Boseley 2020). While this unfounded allegation was later critiqued by migration experts, it seemed to be arising from the unspoken assumption regarding the apartness of non-white migrants from the white mainstream.

What COVID-19 has also triggered is a series of experts responding to calls for reform in not just immigration policy, but also broader local planning issues involving housing and infrastructure. In one such piece for The Guar-dian, Michael Fotheringham, the executive director of the Australian Housing and Urban Research Institute is cited as saying that this is an oppor-tune time to create more social housing in Australia (cited in Ryan 2020). He elaborates that this is because supply is usually falling behind demand, thereby pushing prices up, and affordability as well as construction jobs could be assured through the solution he proposes. At the same time, the article also talks about careful planning of Sydney, Melbourne and Brisbane as they are major migration hubs without directly addressing the controversial issue of migration numbers. Although the earlier half of the article foregrounds the stories of one migrant who just made it as a permanent resident in time, and an international student who has been stranded offshore, the broader question of planning and the hit to the economy post-COVID-19 in the article is still centred on the impact on the longer-term, presumably white resident-citizen.

In other expert contributions, such as a media release from the Committee for Economic Development of Australia (CEDA), it is suggested that the pandemic payments be extended to overseas students and those on skilled work visas (2020). This is to bring Australia in line with the approach of other OECD countries to temporary migrants. Although the rationale for doing so is again primarily economic, it does foreground how Australia's legacy of white nationalism (Hage 1998) continues to impact migrant welfare policies in the post-COVID-19 context when nations with fewer resources are doing more. Most crucially, as Hage points out in his seminal work, it is still the case that 'White Australians' enjoy having ritualistic 'immigration debates' in which 'migrants' and 'ethnics' are 'welcomed, abused, defended, made accountable, analysed and measured', and thus turned into passive objects to be governed (1998, p. 17).

Aspiration and affective congestion

An important demographic group that is still rendered passive in the debates about population density and congestion are Australia's so-called skilled migrants who may already be citizens or permanent residents. This group is not as socio-economically disadvantaged as the working class migrants, those on temporary work visas, and refugees living in public housing, but is still impacted by housing affordability in the capital cities. At the same time, what really distinguishes them is their sense of aspiration in material terms, and with regards to their desire for social mobility (Ho 2020). This section attempts to unpack what congestion means for them, whether and how their concerns are represented in the public sphere, and the impact of COVID-19 on the debates about skilled migration and the 'capacity' of our cities.

According to an ABC news article that looked at the past 30 years of planning data during the NSW state election campaign, most of the 'over-development' is occurring in the migrant-dominated western suburbs (Nguyen 2019). In suburbs like Footscray in Melbourne, there are some instances of second-generation migrants actively facilitating gentrification through food and retail businesses, as well as property development (Parkhill 2017). Despite this, the latest generation of migrants and their representatives is also active in identifying aspects of over-development that do adversely impact their communities. For instance, in the NSW state election, diasporic media publications wrote about the campaigns of second-generation migrant candidates such as Durga Owen who was representing the western Sydney seat of Seven Hills for the Labor Party and campaigning on over-development in her electorate (Badhwar 2019). Another candidate, Charishma Kaliyanda standing from the south-west Sydney seat of Holsworthy also referred to over-development as a significant local issue in her multicultural constituency: 'People are worried about overcrowded schools, cost of living, hospital waiting time, impact of road tolls' (cited in Badhwar 2019). From these accounts, it is evident that all inhabitants of growing middle-rung and outer suburbs are impacted by congestion, despite the mainstream media and politicians' centring of longer-term white residents.

In the wake of the COVID-19 pandemic, the conversation around migration and population is similarly couched in terms of focalizing the concerns of (presumably white) Australians who have been here longer than recent waves of non-white migrants. The only difference is that calls to cut immigration numbers are now based on economic and employment rationale, rather than lifestyle and quality of life reasons alone. For instance, in an opinion piece for *The Sydney Morning Herald*, Labor Opposition Spokeswoman for Home Affairs Kristina Keneally argued that the pandemic was an opportunity to re-think Australia's 'high levels of migration' which in recent years had 'hurt many Australian workers, contributing to unemployment, underemployment and low wage growth' (2020). While this was critiqued in some quarters, it received support from those in government such as West Australian Liberal Dean Smith who suggested a 'comprehensive' debate about 'the composition, geographic spread and the skill components of our population' (Wright 2020). These comments suggest that population density remains a concern in the wake of COVID-19, albeit with a greater focus on overall economic recovery over the infrastructure needs of growing suburbs largely inhabited by new migrants. What is also unchanged is the conflation of 'Australian jobs' with the issues of long-established settlers (whether middle-class or working class 'battlers').

Conclusion: an effective/affective mobility justice response

Finally, in the Australian settler colonial context, it is also vital to ask – what do the original custodians of this land make of this affective politics of congestion? In their study of a rapidly changing part of southern Sydney in 2009, Bloch and Dreher pointed out, 'it is imperative that investigations of place-sharing do not simply reproduce the original and ongoing dispossession of Indigenous ownership and belonging, but rather centre Indigenous knowledges of home and place'. Similarly, in their recent work on re-imagining

Parramatta, Barns and Mar highlight how the area may have been used as a gathering place for at least 5,000 years, and its narrative of 'waves of migration' needs to be foregrounded amidst the thicket of new towers (2018). These pointers towards recognizing and centring Indigenous and subsequent migrant histories in new urban patterns suggest that an overall justice orientation is pivotal when considering an equitable approach to dealing with congestion and its impact on mobility, density and growth. If COVID-19 is being painted as an opportunity to rethink policy with regards to immigration, housing and urban infrastructure, then mobility justice rather that economic considerations alone ought to be foregrounded.

Before unpacking this justice orientation in detail, it is imperative to understand the relationality of certain everyday urban practices, such as transit. This is because on the one hand, they generate the kind of affective experience of congestion that is felt by bodies as a state between mobility and immobility. At the same time, they can also be sites where new bodily dispositions, habits and ethical relations are cultivated. According to Bissell, 'One of the central themes running through research on mobilities is how being mobile with other people mobilizes a series of relational practices' (2010, p. 270). This means that the figure of the passenger should not be considered through assumptions that render them inert and lifeless. Rather, it is important to begin from the perspective of affect as it allows us to account for 'the affective relations that emerge between passengers and, consequently, the capacity of different passengers to affect and be affected' (Bissell 2010, p. 272). Finally, it is this capacity to be affected that can lead to spaces of negotiation between passengers from vastly different socio-economic, racial, educational and other backgrounds. Bissell refers to these spaces as 'sites of ethical responsibility' that can orient us towards a justice approach and enhance our affective capacities (2010, p. 286).

The above-mentioned figure of the passenger and the sites for ethical responsibility can be more broadly applied to white and non-white bodies in congested spaces in our cities. Sheller has coined the term 'mobility justice' to encompass such as approach when referring to rapid urban changes and responses to them in the pre-COVID era:

> Mobility justice is an overarching concept for thinking about how power and inequality inform the governance and control of movement, shaping the patterns of unequal mobility and immobility in the circulation of people, resources, and information. We can think about mobility justice occurring at different scales, from micro-level embodied interpersonal relations, to meso-level issues of urban transportation justice and the 'right to the city', to macro-level transnational relations of travel and borders, and ultimately global resources flows and energy circulation (2018).

The question then remains as to whether this approach can also be applied to the specific urban, density and mobility crises created by COVID-19 in the

Australian context? What is the 'right to the city' of disadvantaged suburb dwellers who are facing harsher restrictions? Are their affective experiences and communication needs being adequately taken into account in policy responses?

The answer, following Pedwell's work on affect and social change, may lay in combining affect with the force of habit. In other words, those in positions of privilege (that is, those who could move to less-congested suburbs pre-COVID-19, or those who can work from home during COVID-19) must focus on managing the self over managing the other. According to Pedwell, any affective discomfort ought not to be avoided as it is in

> learning how to inhabit (rather than transcend) ambivalence, conflict and com-
> plexity that we might move from simply diagnosing "bad habits" to the difficult
> and productive work of creating new tendencies – ones that might take us to a
> different (and more affirmative) intellectual and socio-political place. (2017,
> p. 109)

This new place can in turn be one where social change is mobilized through 'mind–body-environmental assemblages' (Pedwell 2017, pp. 107–108). Butcher also emphasizes how the management of congestion requires developing skills, and not just creating material infrastructure (2014, p. 464). In the post-COVID-19 world, it remains to be seen how these competencies will be prioritized alongside economic recovery. If the trajectory of Australia's debates on population and migration management are any indication, what is required is not so much a comprehensive debate on the 'quantity and quality' of new migrants, but an ethical overview of who is being pushed out to the fringes, what services they have access to, and what impact this has on everyone's public health and well-being. In other words, COVID-19 may have given rise to a new set of relational practices where we realize that everyone could be potentially affected by a new cluster of the virus, even when not travelling together at the same time. Some borders remain permeable, and congestion embodies a more potent threat. Therefore, the affective politics of congestion can only be undone through a collective post-COVID-19 approach to urban space and mobility that is justice-oriented.

Disclosure statement

No potential conflict of interest was reported by the author(s).

Further information

This Special Issue article has been comprehensively reviewed by the Special Issue editors, Associate Professor Ted Striphas and Professor John Nguyet Erni.

ORCID

Sukhmani Khorana ⓘ http://orcid.org/0000-0002-7273-1393

Works cited

Ahmed, S., 2004. Affective economies. *Social text*, 22 (2), 117–139.

Albeck-Ripka, L. 2020. Australia Thought the Virus Was Under Control. It Found a Vulnerable Spot. *The New York Times*. Available from https://www.nytimes.com/2020/07/02/world/australia/melbourne-coronavirus-outbreak.html?smid=fb-share&fbclid=IwAR1ydYDJmf4bGxl7-QBsAD5CzJXuzsE0Zauk2uLdNzhoPBoKz229nCP5l44 [Accessed 20 July 2020].

Avila, E., 2004. *Popular culture in the age of white flight: fear and fantasy in suburban Los Angeles*. Berkeley, Los Angeles, London: University of California Press.

Badhwar, N. 2019. Our four women with diverse agendas standing in elections on March 23. *The Indian Down Under*. Available from https://indiandownunder.com.au/2019/03/four-indian-women-with-diverse-agendas-standing-in-elections-on-march-23/ [Accessed 24 July 2020].

Barns, S., and Mar, P. 2018. Reimagining Parramatta: a place to discover Australia's many stories. *The Conversation*. Available from https://theconversation.com/reimagining-parramatta-a-place-to-discover-australias-many-stories-100652 [Accessed 27 July 2020].

Bissell, D., 2010. Passenger mobilities: affective atmospheres and the sociality of public transport. *Environment and planning D: Society and space*, 28 (2), 270–289.

Bloch, B., and Dreher, T., 2009. Resentment and reluctance: working with everyday diversity and everyday racism in southern sydney. *Journal of intercultural studies*, 30 (2), 193–209.

Boucher, A. 2020. Covid-19 is not only a health crisis, it's a migration crisis. *The Interpreter*. Available from https://www.lowyinstitute.org/the-interpreter/covid-19-not-only-health-crisis-it-s-migration-crisis [Accessed 13 July 2020].

Butcher, M., 2014. Congestion. In: Peter Adey, David Bissell, Kevin Hannam, Peter Merriman, and Mimi Sheller, eds. *The Routledge handbook of mobilities*, 460–467. New York: Routledge.

CEDA. 2020. Migration must be central to Australia's post-COVID-19 economic recovery. Media Release. Available from https://www.ceda.com.au/News-and-analysis/Media-releases/Migration-must-be-central-to-Australia-s-post-COVID-19-economic-recovery-CEDA [Accessed 6 January 2020].

Clift, T. 2019. NSW Labor Leader Michael Daley Slammed For "Racist" Video On The Eve Of The State Election. *Junkee.com*. Available from https://junkee.com/michael-daley-asian-video/198267 [Accessed 22 July 2020].

Davey, M., and Boseley, M. 2020. Coronavirus Victoria: experts warn against blaming migrant communities for spreading misinformation. *The Guardian*. Available from https://www.theguardian.com/australia-news/2020/jun/28/coronavirus-victoria-experts-warn-against-blaming-migrant-communities-for-spreading-misinformation [Accessed 23 July 2020].

Davies, A. 2018. Luke Foley apologises for "white flight" comment, saying he now knows it's offensive. *The Guardian*. Available from https://www.theguardian.com/australia-news/2018/may/24/luke-foley-defends-white-flight-comment-but-denies-dog-whistling [Accessed 22 July 2020].

Gordon, J. 2010. Rudd backflip on "big Australia" vision. *The Sydney Morning Herald*. Available from https://www.smh.com.au/national/rudd-backflip-on-big-australia-vision-20100404-rl3l.html [Accessed 22 July 2020].

Gorton, K., 2007. Theorizing emotion and affect: Feminist engagements. *Feminist theory*, 8 (3), 333–348.

Gothe-Snape, J. 2018. What's the link between immigration and population? *ABC News*. Available from https://www.abc.net.au/news/2018-11-20/permanent-migration-cut-and-population/10513860?nw=0 [Accessed 13 July 2020].

Hage, G., 1998. *White nation: fantasies of white supremacy in a multicultural society*. New York: Routledge.

Ho, C., 2020. *Aspiration and anxiety: Asian migrants and Australian schooling*. Melbourne: Melbourne University Press.

Kehoe, J. 2018. Australia, pop. 50 million: Migration, congestion fears also growing fast. *The Australian Financial Review*. Available from https://www.afr.com/politics/federal/australia-pop-50-million-migration-congestion-fears-also-growing-fast-20181122-h187ze/ [Accessed 13 July 2020].

Keneally, K. 2020. Do we want migrants to return in the same numbers? The answer is no. *The Sydney Morning Herald*. Available from https://www.smh.com.au/national/do-we-want-migrants-to-return-in-the-same-numbers-the-answer-is-no-20200501-p54p2q.html [Accessed 24 July 2020].

Maios, T. 2018. Migrants banned from Australia's major cities. *Neos Kosmos*. Available from https://neoskosmos.com/en/122644/migrants-banned-from-australias-major-cities/ [Accessed 22 July 2020].

Nguyen, K. 2019. Sydney development is a NSW election issue, so we crunched 30 years of government data. *ABC News*. Available from https://www.abc.net.au/news/2019-03-11/nsw-election-puts-spotlight-on-sydney-development/10887366?nw=0 [Accessed 23 July 2020].

No Author. 2019. Migrant visas fast-tracked for regional Australia in $19 million plan. *SBS News*. Available from https://www.sbs.com.au/news/migrant-visas-fast-tracked-for-regional-australia-in-19-million-plan [Accessed 13 July 2020].

No Author. 2020. Coronavirus pandemic gives us a chance to take stock on immigration. *The Sydney Morning Herald*. Available from https://www.smh.com.au/politics/federal/coronavirus-pandemic-gives-us-a-chance-to-take-stock-on-immigration-20200515-p54th9.html [Accessed 13 July 2020].

Packham, B., and Baxendale, R. 2019. States to pressure Frydenberg over capital city congestion. *The Australian*. Available from https://www.theaustralian.com.au/national-affairs/treasury/frydenberg-under-fire-over-capital-city-congestion/news-story/c3d50811877215161de55ee09fa770b8 [Accessed 22 July 2020].

Parkhill, C. 2017. Who are you calling a hipster? *Overland Literary Journal*. Available from https://overland.org.au/2017/01/who-are-you-calling-a-hipster/ [Accessed 24 July 2020].

Pedwell, C., 2017. Transforming habit: revolution, routine and social change. *Cultural studies*, 31 (1), 93–120. doi:10.1080/09502386.2016.1206134.

Ryan, H. 2020. Migration to Australia has fallen off a cliff – will it take the economy with it? *The Guardian*. Available from https://www.theguardian.com/business/2020/aug/02/migration-australia-cliff-economy-international-students-covid-19-coronavirus [Accessed 5 January 2020].

Saulwick, J. 2018. "Sydney's not full": Alliance formed to combat anti-population push. *The Sydney Morning Herald*. Available from https://www.smh.com.au/politics/nsw/sydney-s-not-full-alliance-formed-to-combat-anti-population-push-20181126-p50ia7.html [Accessed 13 July 2020].

Saulwick, J. 2019. Housing not matched by infrastructure - says government review released in comments. *The Sydney Morning Herald*. Available from https://www.smh.com.au/national/nsw/housing-not-matched-by-infrastructure-says-government-review-released-in-comments-20190305-p511y9.html [Accessed 22 July 2020].

Sheller, M., 2018. Theorising mobility justice. *Tempo social*, 30 (2), 17–34.

Untokening Network. 2020. Mobility Justice and COVID-19. Available from https://static1.squarespace.com/static/579398799f7456b10f43afb0/t/5e8f71cedecf77629b6eedc1/1586459086601/Untokening+Mobility+Justice+and+COVID-19.pdf [Accessed 5 January 2020].

Wahlquist, C., and Simons, M. 2020. Melbourne's "hard lockdown" orders residents of nine public housing towers to stay home as coronavirus cases surge. *The Guardian*. Available from https://www.theguardian.com/world/2020/jul/04/melbournes-hard-lockdown-orders-residents-of-nine-public-housing-towers-to-stay-home-as-coronavirus-cases-surge [Accessed 7 July 2020].

Wright, S. 2020. "Put Australian jobs first": Labor calls for migration overhaul after pandemic. *The Sydney Morning Herald*. Available from https://www.smh.com.au/politics/federal/put-australian-jobs-first-labor-calls-for-migration-overhaul-after-pandemic-20200501-p54p0i.html [Accessed 24 July 2020].

The long and deadly road: the COVID pandemic and Indian migrants

Raka Shome

ABSTRACT

This essay focuses on the Indian migrant crisis in the context of the state's handling of the pandemic. It argues that the migrant situation in India pries open 'problem spaces' that, if attended to, reveal how many of the now normative solutions for governing and containing the virus are exceeded by bodies – of migrants in particular – that cannot be kept safe by solutions in place to check the contagion. The essay first raises questions about the unequal distribution of 'saveability' in the Indian context (but this can also apply to others). It asks who cannot be included in the frame of 'human life' that underlies the solutions offered for protecting lives in the pandemic. Second, the essay offers a description of the migrant crisis in India that has ensued in the pandemic. Following that description, the essay focuses on three problem-spaces or aporias that the pandemic has pried open and that call for a more politically complex, contextually sensitive, and humane response to the management of the virus: unequal temporalities, the dilemma of im/mobility, and the challenge of recording death.

The Covid 19 pandemic has functioned as a window to some of the world's most precarious conditions that typically remain hidden from our eyes. In particular, it has called attention to the crisis of migration, the dispossessions accompanying migration, including internal migrations within nations, especially in the Global South. And most painfully it has revealed terrible economic divides in the world such that the very solutions offered for containing and managing the virus--social distancing, hand washing, masking, and sheltering 'in place' or 'at home' – actually eludes swaths of populations whose perilous lives cannot meet or be saved by those dictates.[1] To that extent, the protocols through which the virus is being managed reveal a 'problem space' (Scott 2004) that exposes how many of the 'solutions' offered, and can even be offered scientifically, for checking the spread of the virus, foreclose the possibility of asking (and deriving solutions from that asking) other questions that need to be asked in order to secure disposable lives (of migrants, refugees, slum dwellers and stateless populations) that cannot be incorporated into the folds of these now normative solutions for checking the virus. At the very least, the management of the virus, the world over, has made visible how it is primarily the middle and upper class that can be kept 'safe' with the solutions offered to contain the virus, while the everyday conditions of rest of the world's dispossessed and disposable populations exceed such logics of safety. For instance, a report (Rolloston and Galea 2020) published by *Harvard Medical School* noted that ' those who are most at risk are those who are already vulnerable by way of the social and economic disadvantage that characterize their lives' (see also Spivak 2020). This is not to say that the solutions offered (such as stay at home or masking) are wrong. Clearly, they are science-based. Rather, it is to say that we live in such a time of glaring inequalities in our history that more populations than not, fall outside the figure of 'human' that underlies scientific and administrative efforts to protect 'humans' from the virus.

This yields an important question: What forms of life can be potentially saved and protected through the normative solutions set in place for managing the virus and what forms of life cannot be secured by these frames of 'saveability', thus rendering such lives outside of the frame of 'human life' that can be saved? It has become commonplace for journalists, politicians, and medical personnel to state that the Covid 19 virus is egalitarian – it does not care about who you are, or who it attacks. Yes, and no. Its potential to attack is certainly egalitarian. But a virus while biological is also social. The social spaces (and the bodies that inhabit those spaces) through which the virus moves, and can move, bear an unequal relation with each other and are thus unequally recognized (and often not even recognized) by state machineries attempting to safeguard national space. For instance, weak housing situations (which are common for migrant labour and which in most nations tends to represent ethnically marginalized groups) that lead to overcrowding and poor sanitation – making social distancing impossible– or the reliance on public transport, or the need for hourly-wage workers to constantly find jobs in an informal economy – such as house cleaning, construction, maids, street vendors–or, the homeless who do not have a 'home' in which to retreat, or refugees such as Rohingyas cramped in camps have provided voluminous examples of how the contagion potential of covid-19 is directly related to socio-economic (and in many cases as in India also religious) vulnerability.

In order to explore the theoretical and political implications of such issues, I specifically turn to the migrant situation in India in the context of the covid pandemic. I choose this example not only because it made national and global headlines but also because it significantly calls attention to the precarity of (disempowered) migrancy when disaster hits us. The covid situation (in

India and other places) provides us with an example that highlights the necropolitical fragility of precarious migrants – their lives always hanging between survival and potential death. Covid simply amplified this already existing state of things. As the Indian public intellectual Arundhoti Roy (2020) noted, the covid situation in India is like 'the wreckage of a train that has been careening down the track for years'. I do not suggest that the precarity of migrancy is a monolith; migrants in different contexts and in different nations (including within those nations) experience their precarity differently. Thus migrant precarity in covid times must be understood contextually where a context is not simply the event (of covid) but larger relations and struggles that exceed the event and also construct it (Grossberg 2019). In what follows, I first offer a description of the precarity of the migrant situation in India in relation to the management of Covid 19 by the state. Then, I raise some political and theoretical challenges and complexities that the migrant situation in India bring to the fore.

Pandemic and the migrant situation in India

In India, there is a vast informal economy constituted by internal migrant workers – estimated at 139 million– who come from rural areas to work in big cities such as Delhi and Mumbai (Mishra 2020). Many of them are short-term migrants and are significantly comprised of Dalits (Scheduled Caste), Indigenous groups (Scheduled Tribes) and lower class Muslim populations. They do not have any fixed permanent work. Usually, their daily wage is earned from migratory work–that is working in one location in the city one day and another another day. So, when they move from one site to another in the city, they carry their belongings on their bodies. Many of them sleep at night in groups in one room or a few rooms that may have been collectively rented out for a day by them. Constant mobility is their norm, their 'ordinary'. And if they do have a semblance of a permanent home in their migratory lives, it is their body. The body is their home.

On 24 March 2020, Narendra Modi, the Hindu nationalist Prime Minister (PM henceforth), announced a three-week nation-wide 'lock down' (note the military metaphor) of roughly 1.3 billion people in India. (Later more phases of lockdown would follow.). Modi announced to the nation in a televised address that '[t]o save India and every Indian, there will be a total ban on venturing out of your homes' (Associated Press 2020). Never failing to miss an opportunity to invoke Hinduism, the PM referred to the ancient Hindu epic Ramayana to state to the citizens, that 'a Lakshman Rekha has been drawn outside your doors'.[2] Lakshman is the mythological brother of Lord/God Ram in the epic. *Lakshman Rekha [Rekha* means a line] is a sanctified boundary line that Lakshman drew on the ground around the abode of Goddess Sita, his sister in law, to protect her from evil spirits and enemies who could kidnap her. They would now be prevented from doing so by the boundary line. Within four hours of the speech, from midnight the country locked down. In the government's handling of things, there was no consideration or even recognition of the impossibility of thousands of migrant workers in cities to adhere to the protocols of this immediate lockdown. 'Home' became a dangerous flash point revealing the state's (and most people's) inadequacy to think *beyond* conventional notions of 'home' as a way to offer safe solutions for these migrants for whom mobility is their means of survival. Indeed, the covid situation has foregrounded strongly the conflicting meanings of 'home' (some that are visible and others not) that are at play geopolitically, nationally, economically and culturally in our highly unequal global and national spaces. As I hope to highlight in this essay, rethinking 'home' beyond its conventional notions –which is needed in this covid conjuncture – calls for innovative, highly contextual, reflexive, and multiple approaches to issues of temporality, space and mobility through which we tend to normalize the relations between home, safety and life/survival. This is not an easy task admittedly but this is precisely the challenge the covid has yielded, inviting a recognition that covid is not simply a health issue but one that is intimately woven into the economic, cultural and geopolitical fabrics of our lives that often determine the meaning of 'home' differentially across populations. Covid is an overdetermined phenomenon. And covid times are un/homely times.

In India, as the nation locked down following Modi's speech, the migrants did what they only could do in this situation – try to return to their villages. As the economy shut down, they did not have their daily work in the cities. Not only were they often without a place in which to sleep at night, they also had little or no money for food, as their minimal savings had dried up in a matter of days. It is only much later that some state governments arranged for shelters but many of these were cramped shelters – for instance according to some reports some of the Delhi shelters were often porta cabins designed to accommodate only 50 people with each person getting about 15 sq feet. This meant that thousands of migrants could not be sheltered (in Iman 2020). All public transportation had been frozen by this time. And because the migrants were never a part of the national imaginary of 'the people' invoked by the PM in the first place when he spoke of keeping Indians safe (although if a large number of these migrant had been primarily caste Hindus the story might have been different), no public transportation had been arranged for them by the government to return them home to their far away rural villages (it is only much later that transport was arranged but it was too late). So, with their sparse belongings, young children on their shoulders and, in some cases, even elders, the migrants started walking (or in some cases cycling) back 'home' (Image 1). The journey was often hundred, two hundred, and even six hundred miles. The Economic Times reported

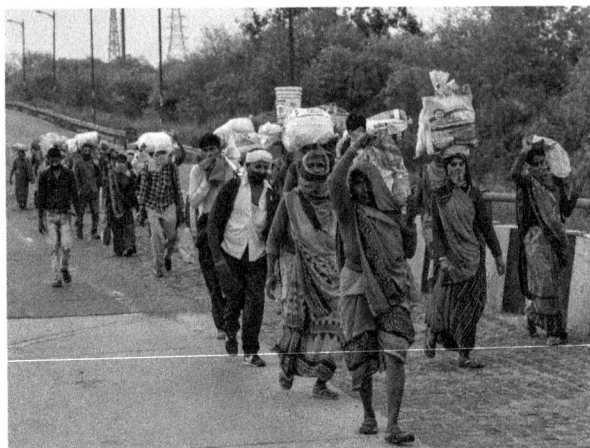

Image 1. Migrants walking home. ©Reuters, Photographer Danish Siddiqi. Reproduced with permission.

that one '[o]ne desperate group [even] travelled inside the cavity of a cement mixer' (Pradhan and Sen 2020). Some gave birth while walking back to their villages. Many starved due to lack of food and water. Many fell ill, many died. But still they walked –desperate to return to their families in villages. The Guardian called this the 'greatest exodus [in India] since partition' (Petersen and Chaurasia 2020). And Indian historian Ramchandra Guha referred to it as the 'greatest manmade [sic] tragedy in India since Partition' (Times of India 2020).

But the plight of the walking migrants did nothing to soften a callous government. In fact, as the migrant body became a 'threatening' and 'reckless' body – threatening national space by their endless walking, thus flouting safety guidelines of the lockdown and thus 'refusing' to be a 'responsible' national subject – they now had to be bordered, put back 'in place' through policing tactics and forceful sanitization. The attitude of the Modi government, noted a Congress (oppositional party) spoke person Manish Tewari, was that '[y]ou broke the lockdown, now go to hell' (Pradhan and Sen 2020). The police lathi-charged (lathi roughly translates to baton) many migrants in order to split them up or disperse them or even force them to be in one place (and not move) so that they would not be at risk of spreading the virus. In one instance, police in the state of Uttar Pradesh, as a way of punishing migrants and enforcing the lockdown, forced some migrants to squat and then hop on the road for several yards. In other instances, migrants (or other poor who could not stay at 'home') were punished by the police who made them hold their ears and squat up and down – as though disciplining wayward children. In other states such as Gujrat in western India, about 500 migrants were teargassed by the police in the city of Surat when they demanded that they be allowed to return to their homes in other parts of the country (Miglani and Khanna 2020). In Bandra in the city of Mumbai, police lathi-charged migrants as they congregated near Bandra bus station protesting an extension of the lockdown. In the city of Bareilly in the northern Indian state of Uttar Pradesh, a group of hundred migrants squatting at a bus station were forcibly hosed down by officials in protective suits. The Telegraph noted that '[t]he disinfectant, a sodium hypochlorite solution, is often used to keep swimming pools sanitised' (Srivastava and PTI 2020). Many migrants experienced a burning sensation in their eyes. Dr. R.N. Singh, a doctor in the state where this incident took place, condemned this brutality and this manner of containing migrant bodies exclaiming that 'I have not seen such a method of sanitization (by spraying humans with the chemical) in my 72 years of life' (in Srivastava and PTI 2020).

Perhaps the most alarming instance revealing the state's necroimaginary informing the containment of the virus was evident in the state of Haryana. The Director General of Police in Haryana issued a notification that large indoor stadiums in the state could be transformed into 'temporary prisons' for those who disobeyed the lockdown orders. In the southern state of Tamil Nadu, a father–son duo was arrested by the police for keeping their mobile phone shop open fifteen minutes beyond curfew time. They were allegedly tortured while in police custody and died in a hospital days later. Relatives of this duo demanded murder charges be brought against the sub-inspectors who tortured them.

Sometimes the migrants, in order to avoid police on regular roads for fear of being arrested or beaten, walked on rail tracks as there was a lesser chance of being apprehended since, other than freight trains, trains were not running. One of the most horrific incidents occurred when eighteen migrants, who had been walking for days, rested by the rail tracks. They did not know when they fell asleep. These migrants were soon run over by a freight train.

These instances reveal how the use of science ('social distancing') in crafting and enforcing (poorly conceived) public policies around covid management converged with the legal power of the state exposing the state's necro-orientation in keeping people 'safe'. The covid situation has revealed in places such as India how the protection of 'life worlds' for the many are intimately linked to the production of death worlds for others. It is an exemplary situation that exposes how the potential for necropolitical governmentality can easily underlie the enforcement of science to execute health policies about 'keeping people safe'.

A national outrage over the migrant situation finally led the government to promise transportation to migrant to aid them to return to their villages. While many migrants felt hopeful with this news, they soon learned that they would have to pay for such government arranged train and bus services. The fact that most such walking migrants had no money – they had used up whatever they had on food, water or trying to hitch a ride (on whatever minimal private transportation was running) – fell on deaf years. Many migrants were thus unable to use these services while many others, having lost trust in the Prime Minister words, chose to continue walking (often by rail tracks) willing to risk apprehension by the police. Some however found a way to organize money to buy train tickets.

Theoretical concerns

The Indian migrant situation reveals problem spaces that, if considered, would (and should) invite a greater ethical and political reflexivity towards what keeping 'people' safe and governing in these pandemic times might mean and what the stakes are. At the least, they should challenge us to ask which people cannot be brought into the imaginary of the 'people' and 'safety' invoked by governments in their pledge to fight covid.

In the following sections, I address some of these challenges and aporias that need attention so that a more complex conversation around 'safety' in pandemic times can (and should) ensue. I do not pretend to have all the answers. Nor do I wish to suggest that what I offer are perfect suggestions. Indeed, the covid pandemic has thrown up such complexities (many of which have remained unaddressed thus far) that our responsibility as intellectuals is to bring to the fore such complexities in the hope of producing and contributing to a much more multifaceted conversation about covid governance than what has prevailed. As cultural studies scholars, we know that any political solution is always without guarantees as Stuart Hall has taught us. So, my discussion offers suggestions without any guarantees of its political success. But it is imbued with the conviction that a more complex engagement with covid governance is absolutely necessary.

Unequal temporalities

The management of any disaster, any emergency, produces a state of exception in which the governance of temporality often becomes central (Adey 2016).[3] There is a need to do things in a hurry, to organize time and timelines in a way that speaks to (whether deliberate or not) the needs and protection (usually) of economically and culturally dominant populations. Forgotten are lives not seen as valuable or lives that exceeds the frame of the 'national people'. One common complaint of the migrants in India and the reason for their anger against the Modi government was that they were not allowed enough time to prepare. Their argument was that if the government had announced that there would be a lockdown a few weeks or even a few days earlier, they would have had time to organize their travels and money for their travel back to their villages. They would not have been stranded without a livelihood or forced to a death walk.

This argument (among others) of the migrants reveals the multiple and unequal temporalities that are actually at work in the Covid 19 situation (and in fact any disaster situation) and that in the management of that situation the state typically ends up governing through one time. Temporality, like resources, was unequally dispensed. So, those who could adhere to the temporal dictates of the lockdown –typically middle and upper class – could, without much trouble, enter the national or sovereign time of Covid management, while others, such as these disposable migrants, were simply out of time, or managing themselves through another deathly time – a slow walk home. Or some were 'stuck' in time as they waited in the cities to collect enough money to buy food in order to walk home.

I would like to suggest that a more complex response to the challenge of 'saving' lives in the pandemic requires us to expand our notion of time and admit into the sovereign time of pandemic management (thus troubling that time) other times – the time of the migrant, the time of stateless populations (such as stateless Rohingyas, an issue that space does not allow me to address here but one that requires a separate and fuller treatment). This is critical if we do not want the management of the Covid pandemic only to be a management of lives that can be incorporated into the 'national' time of that management.

My argument is that state machineries (in India but also other parts of the world) have not paid enough attention to the chronopolitics informing their management of the virus. Indeed, it is important that we attend to, and trouble, the 'power chronography' (Sharma 2014) informing the governance of the pandemic. The notion of power chronography recognizes that temporalities 'exist in a grid of temporal power relations [...] [Temporality] operates as a form of social power and a type of social difference' (Sharma 2014, p. 9). Sharma argues that the 'social fabric is composed of a chronography of power where individual's and social groups' sense of time and possibility are shaped by a differential economy' that informs how 'they find themselves in and out of time' (p. 9) and the differential and unequal social possibilities and agency that emerge from that. Attending to the power chronography of covid governance expands the scope of approaches that can be potentially utilized to protect lives– approaches that, especially in contexts of vast economic inequalities in the Global South, might better save lives whose very conditions of being and survival, whose very needs and demands, reflect and demand different orientations to time.

Im/mobility

This issue of temporality connects to the politics of im/mobility that have arisen in the pandemic. The challenge, as some have already recognized, is this: what do we do with bodies for whom being 'stuck' at home (or in some other shelter) is an impossibility? For the migrant, 'home' functions as a fluid zone as many live in make-shift shelters, reminding us that the boundary between home and home-less-ness for them (as for many in the world) is a false binary to begin with. Given that their lives are always positioned in that tense in-between space between home and home-less ness, between mobility and immobility, the migrant situation (but not only) yields a political challenge to the logic of immobility (or restricted mobility) that has been enforced in the pandemic.

In fact, what is needed in this pandemic is a multiscalar approach to im/mobility (I place a slash in the word 'im/mobility' to suggest that mobility and immobility are not binaries but intricately linked) (Cresswell 2006, Sheller 2011). What is needed is a political consideration of when and what kinds of immobility might keep certain populations safe and when and what kinds of mobility are needed to keep other populations safe. The migrants in India had to move, despite the state's best efforts to close down borders to contain them. And since they had to move, a political calculation could have been made by the government where the state could have aided them to move safely *before* locking down the nation (by distributing food, masks, sanitizers and arranging for transportation which it did only too late) instead of forcing so many of them into an endless death walk.

Similarly, the Rohingya Muslims in India are stuck in place, in their refugee camps. Immobility does not protect them from the virus. Living in cramped horrific conditions that lack adequate hygienic sanitation, toilet and water supply, hand washing and social distancing do not work for them. Soap and sanitizers are luxuries. To protect them, movement is necessary – they have to be moved to some other place where social distancing may be possible and such cramped living conditions would not exist. However, because these camps have been labelled as 'corona bombs', and because they are identified as illegals by the state (as they are seen as threatening the Hindu social order being implemented by the Modi government unlike persecuted Hindu refugees from other parts of the world who are welcome in India) they not allowed to move, even on an 'ordinary' day – a point that reminds us that where refugees and migrant populations are concerned, the binary between an 'exception' (the pandemic) and 'ordinary' is an artificial one. In addition, the government's relief package does not include the Rohingyas as also many internal migrants. As many internal migrants lack proper id cards, working as they do in an informal economy, they lack a digital presence in the state's database.

The lack of attention to the Rohingyas has been mirrored by the ways in which Muslims overall have been targeted by the government, by social media and Hindu nationalists, demonstrating how Islamophobia intersected with governance of (covid) time and (covid)space in India. The Islamophobic covid landscape in India first revealed itself when authorities discovered a number of positive cases amongst Muslims who had attended the early March meeting of *Tablighi Jamat*, an international Islamic missionary movement that congregated in Delhi in its mosque headquarters known as Nizamuddin Markaz. This meeting occurred prior to the announcement of national lockdown. The BJP Minister of Minority Affairs, a Muslim by the name of Mukhtar Naqvi – who functions more as a spokesperson for the Hindu nationalist BJP government to the Muslim community instead of vice versa – attacked the congregation of committing a 'Talibani crime' (in Sarkar 2020). Amit Malviya, head of the BJP's information technology, stated in a tweet that the Tablighi gathering was 'illegal' and made allegations about an 'Islamic insurrection' underway (in Jain 2020). Hindu nationalist groups quickly took up the bait and social media swelled up with hate filled Islamophobic hashtags such as #CoronaJihad that began actively trending on twitter. The authorities compelled over 3000 members of the *Tablighi Jamaat* congregation to quarantine for more than 40 days refusing to release them prior to this, despite many negative reports of covid 19. These forceable quarantine centres for Muslim members of the congregation began to function like detention centres. A petitioner and social worker for these Muslims alleged that 'many people have been illegally lodged in quarantine centres and submitted that several persons who are staying in those centres have written letters to the authorities but they have not been considered' (India Today 2020). Finally, pressure from a petition resulted in the Delhi government releasing those members without covid symptoms.

While this congregation might have acted irresponsibly (as did so many others) they did so before the lockdown and before the world had much knowledge about covid and containment strategies such as social distancing. What is to be noted, in contrast, is that following the lockdown orders there were many Hindu groups who flouted social distancing rules as they visited temples for Ram Navami – which commemorates the birth of Hindu god Lord Ram – in April. But a similar demonization or locking down their bodies in so called 'shelters' did not occur. Muslims also faced violent and discriminatory treatment in many parts of the nation – for instance a Muslim man was beaten up by a mob in Delhi and some Muslim vendors were prohibited from entering various localities to sell their goods. In the city of Meerut in the northern state of Uttar Pradesh a hospital required Muslim patients and their caregivers to provide evidence of negative testing of covid since Muslims by this time had already been labelled as corona jihadis. This requirement was not extended to patients of other religions (Sullivan 2020). The government's restriction of the mobility, and containment, of members of Tablighi Jamat led to an admonishment by the World Health Organization (WHO) which emphasized the importance of not profiling covid cases based on 'racial, religious and ethnic lines' (Downtoearth 2020).

All this provides an example of how the governance of mobility in covid times converged with the governance of Muslim bodies and their move-ments – especially as Muslims began to be seen as engaging in some bio-jihad against the nation. This politics of Muslim im/mobility that converged with Islamophobia and Hindu nationalism take on special meaning against the background of the 2019 lockdown of Kashmir – the only Muslim majority state in India– by the central government when restrictions were placed on movement and on communication (phone lines and internet connections) in Kashmir for several months. This followed the central government's over-turning of Kashmir's long-held semi-constitutional autonomy since post-inde-pendence days. With this overturning, Kashmir came under direct central government rule and people from other regions of India could now buy prop-erty in Kashmir thus creating a situation where Muslims in Kashmir could be forced out of their lands unable to compete with the real estate dreams of corporate and other elites. This also takes special meaning against the back-ground of the highly controversial Citizenship Amendment Act introduced by the central government where persecuted non-Muslims (and primarily Hindu) refugees from other neighbouring nations would be given amnesty in India but not Muslims being persecuted in other nations.

Cultural Studies has been invested in the notion of 'radical contextualism' (Grossberg 1997) in order to analyze a situation or a conjuncture. The pan-demic, especially in relation to the migrant crisis in India (but also else-where), calls for such a radically contextual approach to im/mobility. Instead of positing immobility and restricted mobility as primary solutions to keep 'us' safe, what is needed is a political sensibility informed by what Mimi Sheller has termed 'mobility justice' (2018). A 'mobility justice' stance would consider im/mobility from the framework of justice, rights, (social) responsibilities (especially towards the dispossessed) and historical inequalities. This is not about going against science. Rather, it is about recognizing that in the deployment of science to govern in pandemic times, a radically contextual approach to im/mobility is needed, one and can wed the safety protocols around im/mobility to a justice orientation and can recognize that mobility itself is an overdetermined phenomenon whose relations far exceed a particular event or moment (in this case covid) in which it is being comprehended.

But what might a mobility justice approach mean or look like in this Indian situation? Instead of a top-down approach to restricting mobility – that assumes universal needs of the population – a mobility justice approach would be contextually attentive and decisions about mobility should emerge from connecting mobility (and who needs to move and how) to structural relations – of historical, cultural and economic inequalities that have been exacerbated by neoliberal (and even religious) policies in India in the last two decades that have today resulted in a huge floating migrant population without fixed income or a permanent situatedness in the formal economy. For instance, as many migrants were initially confined in over-crowded shelters hastily built by state governments and civil society groups– despite many migrants complaining of unhygienic conditions as well as asserting their need to return home so as to have some semblance of livelihood, for in their villages they could at least get some farming or other local jobs as the cost of living would be so much lower – there was no desire to connect this migrant situation to larger relations of neoliberal economy that has governed India in the last two and more decades and that has exacerbated migrant precarity. Of course, government's don't care to admit or recognize the economic horrors of neoliberalism for the most vulnerable in society. But this is precisely where a mobility justice stance would be helpful in connecting the urgency of migrant mobility in covid times to larger structural issues of neoliberal logics that have already moved many migrants towards death zones (given the poor wages and fragile livelihood that characterize their lives in an informal economy). As the executive director of the Kerala-based Center for Migration and Inclusive Development noted in a *National Geographic* report that 'They needed to go home because it means a roof over their heads, food, and the comfort of a community' (in Bhowmick 2020).

Before implementing the lockdown, the government could have arranged for unlimited supply of public transportation for the migrants – but that requires a much larger relief package to spend on the poor than what the government was willing to shell out. It was more cost-effective to try to contain migrants. Arundoti Roy labelled the government's handling of things as a 'crime against humanity' (Bezzi 2020) and suggested that a human rights court should investigate India's handling of covid while Indian Nobel economic laureate Abhijit Banjeree chastised the government for its tight-fisted stimulus relief package in relation to many other nations such as the US (Press Trust of India 2020).

That there was no mobility justice framework even remotely informing the policymakers came to the foreground most visibly when the central government began arranging flights to return stranded overseas Indians home –students, professionals, guest workers and overseas migrants (even though they had to pay for airfare) with priority given to asymptomatic individuals revealing again how a neoliberal imaginary informed the governance of covid. Overseas Indians are a valuable population who through remittances bring in foreign capital into the nation. In contrast, internal migrants work in an informal economy and there are no records of their contributions to the national economy. Thus they are disposable in the national imaginary. This is what I meant earlier when I posited that a mobility justice stance can only emerge when we connect the diverse needs of im/mobility to larger structural issues – in this case of neoliberal economic structures in India working differentially for different populations and highlighting their differential economic value to the state.

Similarly, where containment of Muslim bodies are concerned, a mobility justice stance would emerge from a recognition of history's wrongs where Muslim mobility in India is concerned: the fact that ever since independence, the restrictions on Muslim mobility has been a pervasive feature of the nation – for example, denied equal housing access (many landlords do not rent to Muslims), or being made unwelcome in neighbourhoods and, as indicated earlier, the total lockdown of their lives for several months in Kashmir in 2019. If this had been taken into account when forcefully restricting and quarantining Muslims for over 40 days – that simply repeats larger historical patterns – a far more sensitive approach to Muslim mobility could and should have emerged (for instance, only those who tested positive after the Tablighi Jammat meeting should have been quarantined and only for 14 days as dictated by science). Instead, an entire community was thrown into a detention like centre. Indeed, as Peter Adey (2016) reminds us the kinds of mobility (or immobility) that are enforced in emergency governance are rarely symptoms of the emergency but are often 'productive of the emergency itself' (p. 33). The 'emergency' situation of covid thus becomes not just about the 'covid event' but about how the covid event is/was being constructed in ways devoid of attention to larger relations (such as but not only historical, religious, economic) that charged up and exceeded the event of covid producing a multilayered emergency situation in which covid became just one factor.

Tracking death: statistical illusions

One of the most sobering aspects of the pandemic has been the marking of death. How many died every day, in our nation, and in the world? We learn of this every day, and every few hours, as governments update their databases and television screens communicate these statistics. These are the numbers that will go in history books. And when future societies look back to this moment decades later to comprehend the devastation caused by the pandemic, these numbers will serve as important optics. Thus, the recording of death becomes an important issue challenging us to ask: 'Are we to count deaths only in relation to bodies that have been directly infected (and thus died of that infection) by the virus? Or should we also count the numerous deaths that occurred not due to a direct infection but because of the inability of our times to secure precarious lives that were devastatingly impacted by insensitive and simplistic governance of the pandemic by many states – such as the Indian state'? The migrants in India who died in an effort to walk hundreds of miles to return home – what of their deaths? Are they Covid deaths? How to 'mark' their deaths? Should they be included in the databases of Covid deaths? Most people would probably say 'no'. But that is a narrow way of marking deaths – producing a statistical illusion– where death by covid merely takes on a biological frame (the death of the body due to a biological infection) instead of also a *social frame* that exposes a larger necro-landscape produced by inadequate governance of the pandemic. The Indian situation reveals that the state of the migrants in the pandemic was not an exception (for them) but rather reflected the continuing politics of everyday disposability and non-recognition (by the state) within which their lives are situated. When a disaster such as the pandemic strikes, this non-recognition simply becomes more evident as the migrants' already insecure conditions begin to dangerously interact with the necropotential of the pandemic.

What I am arguing is that we need a more complex sensibility in tracking Covid deaths, for the death counts that flash on our screen are statistical illusions. Illusions not in the sense that they are lies but in the sense that they are partial. They do not tell us the whole necropolitical impact of the pandemic. When future generations look back to this moment, it is important that they recognize (so as not to repeat history) that the necropolitics of the pandemic was not just a matter of the biological body being infected and then dying. Thousands of deaths occurred because those lives were already so precarious that they could not surface up to the registers of safety being instituted by the State. Thus, an honest accounting of death by Covid 19 needs to consider the ethics and politics of *how* we are recording death.

This also brings up the related issue of how covid survival is being recorded. We hear little about the conditions under which someone survived covid. Like the statistical illusions marking covid deaths, here too, in recording covid survivals we do not typically get the full story. Many migrants walking back home to their villages might have survived and not died of covid. But how do we give meaning to that survival? Does it just enter our recording books of how many survived covid without an attention to the horrific near-death walks into which migrants were thrown by a callous government. For instance, compare the 'survival' of covid by a rich elite individual who could have afforded the best medical care to that of a precarious migrant who may just have been lucky to survive covid in their death walks, without any medical attention. So *how* one survived covid, under what conditions is important to consider as well so that covid survival does not just freeze into a statistical figure devoid of con-textualism – a contextualism that would call attention to larger structural inequalities that both precede and inform covid survival.

All this is important to foreground so that future generations recognize (hopefully) that it is not just the virus that directly killed many. Non-recognition of, or negligence towards, lives that exceeded the frame of 'human life' invoked by the state also killed many. Or forced them into conditions of survival where their lives hung in that precarious space between death and near death.

Notes

1. Arundhoti Roy makes a similar point noting that both 'lockdown and social distancing cannot be applicable in India, if we think of the tens of millions living in the slums'. See Bezzi (2020).
2. New Delhi Television (2020). Watch Modi's Full Speech. Available from https://www.ndtv.com/video/news/news/watch-pm-modi-s-full-speech-no-one-must-cross-lakshman-rekha-543843.
3. An emerging body of work in critical geography has begun to study what is being call 'emergency mobilities'. See Aday 2016, Anderson 2016, Anderson *et al.* 2020. The insights of these works have furthered my thinking on issues of mobility in this Indian situation.

Disclosure statement

No potential conflict of interest was reported by the author(s).

Further information

This Special Issue article has been comprehensively reviewed by the Special Issue editors, Associate Professor Ted Striphas and Professor John Nguyet Erni.

References

Adey, P., 2016. Emergency mobilities. *Mobilities*, 11 (1), 32–48.
Anderson, B., 2016. Governing emergencies. *Transactions of the institute of British geographers*, 41, 14–26.
Anderson, B., *et al.*, 2020. Slow emergencies: temporality and the racialized biopolitics of emergency governance. *Progress in human geography*, 44 (4), 621–639.
Associated Press, 2020. India will begin 21-day lockdown to curb virus. *PBS Newshour*, March 24. Available from: https://www.pbs.org/newshour/health/india-will-begin-21-day-lockdown-to-curb-virus [Accessed 31 December 2020].
Bezzi, D., 2020. Arundhoti Roy: Indian Muslims facing genocidal climate amid pandemic. *Open Democracy*, June 11. Available from: https://www.opendemocracy.net/en/arundhati-roy-indian-muslims-facing-genocidal-climate-amid-pandemic [Accessed 4 January 2021].

Bhowmick, N., 2020. 'They treat us like stray dogs': Migrant workers feel Indian cities. *National Geographic*, May 27. Available from: https://www.nationalgeographic. com/history/2020/05/they-treat-us-like-stray-dogs-migrant-workers-flee-india-cities. [Accessed 4 August].

Cresswell, T., 2006. *On the move*. New York, NY: Taylor and Francis.

Downtoearth, 2020. Refrain from religious profiling of COVID-19 cases: WHO in context of Tabligh. *Downtoearth*. April 7. Available from: https://www. downtoearth.org.in/news/health/refrain-from-religious-profiling-of-covid-19-cases-who-in-context-of-tabligh-70262. [Accessed 2 January 2021].

Grossberg, L., 2019. Cultural Studies in search of a method, or looking for conjunctural analysis. *New formations*, 96–97, 38–68.

Grossberg, L., 1997. *Dancing inspite of myself*. Durham: Duke University Press.

Iman, A., 2020. India's migrant crisis pointed to another problem-its lack of shelter homes. *Scroll.In*. July 31. Available from: https://scroll.in/article/968374/indias-migrant-crisis-pointed-to-another-problem-its-lack-of-shelter-homes. [Accessed 1 September 2020].

Jain, R., 2020. Covid-19: How fake news and Modi government messaging fuelled latest spiral of Islamophobia. *Scroll.in*, April 21. Available from https://scroll.in/article/959806/covid-19-how-fake-news-and-modi-government-messaging-fuelled-indias-latest-spiral-of-islamophobia. [Accessed 5 August 2020].

India Today. 2020. Petition seeks release of 3300 Tablighi Jamaat members detained for 40 days in quarantine centres. *India Today*. May 14. Available from https://www. indiatoday.in/india/story/petition-seeks-release-of-3-300-tablighi-jamaat-members-1677933-2020-05-14 [Accessed 5 August 2020].

Miglani, S. and Khanna, S., 2020. Indian police fire tear gas at jobless workers defying coronavirus lockdown. *Reuters*, March 30. Available from: https://www.reuters. com/article/us-health-coronavirus-southasia/indian-police-fire-tear-gas-at-jobless-workers-defying-coronavirus-lockdown-idUSKBN21H0OR [Accessed 4 August 2020].

Mishra, K., 2020. We need to provide undivided attention to the working conditions of migrants. *Indian Express*. June 20. Available from: https://indianexpress.com/article/opinion/columns/migrant-workers-india-lockdown-up-bihar-6467104 [Accessed 1 September 2020].

Pradhan, B. and Sen, S., 2020. Anger grows against Modi among worker hits hardest by lockdown. *Economic Times*, June 11. Available from: https://economictimes. indiatimes.com/news/politics-and-nation/anger-grows-against-modi-among-workers-hit-hardest-by-lockdown/articleshow/76315132.cms?from=mdr. [Accessed August 2020].

Petersen, H. and Chaurasia, M., 2020. India racked by greatest exodus since partition due to coronavirus. *The Guardian*, March 30. Available from: https://www. theguardian.com/world/2020/mar/30/india-wracked-by-greatest-exodus-since-partition-due-to-coronavirus.

Press Trust of India. 2020. India needs big stimulus package to mitigate the impact of Covid-19. *Firstpost*, May 5. Available from: https://www.firstpost.com/india/india-needs-big-stimulus-package-to-mitigate-impact-of-covid-19-on-economy-give-money-to-bottom-60-says-abhijit-banerjee-in-live-chat-with-rahul-gandhi-8334841.html. [Accessed 5 August].

Rolloston, R. and Galea, S., 2020. The coronavirus does discriminate. *Harvard Medical School*. Available from: http://info.primarycare.hms.harvard.edu/blog/social-conditions-shape- covid. [Accessed 1 January 2021].

Roy, A., 2020. The pandemic is a portal. *Financial Times*. April 4. Available from: https://www.ft.com/content/10d8f5e8-74eb-11ea-95fe-fcd274e920ca.   [Accessed   5 November 2020].

Sarkar, S., 2020. Religious discrimination is hindering the covid-19 response. *BMJ*, June 29. Available from: https://www.bmj.com/content/369/bmj.m2280. [Accessed 5 August].

Scott, D., 2004. *Conscripts of modernity*. Durham: Duke University Press.

Sharma, S., 2014. *In the mean time*. Durham: Duke University Press.

Sheller, M., 2011. Mobility. *Sociopedia.isa*, 1–12.

Sheller, M., 2018. *Mobility justice: The politics of movement in an Age of extremes*. New York: Verso.

Spivak, G.C., 2020. The left reflects on the global pandemic and speaks to transform!. *Journal of bioethical inquiry*, 17, 479–482.

Srivastava, P. and PTI. 2020. Migrants sprayed with chemicals. *The Telegraph Online*. March 30. Available from: https://www.telegraphindia.com/india/migrants-sprayed-with-chemical-in-bareilly-town/cid/1760720#:~:text=A%20group%20of%20about%20100,they%20had%20gone%20too%20far.&text=The%20disinfectant%2C%20a%20sodium%20hypochlorite,to%20keep%20swimming%20pools%20sanitised. [Accessed 20 August 2020].

Sullivan, R., 2020. Muslims turned away from hospital in India 'unless they can prove they are coronavirus free'. *The Independent*. April 20. Available from: https://www.independent.co.uk/news/world/asia/coronavirus-muslims-rejected-indian-hospital-a9474161.html. [Accessed 4 August].

Times of India. 2020. Migrant woes greatest manmade tragedy in India since partition, May 24, 2020. *The Times of India*. Available from: https://timesofindia.indiatimes.com/india/migrant-woes-greatest-manmade-tragedy-in-india-since-partition-ramchandra-guha/articleshow/75938611.cms

Media, Data, and Fragments of the Popular

New normals, from talk to gesture

Chris Ingraham ⓘ

ABSTRACT
Despite all the news coverage and online chatter about the repercussions of COVID-19, the pandemic has underscored the material limitations of public discourse to redress a health crisis of such magnitude. No amount of talk or deliberation will cure a virus of this scale. If part of the work of cultural studies is to identify the ways a given conjuncture shapes and delimits the felt experience of everyday life, then one charge of our work now is to examine the emergence of those 'new normals' that the novel coronavirus has spawned. One of these emergent new configurations of the everyday has been the spread of concerned gestures as a counterpoint to the usual *talk talk talk* of communicative capitalism. Gestures of concern, from chalking sidewalks to applauding essential workers, build the affective commonwealths that cultivate solidarity in times of protracted precarity. Exceeding Raymond Williams's notion of 'structures of feeling,' affective commonwealths are a resource built from ordinary people whose gestural rituals enact the sorts of worlds that talk alone just can't bring about. This essay makes a case for the importance of such gestures and suggests they deserve further attention in and beyond the context of the pandemic.

The pandemic has underscored the material limitations of public discourse to redress a health crisis of such magnitude. Unfortunately, there's no 'talking cure' for COVID-19. More than ever, we need the guidance of epidemiologists and other scientists whose expertise can teach us best-practices for safe collective action. Yet, in a time when digital media have, at least in specific contexts, sought to democratize communicative participation in public affairs, the evidential knowledge of experts is often held as coeval with the conviction of anyone's bald opinion. Under such circumstances, public discourse comes to be seen as ever more essential to democracy at the same time that its shortcomings become ever harder to ignore. Though this problem now exists in all liberal democracies – and has long been evident in aspiring or threatened ones, wherever citizens rely on communication to express their will to one another but hit obstacles when they express it to those in power –

America's valorization of such communication makes it particularly suited for scrutiny.

American democracy, like many others, has generally faced the challenge of living interdependently among others with an insistence that communicative participation in public life is what helps societies to form the public opinions that, in principle, serve to guide state action according to the will of the people. Regardless of where you stand on whether that principle has lost its shine in the age of corporate governance, executive orders, and above-the-law leadership, even its optimal version would be insufficient to deal with the catastrophe of a public health crisis as massive as the one caused by the novel coronavirus. The idea that citizens should deliberate about issues of collective import, and that governments should codify whatever 'public opinion' determines, may sound like representative democracy at its boilerplate best if we're talking about adding new parking meters downtown. During a pandemic, though, when even minor administrative delays or failures in response can lead, as they did in America, to at least 130,000 unnecessary deaths by October 2020 alone (Redlener et al. 2020), the limitations of citizen talk to guide state actions is difficult to deny.

In all cultures and societies, regardless of their governing system, decisions with wide ramifications sometimes need to be made quickly, and ideally made using the insight of those whose expertise typically exceeds even the informed opinions of politicians and invested citizens. One of the great challenges of democracy is to vouchsafe that decisions of urgent consequence can be made swiftly from the top while also maintaining the 'checks and balances' needed to ensure that such privileges will not be misguided, abused, or follow a slippery slope toward authoritarianism. In light of this challenge, political theorists and scholars of social change have been noticing the shortcomings of (American) democracy for some time, whatever name its recent iteration might take: neoliberalism (Dean 2009), late liberalism (Povinelli 2011, p. 25-42), technocapitalism (Suarez-Villa 2009), surveillance capitalism (Zuboff 2019), or something else. One theme of such critiques is a strident concern that the role of discourse in democracy has been supplanted by the machinations of power and corporate interest. What Jodi Dean (2009, p. 17-18) calls the democratic fantasy of 'communicative capitalism' captures the fundamental problem with its supposition that the mantle of democracy now 'fetishizes speech, opinion, and participation' to such a degree that 'conviction is indistinguishable from knowledge and certainty triumphs over evidence.'

Though Dean formulated these ideas in 2009, during the aftermath of the Bush-Gore election fiasco, the trends she identified then are all too familiar now. Consider the tension that played out publicly during the pandemic's American onset between President Donald Trump and Dr. Anthony Fauci, the nation's chief infectious disease expert, over the appropriate public health response. As Trump asserted with no basis beyond his own certainty that face masks weren't needed to prevent the spread of COVID-19, that hydroxychloroquine could effectively treat the virus, even that injecting household bleach might do the trick, Fauci's more modestly articulated yet genuine expertise became positioned as just another communicative counterpoint to the President's own: an opinion, merely, and perhaps a biased one at that. Such is the quintessential move of communicative capitalism: to render complexity vulnerable to conviction, and to make conspiracy a legitimate currency.

Pandemics aside, the United States need not have reached this point. Nearly a century earlier, two prominent American public figures of their own time – Walter Lippman and John Dewey – clashed over their own not-unrelated concerns, in their case whether or not the complexity of modern, technological life made it impossible anymore for ordinary citizens to have the competence needed to decide about issues with wide societal ramifications. The question for Lippman and Dewey was whether ordinary citizens could viably (or should axiomatically) be involved in the public discussion of how to redress human actions that impact them despite their having no direct impact on those actions themselves.[1] For Dewey (1927), the answer was affirmative: only by participating in the discussion of shared issues would the promise of democracy be achieved for its citizens. For Lippmann (1925), the answer was no: governments shouldn't listen to the opinions of inexpert citizens to guide important decisions better left for those with the competence to chart informed courses forward.

Though history seems to have favored Dewey for now, the rise of digital culture as an essentially commercial enterprise – especially through the participatory ethos wrought by so-called Web 2.0 and its successors – has 'democratized' public communication in ways that enable the spread of falsities without bothering to curb them, because to do so would run counter to the spirit of capital gain that charges the whole enterprise. 'User-generated content' is just too good to curtail. It drives traffic, gets clicks, and glues eyeballs to the screen. Advertising and subscription revenues grow from unpaid labor while the ones and zeros that drive it all remain cleanly indifferent to the truths or fabrications on the surface – though these features of course do influence human perceptions of broader public feelings, roiling as they do the ordinary experience of being alive at this particular moment.

Part of the work of cultural studies is to identify how a given conjuncture maps affectively onto the texture of everyday life.[2] Insofar as the pandemic has brought forth an array of 'new normals' around work, education, domesticity, dating, shopping, travel, recreation – virtually everything in the ambit of ordinary experience – the importance of cultural studies to help chart and navigate these emergent tremors is as urgent as ever. The modest point I wish to make in this essay is that some of the most fertile scenes of investment in the formation of new ordinaries during the pandemic are not where it might be most tempting to look: in the fracas of national politics and policy, in the advice of presidents and epidemiologists, or even online where so much of public discourse now transpires. Though these are all among the valuable sites of attention for studying the pandemic's monumental influence on everyday life – and on the workings of politics and democracy – the deployment of symbolic communication to advance assertions or arguments alike is secondary to the more constitutive role of expressive acts whose force registers affectively more than meaningfully or logically.

In my recent book, *Gestures of Concern* (2020), I argue that focusing principally on the role of discourse in democracy neglects the more primary role of concerned gestures for building affective commonwealths. Written before, but published during, the pandemic, the book doesn't take on the many examples of concerned gestures that COVID-19 has inspired. If the pandemic has illustrated anything, however, it's just how essential such gestures are for the building and maintenance of communities and coalitions that foster the resilience needed to endure prolonged precarity. The prototypical gesture of concern is a 'Get Well' card. Such cards are expressive acts performed in full recognition, by sender and receiver alike, that the card will do nothing to cure the ailment that it exists to acknowledge. Yet, people do send these cards, and they do make a difference, though that difference is analogous to the difference between their 'effects' and 'affects.' To be sure, the *effect* of 'Get Well' cards is minimal. They certainly won't cure COVID, if that's the idea. The capacity of such gestures to *affect* a social relation, however, is inseparable from their purpose, despite such affects defying quantification or interpretability according to the logic of use-values.

Readers of this journal will likely be familiar with Raymond Williams's concept, 'structures of feeling.' What may be less remembered is how much Williams, in his constant sensitivity to the historical baggage of words, hesitated over the inadequacy of his term. Even when he first introduces it in *Preface to Film* (1954, p. 33), he hedges over the concept's shortcomings but says that his term is more accurate 'than *ideas* or *general life*,' because there is a difference between how we *study* particular aspects of life and how we *experience* them (Williams wanted to understand the latter). Some two decades later, though, in *Marxism and Literature*, his most extended treatment of the topic, his misgivings remain: 'The term is difficult,' he writes, 'but 'feeling' is chosen to emphasize a distinction from more formal concepts of 'world-view' or 'ideology'' (Williams 1977, p. 132). He goes on to say that, actually, 'experience' would make 'the better and wider word' (Williams 1977, p. 132). In this way, over time, by situating the structure of feeling concept within this constellation of related terms – *ideas, general life, world-view, ideology, experience* – Williams offers an associative map of its contours. Doing so marks the concept, paradoxically, as at once both excessive and insufficient.

This liminal position – between too much and not enough, between past and future, between the complex whole of a social totality and the particular forms of its materialization – is what makes the concept alluring as a heuristic for cultural inquiry. By promising only speculation, it never reduces the cultural field to 'belief-systems, institutions, or explicit relationships,' though these are part of what a structure of feeling means to designate (Williams 1977, p. 133). Instead, Williams expands the range of cultural analysis by identifying a felt register of sociality that, as both a traceable structure and elusive register, can accommodate materialist projects invested in more than mere talk or theory. The lingering trouble – for him, as for those of us inspired by his insights – remains that identifying the 'felt sense of the quality of life at a particular place and time' is exceptionally difficult to do (Williams 1975, p. 47).[3] Our best hope, Williams wagers, is to find the residue of a structure of feeling left behind in art and other artifacts of cultural production. My wager is that a structure of feeling can become a resource, not just a residue – that is, it can become an *affective commonwealth* – when we identify its expression through concerned gestures that do some work to close the differential between what lived experience feels like and our ability to articulate it.

Living through the novel coronavirus pandemic has felt like lots of things, and no doubt different things for different people living in diverse geo-political contexts. But one of the ways to draw upon the affective commonwealths that this strange conjuncture has built is not to focus on the *talk talk talk* that attends digital culture and public affairs, but rather to treat gestures of concern as the 'mattering maps' that highlight what Lawrence Grossberg would call the 'things that do and can matter to those living within the map' (1992, p. 398). By enacting the sort of worlds one would like to make a home in, gestures of concern embody the principle of Gandhi to 'be the change.' Though such a principle, as Auden says of poetry, 'survives / in the valley of its making where executives / would never want to tamper,' its expression through concerned gestures need not be leveled-up to something more effectual: to a changed policy, say, or to overt political action. Rather, these gestures are their own reward, a resource for building the shared dispositions and fellow-feeling that sees even individual struggles within a community as mutual struggles.

Examples of such gestures have been all over during the pandemic. In New York, for instance, the city with the highest urban density in America, gestures of concern became regular acts of solidarity, from the nightly playing of the national anthem over electrified guitar off an East Village apartment balcony (à la Jimi Hendrix at Woodstock) to the applause given across the city to healthcare and other essential workers as they got off work around 7:00 each night. Manhattan's unenviable position as the American epicenter of the pandemic during its first peaks in April 2020 gave these gestures an affirmative quality of in-this-togetherness despite most people living holed up in their apartments (except, in many cases, for the rich, who were privileged enough to leave the city altogether). For those who stuck around, by choice or not, the on-cue hoots and claps and banging pots ricocheting down the city's chrome canyons offered an aural, embodied counterpoint to the all-online interactions that were beginning in their new normalcy to affirm Shelly Turkle's (2012) thesis about technology making us 'alone together.' Though initially acts of gratitude for the essential workers risking their own lives to help the afflicted – particularly the many who had come from out-of-state to do so – the nightly applause evolved into a performance of something bigger. Amanda Hess (2020), writing in the *New York Times* during the phenomenon's height, called the marvel 'a communal outburst,' noting that 'the more the ritual is repeated, the more it feels as if it's for the rest of us, too.'

Far away on the front range of the Rocky Mountains in the state of Colorado, concerned citizens Shelsea Ochoa and Brice Maiurro offered their own small gesture through a Facebook group called 'Go Outside and Howl at 8 pm' Soon they spawned a ritual that caught on in all 50 states and 99 other countries. Although hearing yips and bays through your neighborhood as the sun went down had its charms (just as making them had its primal joys), the howling of course did nothing to abate the pandemic, to reduce one's risk of exposure, or to push health policy in a particular direction. But that did not make the gestures useless, at least not in a pejorative sense. In the context of stay-at-home orders and a looming fear of contagion, a good nightly howl makes a fine equivalent to what James Carey must have had in mind when he wrote about the ritual view of communication. 'A ritual view of communication is directed not toward the extension of messages in space but toward the maintenance of society in time; not the act of imparting information but the representation of shared beliefs (Carey 2009, p. 15). The purpose of these nightly howls wasn't to transmit messages with readily interpretable meanings; it was to enact a shared sensibility, to draw 'persons together in fellowship and community,' as Carey described ritual communication's archetypal function (2009, p. 15).

In my neighborhood in Salt Lake City, Utah, all kinds of ritual gestures were also on display, each of which subtly shifted the felt experience of living in that time and place. Kids and grown-ups alike had suddenly become chalk artists, leaving messages of encouragement on sidewalks – *Stay safe! We got this!* – as well as the occasional drawing, hopscotch course, or walking maze for pedestrians to play along with and enjoy. Many houses now had teddy bears and other stuffed animals in their windows: part of a global trend, during the pandemic, to give children something to do during lockdown in communities in which walking around outdoors was safe but undirected enough to benefit from being gamified with a scavenger hunt. Find the bears! Odd sightings of painted river rocks also began showing up in strange places. Here on a fire hydrant, there on a mailbox, elsewhere tucked amid ordinary stones in a xeriscaped yard or at the base of a street sign. These too had a communal function. Alongside stones painted with hearts or trees were others with a message of support and solidarity. 'SLC.' 'Love.' 'Science.' Some stones were painted to look like animal or human faces – wearing a facemask. Juvenile or trite they may have been, but the point wasn't art or poetry. It wasn't even inspiration. The painted stones, the teddy bears, the chalk art: all were concerned gestures that built an affective commonwealth for strangers to share through challenging times Figure 1.

Yet, if the shared quality of affective commonwealths built through concerned gestures is a resource, it's not one that can be taken to market. Carey's apparent interest in ritual models of communication was based on a similar observation. If we understand communication as mere transmission, we also understand it to produce a more or less clean ledger of exchange, to begin and end in finite and measurable terms. Transmission models see communication as being 'for the purpose of control' and characterized by 'instruction and admonition' (Carey 2009, 15). Though Carey didn't quite put it this way, it's not hard to see conceptually that there's an imposing, patriarchal and economic aspect to this sort of understanding. By contrast, ritual models, grounded in repetitive or ongoing acts like gestures of concern, serve to maintain communities over time, building fellowship in the process. They don't expire in the same way – or yield the same calculable effects. And it's in this sense that gestures of concern can become a resource,

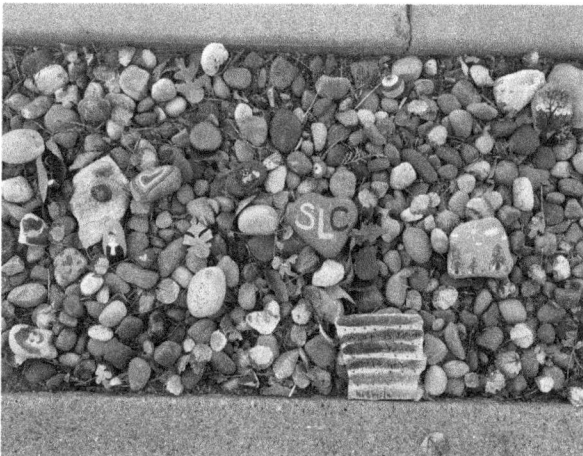

Figure 1. Painted River Rocks, Salt Lake City, UT. December 2020. Photo: Author.

if only a qualitative one: they change what it feels like to be living among others under circumstances that might bring isolation or despair without the affirmative gesture of disclosing affective bonds that may otherwise go unnoticed. These gestures say, *Others are in this with you.*

In this sense, even when the chalk art began to disappear, when newly painted river rocks stopped showing up, or when the teddy bears left the windows, my neighborhood was already primed to sustain its affective commonwealth. This became clear near the end of 2020, when anti-mask protesters began showing up in the neighborhood, making tacit threats outside the home of Dr. Angela Dunn, Utah's State Epidemiologist, who had supported a mask mandate given the virus's rising transmission rates in Salt Lake County. The protestors had posted Dr. Dunn's home address online and showed up day and night outside her house, waving their flags and fury, forcing her and her family to stay inside and draw the blinds. But that's when the yard signs started popping up, like clovers, all over the neighborhood: 'We Stand with Dr. Angela Dunn.' Neighbors began parking their cars along the roads, instead of in driveways, so protestors would have nowhere to park theirs. These minor gestures, fraught with concern, went beyond the positional work of the many 'We Believe ... ' signs that professed a list of values about Black lives mattering and science being real, which could be found in yards across different pockets of the city and country. They even exceeded the more gestural yard signs, also not uncommon elsewhere, that expressed some variation of, 'Thank You, Essential Workers.' The overnight yard signs for Dr. Dunn, rather, were primarily limited to our neighborhood, which saw Dr. Dunn not just as a representative of the State, but as a member of our community. They showed a solidarity that operated in a different key than more vociferous protests or public discourse was equipped to do. Though yard signs and river rocks probably can't galvanize or sustain a revolution, they can lead to resilience and togetherness in a more affirmative spirit Figure 2.

The lure of such gestures, of course, does not make them impervious to capture. One example is the work of actor John Krasinski, who created a YouTube series called *Some Good News* from his home office while quarantining. The show's handwritten sign made of poster-board taped on the wall behind him said it all. *Some Good News* was a low budget, DIY news program that reported positive, uplifting stories intended as an alternative to doomscrolling through all the bleak social media content and ominous reporting by the broadcast news. The germinal idea, Krasinski (2020) later reflected, was that the pandemic had made things seem so grim that 'we all just wanted good news to be more fully represented in our everyday lives.' The eight-episode series captured a genuine spirit of coalition and solidarity born from concern. Featuring a reunion of castmates from *The Office*, a performance from *Hamilton*, a virtual prom and wedding, not to mention all

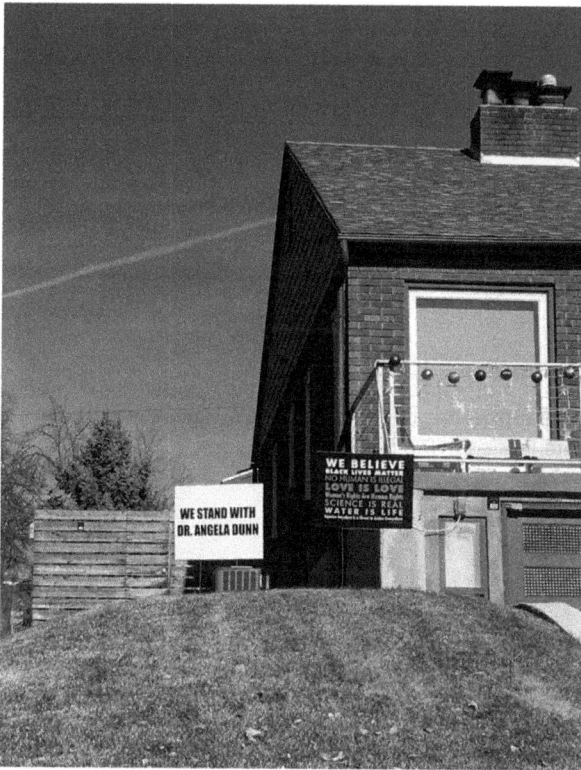

Figure 2. Yard Signs, Salt Lake City, UT, December 2020. Photo: Author.

the dance-moves, laughter, and celebrity guests, *Some Good News* was a feel-good palliative that fulfilled its purpose just by being there.

It should not be surprising, though, that an amateur web-series born as a gesture should soon enough be seized by capital in a bidding war to own the rights to profit from it. Despite a backlash from the show's 2.5 million subscribers, Krasinski eventually sold the concept to ViacomCBS. But this is just what communicative capitalism does: it takes even quasi-counterpublics and swallows them whole, only to be digested and served again to the mainstream, this time for major cash. Communicative capitalism is also what's at work when decisions in the interest of boosting the economy trump more scientifically prudent decisions in the interest of public health. Though the pandemic has underscored the limitations of public discourse alone for resolving a health crisis of such material and life-threatening stakes, it has also given us maps to find and build what matters most in times of precarity and uncertainty: minor affective commonwealths worth sharing and savoring, if only for now.

Notes

1. For more, see Marres 2005, p. 213.
2. See, e.g., Hall 1988; Grossberg 2006.
3. James Aune notes on this regard that, 'The most interesting aspect of studying culture is the most difficult to achieve' (1994, p. 99).

Disclosure statement

No potential conflict of interest was reported by the author(s).

Further information

This Special Issue article has been comprehensively reviewed by the Special Issue editors, Associate Professor Ted Striphas and Professor John Nguyet Erni.

ORCID

Chris Ingraham ⓘ http://orcid.org/0000-0001-9093-340X

References

Aune, J., 1994. *Rhetoric and marxism*. Boulder: Westview Press.

Carey, J., 2009. *Communication as culture*. New York: Routledge.

Dean, J., 2009. *Democracy and other neoliberal fantasies*. Durham: Duke University Press.

Dewey, J., 1927. *The public and its problems*. New York: Swallow Press.

Grossberg, L., 1992. *We gotta get out of this place*. New York: Routledge.

Grossberg, L., 2006. Does cultural studies have futures? should it? (or what's the matter with New York?). *Cultural studies*, 20 (1), 1–32.

Hall, S., 1988. *The hard road to renewal: thatcherism and the crisis of the left*. London: Verso.

Marres, N., 2005. Issues spark a public into being. A key but often forgotten point of the lippman-dewey debate. In: B. Latour, and P. Weibel, ed. *Making things public: atmospheres of democracy*. Cambridge, MA: MIT Press, 231–261.

Hess, A., 2020. In praise of quarantine clapping. *The New York Times*, 9 April. https://www.nytimes.com/2020/04/09/arts/virus-quarantine-clapping.html.

Ingraham, C., 2020. *Gestures of concern*. Durham: Duke University Press.

Krasinski, J., 2020. *Wow who can believe when we started this thing together we all just wanted good news to be more fully represented in our everyday lives.*, Tweet, 22 May

2020, viewed 21 December 2020. https://twitter.com/johnkrasinski/status/
1263859874632474631.

Lippmann, W., 1925. *The phantom public*. New York: Transaction Publishers.

Povinelli, E., 2011. *Economies of abandonment*. Durham: Duke University Press.

Redlener, I., et al. 2020. 130,000–210,000 avoidable COVID-19 deaths—and counting
—in the U.S. *National Center for Disaster Preparedness*. Earth Institute. Columbia
University. 21 October. https://ncdp.columbia.edu/custom-content/uploads/2020/
10/Avoidable-COVID-19-Deaths-US-NCDP.pdf.

Suarez-Villa, L., 2009. *Technocapitalism*. Philadelphia: Temple University Press.

Turkle, S., 2012. *Alone together*. New York: Basic Books.

Williams, R., 1954. Film and the dramatic tradition. In: R. Williams, and M. Orrom, ed.
Preface to film. London: Film Drama, 1–55.

Williams, R., 1977. *Marxism and literature*. Oxford: Oxford University Press.

Williams, R., 1975. *The long revolution*. Westport: Greenwood.

Zuboff, S., 2019. *The age of surveillance capitalism*. New York: Public Affairs.

Everyday life and the management of risky bodies in the COVID-19 era

Jeffrey A. Bennett

ABSTRACT
This essay explores how public reception of, and individual resistance to, public health mandates have reinforced agentic notions of bodily management in the COVID-19 era. Our collective approach to the pandemic continues to secure prevalent understandings of human agency over disease and illness by reifying the concept of personal choice. Notions of risk and shame shape these performances but do little to dislodge cultural frames that reify notions of individualism and the entrepreneurial subject. The wide circulation of viral videos highlighting the defiance of mask mandates is one site where choice and personal autonomy animate these debates. These confrontational acts are not easily segmented from the other cultural apparatuses where the privatization of risk is marshalled for political ends.

Pandemics have a way of drawing attention to the mechanisms of everyday life that were generally obscured prior to their arrival. The appearance of COVID-19 is certainly no exception. The novel coronavirus has refocused attention on our most rudimentary norms and habits: the space we share with others, the invisible infrastructure of supply chains, the risks that accompany publicness, the import of institutions, the necessity of competent leadership, and the dynamic interplay between global circulation and localized experience. The last year has revealed how the reduction of routine practices, such as commuting by car, can swiftly clear the air, while the advent of new conventions, such as wearing a mask, can destroy the oceans. Our homes lives have been put on full display as technologies become more essential to the operationalization of work, education, personal connection, and survival. Not surprisingly, this upheaval of our daily lives has had a disquieting effect on our collective psyche and contributed to skyrocketing rates of depression and anxiety. Scholars of performativity (Butler 1990, pp. 43–44) teach us that our identities are enlivened through the repetition of ordinary acts that 'congeal over time to produce the appearance of a substance, a natural sort of being.' The pandemic's dislocation of these see-mingly unexceptional norms ruptured this presumed familiarity and beset our quotidian lives with uncertainty and alarm.

For many of us, the exposure of the ideological commitments of strangers has been among the most unsettling of these circumstances. As municipali-ties around the United States implemented public health measures to contain the spread of the virus, people visually communicated their support or opposition to these policies by wearing, or disregarding, a mask. This simple non-verbal gesture became an index of who should be trusted and who should be treated as a volatile vector of disease. Masks became a signifier of political allegiances, scientific literacy, and civic obli-gation. Donning a mask, or not, is the confessional medium of the pandemic and its emergence as a site of public controversy has much to teach us about contemporary biopolitical conceptions of disease management. Although mask use has become a marker of political polarization, ideas about personal choice were the major organizing trope of bodily management among those who reject the accoutrements *and* those who shame the agitators. And as we moved deeper into the pandemic, the focus on choice became even more intense and problematic. But with 400,000 people dead in the U.S. as of this writing, it is simultaneously impossible to argue that our collective decisions have been sound and equally challenging to lay blame at the feet of a few select individuals.

In this short essay I explore how public reception of, and individual resist-ance to, health mandates have reinforced agentic notions of bodily manage-ment in the COVID-19 era. The very essence of the pandemic – the materialism of disease in the population – continues to be personified in ways that secure prevalent understandings of human agency over disease and illness. Notions of risk and shame shape these performances but do little to dislodge cultural frames that reify notions of individualism and the entrepreneurial subject. The wide circulation of viral videos highlighting the defiance of mask mandates is one nodal point where choice and per-sonal autonomy animate these debates. These fantastic acts are not simply standalone instances of bravado but also indicators of a pervasive sensibility about sovereignty, sacrifice, and the ethics of care. These out-bursts run contrary to the acceptance of risk privatization where potential hazards are hidden from view, where our personal narratives can be judi-ciously curated, and where structural concerns can be given greater con-sideration. However, these obstreperous performances are not easily segmented from the other cultural apparatuses where risk is marshalled for devious ends. Politicians who have done little to help control the ravages of the epidemic, for example, often adopt reductive notions of choice to blame the citizenry for viral spread and deflect institutional responsibility for the proliferation of disease.

Risky stranger relationality

Public health responses to the pandemic brought to life a series of common-place measures intended to reduce the risk of transmission. Those who hope to avoid infection have been cautioned to wear a mask when necessary, maintain distances of six feet from others, wash their hands, and eschew large gatherings. Early in the pandemic when little was known about the virus methods of circulation people also resorted to 'hygiene theater,' such as disinfecting groceries, to assert more control over their exposure to the virus. We have developed new rituals, such as bumping elbows rather than shaking hands, in order to mitigate risks but also to preserve degrees of human interaction. Of course, none of these exercises provide guarantees. A staple of pandemic writing has included those who remark that they did 'everything right' and were still unable to escape COVID's grip. *The New Yorker's* Carolyn Karmann (2020) referred to her experience as a 'parable' because she followed all public health guidelines but still got sick. She implored her readers to be vigilant: 'Even if you wear a mask, wash your hands frequently, and social-distance, as you must, you might still contract this disease. Call it an atmospheric threat.' The uncertainty posited by this writer was not uncommon, especially during the first six months of the pandemic: most people diagnosed with COVID did not know how they contracted it.

The images that will define this era, however, are far from ambiguous or circumspect. Videos of people refusing to wear masks, often under the guise of claims to individual liberties, were as viral as COVID in the summer of 2020. In one of the most famous clips of the genre, a white woman was recorded having a meltdown in a North Hollywood Trader Joe's after being told she had to use a mask while in the store (Rivas and Bernabe 2020). In another post, a white man wearing a 'Running the World Since 1776' t-shirt assaulted a woman in a Costco after she asked him to wear a face covering (Dorsey 2020). He screamed that he felt 'threatened,' even though he appeared to be armed. In yet another instance, a white woman had a temper tantrum in a Dallas grocery store after being told to leave for not wearing a mask. She callously smashed all of the items in her cart on the floor (Guerrero 2020). These recalcitrant citizens inspired a glut of popular press articles, including those that pondered why so many men refused to wear masks (Abad-Santos 2020, Marcus 2020, Willingham 2020). Although men certainly constitute a sizeable number of people who reject mask-use in the United States, the subjects of on-line videos and commenter discipline were almost always women. The 'Karen' phenomenon took hold and garnered an incongruous amount of attention from the notice given to so-called Chads. The 'extreme whiteness' of these disruptive consumers was glaring and became a marker of power, privilege, and entitlement (Kintz 2010, p. 759).

These conspicuous antagonists, coupled with our inability to document COVID's infectious transmission points, all but ensured that the threat of risky contact with strangers would become a persistent trope of the pandemic. For weeks on end, I would watch my screens as people would parade through stores attempting to pick fights with unsuspecting interlocutors. Indeed, on a trip to a local merchant that requires all customers to wear masks, I encountered a woman loudly proclaiming her right to be in the store without a mask. She was followed by security and eventually escorted out. But her obtrusive objection to the policy was far from an isolated incident. Across the country countless people performed excessive emotionality in public spaces as if they were possessed by the ghost of Ayn Rand and invited the judgment of an exhausted citizenry. Rather than keep risk behaviours to themselves, their bluster was put on full display for all to witness. The ensuing lesson was always the same: these selfish strangers posed life-threatening risks, and they could appear seemingly anywhere in the polity. In this way, COVID inspired its own brand of paranoid surveillance. The virus is simultaneously nowhere and everywhere and all people should be treated as infectious, lest the unsuspecting be caught off guard. This suspicious civic conjecture attempts to uncover peril wherever it may lie to determine which of our fellow citizens pose unfathomable risks.

By most measures, these eruptive denizens of retail are outliers. Upwards of three-quarters of Americans support a national mask mandate (Silverman 2020). Nonetheless, I contend that these nihilists are indicative of how we frame ideas related to bodily control and regulation more broadly. Scripts of management, especially when articulated to ideas about disease and illness, are inevitably bounded by rhetorics of risk that moralize everyday corporeal practices. Public accounts of risk tend to be future-oriented, and a major purpose of these warnings is to mitigate uncertainty. Narratives of risk perform a normative function that signal whose behaviours are acceptable and whose are intolerable. Deborah Lupton (2013, p. 132) asserts that individuals are 'increasingly expected to engage in practices identified as ways of avoiding or minimizing the impact of risks to themselves' and, as a result, 'the concept of risk has become more privatized and linked ever more closely to the concept of the entrepreneurial subject.' Within such a framework, ideas related to choice and personal empowerment stand in as markers of integrity and good character. In the pandemic era, electing to attend indoor gatherings or refusing to wear a mask are at least on par with not wearing an automobile seatbelt.

The development of risk as a central component of bodily management presents a striking paradox: while risks have become more globalized, incoherent, and conceived as a biopolitical project to be monitored and surveilled, risk also continues to be more radically individualized. But if the pandemic has proven anything, it is that the further individuation of bodily management is a poor substitute for institutional oversight or for addressing structural barriers to necessities such as healthcare. An economically-disadvantaged person cannot simply make the decision to stay home from work. A Black man in America cannot always wear a facemask without fear of being racially profiled or violently accosted by the police. People living with chronic conditions that are regarded as 'manageable' know well the disciplinary effects of being told that if they just controlled their bodily urges or made the correct choices then they would live free of disease. People with HIV or those living with type-one diabetes recognize the detrimental practices of being told to reign in their desires or suffer the consequences that await. But these shaming tendencies have never proven to be an effective way of managing disease because such conditions do not exist in isolation. People living with diabetes, for example, know that their disease is complicated by macro-issues such as the high cost of insulin, but also vernacular practices such as the sociality of eating meals with others.

To be sure, the violent outbursts of intractable strangers are products of neoliberalism, ableism, and white supremacy and are actualized by mundane practices like the assumed ownership of public space. But they also exist in an apparatus of risk privatization that has been troubled by the pandemic. Even seemingly innocuous phrases such as 'social distancing' become a barometer of privilege, power, and good citizenship. Social distancing is, in Lily Scherlis' words (2020), 'both a prescription for interpersonal behavior and a way to figure mass inequality.' Scherlis observes that 'social distancing is now a social good. People rarely know if they're a vector or a victim, so we shore up our bodily boundaries to protect the inside from the outside and the outside from the inside.' Even as social distancing is fraught with a history of racism, classism, and colonialism that is often left unmentioned, it imparts commonsense values about sovereignty and choice. Social distancing reflects the complicated interplay of risk as both an individual surveillance practice and a biopolitical metric that gauges behaviour and, by rhetorical extension, morality. Public health guidelines about masks or social distancing certainly reduce rates of infection but they also deliver moral ideas about behaviour and the consequences of not properly performing safety. The binary foretells the existence of good subjects, and the failure to meet those expectations implies poor citizenship.

It is little wonder, then, that the audacious behaviour of public health detractors engendered an omnipresent fear of strangers. As psychiatry professor Jacek Dębiec told *The Independent* (in Bate 2020), the 'stranger on the street could [now], in theory, be deadly, even without deadly intentions.' Sociologists have long documented the social practice of 'civil inattention,' wherein strangers develop methods for overlooking others in public to share space and maintain order (Goffman 1972). However, in doing so, this inattention can have the effect of depleting the moral obligations we have for others. Those resisting mask mandates turn this idea on its head: they feign shock that those in close contact would notice their behaviour, much less correct it, when in fact their flailing displays of whiteness 'under siege' demand an audience (Giroux 2018, p. 4). Perhaps more sincerely, those who refuse to tolerate such digressions are dumbfounded by the idea that they must necessarily notice these martyrs. These tense confrontations also bring to mind Danielle Allen's (2004) contention that in a democracy, strangers are often called upon to sacrifice in the name of the polity. But, sadly, some citizens, including the most economically marginalized, are often called upon to make a disproportionate number of those sacrifices. The pandemic seems to bolster the worst of neoliberalism's impulses by prizing individual choice in avoiding contact with strangers. But those who work in grocery stores or restaurants are passively positioned in regard to risk, having neither the resources nor the power to shy away from obstinate and unruly customers.

These vexed encounters of stranger danger cast a shadow over narratives that more truthfully detailed routes of transmission among intimate contacts. As I wrote this piece, there were countless news stories about the reckless judgment of people who disregarded public health mandates: members of Congress were infected by recalcitrant colleagues who spewed conspiracy theories; thousands of fans celebrated an American football championship by cramming into the narrow streets of a college town; and a professional basketball player was video recorded maskless at a party, violating the league's rules. The repetition of the message is clear enough: those who do not take safety measures seriously are wreaking havoc on the polity. But, importantly, the transmission of the coronavirus by the Congressional representatives, students, and pro-athletes mentioned above did not proliferate because of strangers. These were colleagues and kin. Whereas anecdotes of risk generally warn of unknown hazards brought by strangers in retail spaces, these examples conform to the data that shows gatherings among family, friends, and acquaintances are the most common cause for spreading COVID.

The binary between those who perform public health and those who do not obscures the fact that all us of think we are safe with our risks – it's those 'other people' we need to watch out for. Most of us want to believe that we are making the right choices and that our risks are low. But when couched in a public discourse organized around commendable and shameful choices, these practices become a zero-sum game. This has only intensified as hundreds of thousands of people have continued to die in the United States alone. The shame directed at those not following public health rules may be warranted and feel good in the moment, yet it also has the residual effect of contributing to an atmosphere where risks of all kinds are covered up. Perversely, the viral videos may encourage people to hide risks or make unending disclaimers about the precautions they took to ensure the safety of others so that they are not perceived as being 'one of those people.' Are you ordering groceries for pick-up or actually going into the store? Are you in a secure pod or merely hanging out? Did you enter the salon to get your hair or nails done? Did you leave your car during that birthday parade? Choice becomes the default position in a reductive imagining of the pandemic. Few among us want to be one of the awful people from the viral videos. This dialectic of shame and choice leads to the self-censorship of social media feeds, the selective narration of our outings, and the omission of details that might keep others well for fear of reprisal.

Of course, the pandemic does supersede individual bodies in significant ways. An essay in the journal *Nature* (Maxmen and Tollefson 2020) found that decades of pandemic war games failed to account for the most glaring hole in our response: former U.S. President Donald Trump. His administration dropped the ball on manufacturing and allocation of reliable diagnostic tests, the expansion of personal protective equipment, and vaccine development and distribution. Trump silenced the Centers for Disease Control and Prevention and inhibited coordination at the federal level that has haunted the globe for the entirety of the pandemic. He encouraged state governors to keep businesses open, no matter the risks. For months he chided the use of masks and publicly heckled those who elected to employ them. The decentralization of any kind of federal guidance was built on a house of cards about individual responsibility. The Trump administration continued its relentless campaign to overturn the Affordable Care Act (ACA), which protects at least 133 million people living with pre-existing conditions (Abelson and Goodnough 2020). If the ACA were struck down by the courts, their doing so would raise significant questions about what constitutes a 'pre-existing condition' should one be diagnosed with COVID-19. Further, even as the global pandemic has stratified certain populations into identity categories where some will have access to cutting edge medicines and other will receive remedial care, what Elizabeth Povinelli (2006) calls 'ghoul health,' the White House continued to push an agenda that exacerbates inequalities.

The political uptake of blame

The systemic obstacles I highlight above have been repeatedly displaced by a rhetoric emphasizing personal choice. The mendacity of management discourses has materialized most notably in political communication that castigates the citizenry for the unchecked pandemic. The response of Tennessee Governor Bill Lee is a perfect example. Since the beginning of the pandemic, the governor has refused to implement policies that would keep residents safe. Businesses have largely remained open and no state-wide mask-mandate has ever been issued. These efforts have been sidelined even as studies conducted at the local level found that counties with mask-mandates better contained the spread of the virus than those without them (Allison 2020a). The lack of government accountability came to a head the third week of December 2020, when Tennessee was recording some of the highest coronavirus infection rates in the world.

The explosion of diagnoses coincided with the state's first received allotment of COVID vaccines. That initial supply was less than 1000 doses, miniscule by any measure, but still could have provided vaccinations to the staff of at least one hospital. Rather than distribute the initial doses of the vaccine, however, the governor decided to place it in storage, citing concerns over 'equity.' One aid to the governor, who refused to be publicly identified, told Nashville's paper of record (Allison 2020c), *The Tennessean*, 'There's absolutely no way to equitably choose which facility got the 975 doses.' Lee himself told reporters (Allison 2020c) that distribution needed to take place in 'an equitable way that is safe and that makes certain that the right people with the highest risk in the shortest amount of time can receive this vaccine, and that is our goal.' The fact that Lee's administration had not thought to do the work of laying out a nuanced vaccine distribution plan was not lost on most citizens. 'Equity' meant no one got the vaccine.

Later that week, Tennessee received a more sizable amount of vaccinations to allocate to residents. In a speech announcing its arrival, Lee skipped over any optimistic take on the medication and decided instead to lambast citizens for rising infection rates. He excoriated Tennesseans for their poor decision-making: 'One thing that this vaccine will not solve, one thing that it will not cure, is selfishness or indifference to what is happening to our neighbors around us' (Burnside 2020). Rather than take responsibility for the crisis, Lee scapegoated his own citizens. He argued that 'Tennesseans need to wear a mask. It's important, it works,' but also stopped short of legislating a mandate, leaving that work to local mayors and county executives (Harris 2020). The governor (Lee 2020) completely dismissed the science and turned instead toward the politicization of the virus. He noted: 'Many think a statewide mandate would improve mask wearing, many think it would have the opposite effect. This has been a heavily politicized issue.' Scripts of individualism and personal choice were on standby to provide political cover for the governor's derelict decision-making.

Two days later it was announced that Tennessee's first lady, Maria Lee, had tested positive for the virus (Allison 2020b). The governor did not mention if his wife was selfish or merely indifferent, nor would he. His party laid the groundwork for questioning public health measures while simultaneously insisting that it was a few bad apples who inhibited progress in defeating the pandemic. But with 400,000 dead, we know it is not the individual choices of a few people devastating the country, much less the world. The stark dualism between unacceptable and laudable behaviour has contributed to an atmosphere where risk is not only privatized, but narratively segmented for the worst political ends. Even as the pandemic has cast a spotlight on the invisible mechanisms of our everyday lives, cultural judgments have empowered people like the governor to chastise unnamed residents and then quickly hide from view. For him to admit anything more is to confess an identity constituted by shame. He has none.

Disclosure statement

No potential conflict of interest was reported by the author(s).

Further information

This Special Issue article has been comprehensively reviewed by the Special Issue editors, Associate Professor Ted Striphas and Professor John Nguyet Erni.

References

Abad-Santos, A. 2020. Performative masculinity is making American men sick [online]. *Vox*. Available from: https://www.vox.com/the-goods/21356150/american-men-wont-wear-masks-covid-19 [Accessed 7 January 2021].

Abelson, R., and Goodnough, A. 2020. If the Supreme Court ends Obamacare, here's what it would mean [online]. *New York Times*. Available from: https://www.nytimes.com/article/supreme-court-obamacare-case.html [Accessed 5 December 2020].

Allen, D., 2004. *Talking to strangers: anxieties of citizenship since brown v. board of education*. Chicago: University of Chicago Press.

Allison, N. 2020a. Gov. Bill Lee enacts gathering restrictions, refuses mask mandate as Tennessee COVID-19 outbreak surges [online]. *Tennessean*. Available from: https://www.tennessean.com/story/news/politics/2020/12/20/tennessee-mask-mandate-covid-19-cases-surge-bill-lee/3977135001/ [Accessed 21 December 2020].

Allison, N. 2020b. Tennessee first lady Maria Lee tests positive for COVID-19 [online]. *Tennessean*. Available from: https://www.tennessean.com/story/news/politics/2020/12/19/tennessee-first-lady-maria-lee-tests-positive-covid-19/3978510001/ [Accessed 20 December 2020].

Allison, N. 2020c. Tennessee Gov. Bill Lee touts equitable rollout of COVID-19 vaccine, despite criticism over speed [online]. *Tennessean*. Available from: https://www.tennessean.com/story/news/politics/2020/12/15/tennessee-coronavirus-vaccine-gov-bill-lee-touts-equitable-but-slower-initial-rollout/3911107001/ [Accessed 16 December 2020].

Bate, M. 2020. Stranger danger: when can we stop being scared of other people in a pandemic? [online]. *The Independent*. Available from: https://www.independent.co. uk/life-style/coronavirus-social-anxiety-fear-strangers-how-help-pandemic-a9694201.html [Accessed 12 January 2021].

Burnside, T. 2020. Tennessee governor: 'one thing this vaccine will not solve or cure is selfishness [online]. CNN. Available from: https://www.cnn.com/2020/12/17/us/tn-bill-lee-comments-vaccines-covid-trnd/index.html [Accessed 12 January 2021].

Butler, J., 1990. *Gender trouble: feminism and the subversion of identity*. New York: Routledge.

Dorsey, D. 2020. 'I feel threatened!' viral outburst at Fort Myers Costco costs man his job [online]. Fort Myers News-Press. Available from: https://www.news-press.com/ story/news/2020/07/07/costco-yell-fort-myers-florida-man-video-viral/ 5393247002/ [Accessed 6 January 2021].

Giroux, H.A., 2018. Trump and the legacy of a menacing past. *Cultural studies*, 33 (4), 711–739.

Goffman, E., 1972. *Relations in public: microstudies of the public*. New York: Routledge.

Guerrero, M. 2020. Woman tosses groceries in face mask tirade [online]. NBCDFW. Available from: https://www.nbcdfw.com/news/local/woman-tosses-groceries-in-face-mask-tirade/2397702/ [Accessed 12 January 2021].

Harris, A. 2020. 'This vaccine won't cure selfishness,' Gov. Lee says as vaccine distribution begins in Tennessee amid COVID surge [online]. WVLT Knoxville. Available from: https://www.wvlt.tv/2020/12/17/this-vaccine-wont-cure-selfishness-gov-lee-says-as-vaccine-distribution-begins-in-tennessee-amid-covid-surge/ [Accessed 8 January 2021].

Karmann, C. 2020. How did I catch the coronavirus? [online]. *The New Yorker*. Available from: https://www.newyorker.com/culture/personal-history/how-did-i-catch-the-coronavirus [Accessed 15 August 2020].

Kintz, L., 2010. Performing virtual whiteness: george gider's techno-theocracy. *Cultural studies*, 16 (5), 735–773.

Lee, W. 2020. Remarks as prepared for delivery on the COVID-19 pandemic. Tennessee Office of the Governor [online]. Available from: https://www.tn.gov/governor/ news/2020/12/20/gov–bill-lee-remarks-as-prepared-for-delivery-on-the-covid-19-pandemic.html [Accessed 5 January 2021].

Lupton, D., 2013. *Risk*. New York: Taylor and Francis.

Marcus, J. 2020. The dudes who won't wear masks [online]. *The Atlantic*. Available from: https://www.theatlantic.com/ideas/archive/2020/06/dudes-who-wont-wear-masks/613375/ [Accessed 25 August 2020].

Maxmen, A., and Tollefson, J. 2020. Two decades of pandemic war games failed to account for Donald Trump [online]. *Nature*. Available from: https://www.nature. com/articles/d41586-020-02277-6 [Accessed 1 September 2020].

Povinelli, E., 2006. *Empire of love: toward a theory of intimacy, genealogy, and carnality*. Durham: Duke University Press.

Rivas, K., and Bernabe, A.J. 2020. Video of woman's tirade after refusing to wear a mask in Trader Joe's goes viral [online]. ABC News. Available from: https://abcnews.go. com/GMA/News/video-womans-tirade-refusing-wear-mask-trader-joes/story?id= 71505060 [Accessed 12 January 2021].

Scherlis, L. 2020. Distantiated communities: a social history of social distancing [online]. *Cabinet*. Available from: https://www.cabinetmagazine.org/kiosk/scherlis_lily_30_april_2020.php [Accessed 7 August 2020].

Silverman, E. 2020. STAT-Harris poll: most Americans would support Biden issuing a mask mandate [online]. STAT News. Available from: https://www.statnews.com/pharmalot/2020/12/21/biden-trump-covid19-coronavirus-pandemic-mask-vaccine/ [Accessed 5 January 2021].

Willingham, E. 2020. The condoms of the face: why some men refuse to wear masks [online]. *Scientific American*. Available from: https://www.scientificamerican.com/article/the-condoms-of-the-face-why-some-men-refuse-to-wear-masks/ [Accessed 12 January 2021].

Virus government – A twenty-first-century genealogy of the 'dusk mask' as biopolitical technology

James Hay

ABSTRACT
This essay provides a genealogy of the recent operations of 'virus government' in the United States which followed the early twenty-first-century governmental discourse about and technologization of Homeland Security and a War on Terror. Through the genealogy, the essay asks what has and has not changed during the last twenty years of governmental and biopolitical response to public safety and social security as a personal responsibility. To understand and rethink that history, the essay proposes the usefulness of considering the COVID mask as a technology of virus government and as a Liberal object.

Modern man is an animal whose politics places his existence as a living being into question

Michel Foucault, History of Sexuality, Vol. 1, p. 146

The self-administration of security & preparedness

As a means of addressing 'virus government' and its operation in the response to COVID-19 from the United States, I propose a genealogy. In 2006, *Cultural Studies* published 'Homeland Insecurities', a special issue which I co-edited and which assembled various analyses of the historical circumstances surrounding the formation of Department of Homeland Security (DHS) in the United States in 2002 (Hay and Andrejevic 2006). One of my contributions to the special issue, 'Designing Homes to be the First Line of Defense', provided a genealogy of the birth of Homeland Security through its 2005 proposal for a 'Family Communication Plan' (FCP) and that plan's targeting of 'home' as the *primary* platform for advancing a simple regimen and standard of national security and public safety. In the plan's rationale which circulated as a letter to citizens in major U.S. newspapers, the DHS declared,

'Homeland Security begins at home'. This foundational plan was supposed to make security personal, and personal security more rational and programmatic by following checklists which would allow family members to monitor each other's everyday movements and which would enhance one's awareness of the availability of materials, appliances, and domestic technologies (infamously duct tape) for responding effectively to emergencies and disasters.

The individualized plan for securing one's household was supposed to operate as a technology of government on three registers – the government of oneself, the government of family, house and household, and the government of 'public safety' and 'national security'. Following the attacks of September 11, 2001, these three objects of government and security were frequently aligned, sometimes loosely and sometimes vigorously, through the waging of a 'war on terror'. The DHS, urgently formed and heralded as an unprecedented response to the unprecedented War on Terror, was the newest and largest reorganization of government in over fifty years, overseeing and networking twenty two agencies for securing 'the homeland', a term adopted and governmentalized in the United States through the DHS. The creation of the DHS was accompanied by efforts to mobilize and galvanize citizens through Bush-Cheney administrated initiatives such as 'Ready.gov', the 'Citizen Corp', and private-foundation initiatives such as the 'America Prepared Campaign'.

One of the contradictions on which the DHS and its FCP were predicated was the creation of a massive new federal agency that operated within a deepening (some would call it 'neoliberal') reasoning about the value of 'reinventing government' by 'out-sourcing' the state administration of public services–by developing 'partnerships' with (catalyzing and enlarging the roles of) corporate, non-profit, and volunteer organizations, and citizens in administering services as a matter of public welfare and social security. So, in its justification, design, and operation, the DHS might avoid what libertarians considered to be the trappings of a Super Nanny State (Hay 2007).

The FCP thus was born of a political reasoning about empowerment, catalyzation, and mobilization of citizens whose security would be achieved through the effective materiality and everyday technologies of self-security and whose personal performance of security could be linked with a more abstract but regularly and widely invoked problem of national and social security in the age of a War on Terror. Given the historical contradiction through which the DHS was formed and politically rationalized (as a massive, unprecedented response to an ubiquitous War on Terror through personalized materials and technologies), its FCP was a 'technology of the self' which objectified threats and rationalized a citizen's control of them. In this way the FCP mediated a related contradiction: it was supposedly suited as much to the instabilities and uncertainties accruing from the threats posed by a new War on Terror as by the deepening insecurities of *self*-administered social security (in Agamben's term, the *bare life*) accompanying the creeping libertarian posture about diminishing State-administration (Agamben 1998). In both these respects, the FCP became an instrument for maintaining safety and security in a new regime of welfare *and* warfare.

Reconstructing how a FCP operated as communication technology within the early twenty-first century environment, culture, and economy of media lies beyond the scope of this essay but deserves a few reminders about context. The DHS was created on the cusp of the technological regime of digital media. As a department that oversaw and managed a network of federal agencies, not to mention a host of partnerships with private entities, its website quickly became a crucial means of performing, representing, and growing its network of governance. Government in the U.S., as and through digital networks, was 'reinvented' that way. The DHS's injunction to citizens to secure themselves and their households through a portable 'wallet-sized' emergency-list of contacts and tasks was suited for the ascendant media economy of mass customization and interactivity, and to the attractive assumption in those years that heightened states of interactivity guaranteed a more participatory and thus democratic citizenship – *freeing* the citizen-consumer from various restraints associated with twentieth century media, and empowering us all in that sense (Hay 2011). To that end, the wallet-sized, portable list (reminiscent of a pre-digital medium) soon was replaced by an interactive DHS-designed website, which allowed users to download and archive their personal emergency checklist and, in so doing, their relation to an actively 'prepared', 'Ready.gov-' citizenship, as potential members of a Citizen Corp. The FCP, as part of a growing, interactive, and customize-able information-network overseen by DHS, also was operationalized within the emerging instructional-regime of early twentieth-century Reality TV and lifestyle pro-gramming, some of which was directly about maximizing personal safety and security but much of which was about learning how to administer to oneself and to provide for one's own welfare and social security (Hay 2006, 2007, Ouellette and Hay 2008). The relation between Reality TV and the web presence of certain institutions of state was quite organic, such as the web links and referencing between ABC's *Shaq's Big Challenge* and the Bush administration's 'President's Fitness Challenge' (Hay 2010). As Reality TV contests and challenges demonstrated throughout the 2000s, the FCP as a personal gauge/exam of a citizen's readiness was also a *citizenship test* for calculating preparedness–a test to see whether one 'measures up', and a reminder of the state of risk and insecurity which required assembling new materials, techniques, and technologies for 'passing' the test.

Citizenship, self-testing & the current technological regime of virus government in the U.S.

The genealogy that I charted in my earlier account of the FCP and its networks of government underscored what was and was not unprecedented about the creation, design, and purview of the DHS. I invoke the birth of the DHS and its FCP with a similar aim in mind for thinking about the current networks through which COVID-19 has become a problem and objective of government. To the extent that the FCP was a technology for making rational the management of one's household and self, as a means of improving personal safety and security and of preparing for an emergency, it also served as a measurement and ongoing test of readiness. The test's authorization by and link to the newly created DHS made it doubly a citizenship test – a measure of one's relation to the active, self-responsible model of citizenship valued and valorized by the Bush administration's Ready.gov initiatives and Citizens Corp. If 'homeland security' *began* (as Director Tom Ridge claimed) within and from the communicative space, moral economy, and operation/ management of the early twenty-first-century U.S. household, then the DHS was primarily and from its beginning about implementing 'public safety' as a profoundly individualized, active, responsible form of citizenship.

The DHS's FCP provides a useful point of reference for considering what has and has not changed about the early experiments for COVID-testing in the U.S., particularly the utter lack of a central or federally organized system of testing during and the various proposals and rationalizations about privately administered and self-administered testing during 2020. The U.S. Center for Disease Control (CDC) website during 2020 provided advice and instruction about the state of testing in the U.S. and how to understand the results of a personal test administered privately. The CDC website also included a 'self-checker' – an online questionnaire and checklist for self-diagnosis, and an 'In-home COVID Screening Tool' developed by Apple. Clinics, as the primary though not uniform administrators of testing in the United States, elaborated on-line checklists for prospective patients to self-diagnose, as a *civic service*. The websites of major research hospitals such as Johns Hopkins and Mayo served collectively as a private model for public-service instruction and resources for *self-testing*. (See Hopkins' 'COVID Self-checker' https://www.hopkinsmedicine.org/coronavirus/covid-19-self-checker.html, and Mayo's 'COVID-19 Self-assessment Tool': https://www.mayoclinic.org/covid-19-self-assessment-tool). Smaller, local clinics typically developed versions of this self-test, sometimes with an eye toward maximizing hospital safety and civic responsibility in advance of a patient's visit to the clinic, and these clinics often referred visitors to their websites back to the CDC's self-checking software. So the CDC became primarily a centralized facility for *self*-administered testing and safety.

However, this mentality about self-testing and medical self-information also has acted on and through the technologization of 'self-tracking' and the Quantified Self, which gained momentum during the 2010s (Lupton 2016, Neff and Nafus 2016). By the late- 2010s, self-tracking and the Quantified Self not only referred to devices such as Fitbit and the Apple watch for monitoring and measuring personal movement and bodily functions, as a means of determining normalcy and health, of establishing personal plans and goal-setting, and of improving one's life and lifestyle that way. Self-tracking also referred to the personal management of pets, children, and households. (If so, see appended image. (Figure 1)) In that sense, self-testing and self-tracking (conjoined objectives) for virus monitoring could be rationalized as already available for the most prepared and active citizens – for the most advanced, invested, and self-caring Quantified Selves. One of the promoters of the Quantified Self-movement and -culture, Charles Wolf, thus proposed early in the pandemic the utility of self-tracking devices and regimens potentially to control the virus, or at the very least to develop knowledge-networks for understanding/researching how self-tracking technologies could be deployed to enhance *self-administered* testing (https://quantifiedself.com/blog/self-tracking-for-covid-19/). It is worth recognizing therefore the relation of recent self-tracking appliances to the legacy of the

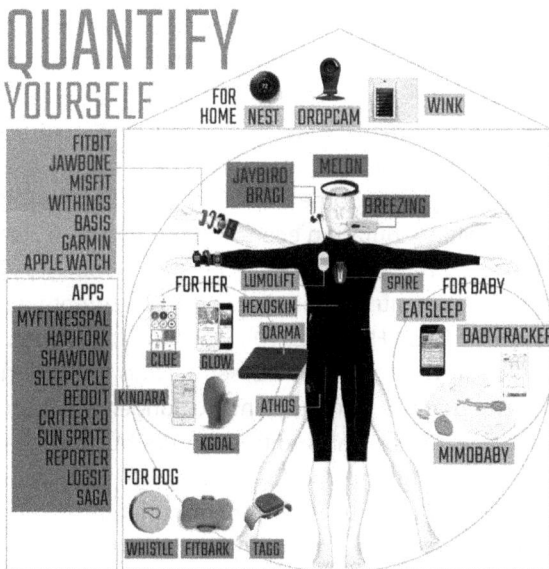

Figure 1. The technological regime of the Quantified Self *at home* has been represented this way: Anne Helen Petersen, 'Big Mother is Watching You', *BuzzFeed* , January 1, 2015.

FCP as the 'primary' and 'original' checklist and testing-tracking technology for self-protection and emergency preparedness.

Due to the deepening and normalization of the self-tracking regime in the U.S. before the onslaught of the COVID virus, it is not surprising that Apple and Google, arguably the two largest manufacturers of self-quantification technology in the U.S., quickly announced a partnership to develop an app for self-administered virus-tracking, and made the system available in May 2020. By late 2020, however, only ten states in the United States had adopted that system. A consortium of academic research and development, whose U.S. base is Stanford University, also quickly unveiled an 'open-source' self-tracking app linked to its 'COVID Watch'-network. Although the apps mentioned above followed the disposition in the U.S. for self-tracking for a population invested in the Quantified Self, and although they were the primary early app-oriented initiatives in the U.S., none of them is suited for a national network or even large-scale networks of self-tracking because the U.S. currently lacked in 2020 a technical means or political commitment for centralizing data from do-it-yourself tracking, and because achieving a national database would have required well over half of U.S. citizens to became voluntarily active in the network. Unlike many countries (such as Britain, China, Germany, Israel) which developed, sometimes through public-private partnerships, a 'national app' that linked self-tracking to a national/central database, the CDC's arrangement with Apple only produced a personal, self-checking app(-lication), and the Apple designed self-checker on the CDC website referred users back to their *local* healthcare facilities. This solution has as much to do with the U.S.'s lack of national healthcare system as its deepening reliance on the increasingly robust technological regime of self-tracking and self-quantification for life/-style management, albeit for those who are and can be most invested in it. This arrangement also accentuates the deepening of 'home care' as the 'primary care'- matrix, location, and governance of the virus – a deepening in that sense of the dictum that 'Homeland Security begins as home'.

The emerging 'digital reputation economy' which Alison Hearn examined ten years ago has become decidedly more pervasive and integral for harnessing the media and communication networks of entrepreneurialist digital labour during the 2010s (Hearn 2010), and the reputation economy is shaping the stakes and utility of COVID self-testing and self-tracking. Over the last decade, reputation management no longer has been oriented to public relations for businesses and entrepreneurs but has been baked into the regime of self-tracking and the Quantified Self – marketed for anyone concerned about the health of their 'net reputation'. As Lee Humphries demonstrates, following Hearn, the reputation economy is predicated on a growing array of technologies for making each of us, but particularly the most active and invested in social networking, *accountants* and *accountable*, and what Humphries terms a 'qualified self' (Humphries 2018). Both Hearn and Humphries gesture briefly and obliquely to how the self-administration of one's reputation through apps and web resources is a matter of citizenship, and not only labour and sociality. Although the initial and uneven development of COVID self-testing and self-tracking technologies in the U.S. has not brought much attention yet to how the self-government of the virus might (likely will) become a matter of monitoring and managing one's reputation (as *in-valid* or as healthy), it is not difficult or far-fetched to imagine how fulfilling the responsibility of accountability through self-testing and self-tracking also can become an index of not only one's ability to work but also of social responsibility as good citizenship, i.e. of being governmentally an 'accountable' and thus Qualified Self. By 2021, some state governments in the United States rationalized their reluctance to adopt the Google-Apple application over concerns about data-privacy.

To the extent that COVID self-testing and self-tracking (medical *self*-information) have operated as what Foucault termed 'biopolitical' procedures and technologies for measuring the health of a population and the social body's reproductive capacity, and to the extent that biopower developed as an early Modern administrative technique of counting as 'state-istics', it is worth grappling with what 'biopower' entails through these practices in the U.S. during the pandemic, and with what does and does not remain in the current context from the counting-technology that Foucault attributed to early Western (particularly French) Liberal government (Foucault 1990, 2003). Self-measurement through COVID self-testing and self-tracking is and is not the technological regime of biopower that Foucault described. Current self-testing for the virus is what he described as a 'technology of the self', but it operates differently within a state apparatus (institutions and technologies) of measurement that is not designed to archive *statistics* (the national count) and that has largely ceded the measurement procedure to subjects who are afflicted or invested (Foucault 1998). Is virus government in the U.S. during the COVID pandemic therefore a deepening of a political libertarianism which attempts to 'deconstruct' and 'wage war' against the administrative institutions of Liberal statehood (Steve Bannon at Conservative Political Action Conference, February 2017), or another reinvention of Liberal government and citizenship? Does it represent on either of these counts a crisis of the history Liberalism? And for whom does that matter?

The COVID mask as Liberal Object – A counter-checklist, or a checklist about checklists

My genealogy of the FCP and its network of government in 2005 was engaged with Foucault's history (genealogy) of the birth of Western Liberalism and with appropriations of Foucault's thought to explain 'neo-liberal' governmentality and technologies of the self. Through that lens, my account of the FCP emphasized the network of government between the state and the FCP's shaping of a responsible, prepared, and secure citizen of a home and 'homeland', and that the FCP operated (simultaneously as a technology of individual liberties and self-control) within a political rationality that valued and valorized an entrepreneurial citizenship. That analysis did not energetically address the materiality of the FCB as 'Liberal object', and how (following Otter 2007) one can chart a history of Liberal agency and government through a history of *objects* and things. One cannot separate that history from the changing regimes of knowledge and acquisition of techniques through which materials become instrumentalized–as objects and objectives, and *technologized* in the Modern sense. However, particularly with respect to an importance placed from cultural studies and critical studies on the role of media representations and of communications through 'media', it is worth not losing sight of how Liberal objects have mattered as and through *the government of things* (Lemke 2015) and as the materiality of Liberal exercises of freedom as well as (self-)control and (self-)security.

One of the accouterments included in the FCP's checklist for home security was a 'dusk mask'. It was extraordinary that the FCP as a foundational technology for the DHS and a War on Terror would misspell 'dust mask' on their standardized personal security plan. Perhaps the misspelling was evidence of the department's lack of care and even seriousness about the protective care that they were instituted to provide or about the real utility of a personal emergency plan or about the practicality of fashioning a citizen-soldier through the most everyday household materials. Including a dust/dusk mask on the standard checklist perpetuated a discourse at that time about the new hazards and risks of 'biological agents' and biochemical warfare. An early bulletin produced by the DHS through the Federal Emergency Management Agency (FEMA) explained and listed potentially dangerous substances and scenarios, but did not elaborate reasons that a simple device such as the dust mask could effectively shield households from radioactive, hazardous chemical, or contagious biological particulate (FEMA 2004).

In the U.S., the face mask became over the first few months of the pandemic as simple and flimsy a technology of self-protection (of the self-government of the virus) as was the dust/dusk mask fifteen years earlier, even as the COVID mask also immediately became a more conflicted and fraught technology of virus government than almost anywhere in the world. There are many ways to analyze the mask. For instance, more than the 'dusk mask' recommended by the early DHS's FCP, the COVID mask not only broke with long-standing semiotic convention/code associated with the outfits of medical specialists or home remodellers, it quickly became a robustly complex as well as an empty signifier, filled with meanings in nothing short of a rapid and intense semiotic guerilla warfare. More than the 'dusk mask', the commodification of the COVID mask also has mattered profoundly, as a means (or not) of protecting or exploiting workers, and as a product whose exchange value and availability the pandemic impacted profoundly and put under stress, particularly through a political rationality in the U.S. that eschewed a national, public provision and coordination of mask production and distribution. However, it is just as helpful to consider (or rethink) the mask within a long and/or recent history of Liberal objects – as an aim and a technology/machinology of Liberal exercises of power, and as the basis for a *new materialist* understanding of virus government.

With that in mind, I pose the following questions – not a comprehensive (check-)list but one that underscores what is useful about examining the mask as Liberal object. Is it possible to wear the mask freely, without always *testing* the limits of its governmental utility? How has the mask operated biopolitically in and through a current Liberal government of things, bodies, and populations? How has the mask problematized a Liberal regime of rules, protocols, laws, and policies? How has it operated, how should we assess its utility, as a technology of freedom *properly* exercised through self-control, discipline, and good, responsible citizenship? How has it been called forth within an *etiquette* (ethics and proper conduct) of preventing the spread of the virus – in that sense, what Nikolas Rose termed, an 'ethico-politics' of virus government (Rose 1999)? What is complicated and problematic, in new ways, about its relation to Liberal ideas of rights and responsibilities of citizenship? Or stated differently, how has the mask operated as a technology of self-protection and security within a lack of rules governing mask-wearing and in states of government where the mask is worn voluntarily? How has it become the point of a binary understanding of individual sovereignty and liberties as the opposite of forms of control, disciplinarity, policing, and security? How has the 'opening of a state' (with the promise of new or returned liberties, folded into a conception of normalcy) been predicated mostly on privatized and personal policing of 'mask rules'? How has the mask become simultaneously a central problem and tool for the orderly operations of governmental legislation and policy in Washington, D.C. and statehouses? What are the rights of consumers, shoppers, and clients (as citizens) to wear a mask in public- but privately-owned spaces, and who should or does enforce those rights? What has been the appropriate or legitimate authority (states, municipalities, proprietors, homeowners, passers-by) for governing appropriate mask-wearing, particularly lacking a national, federal regulation? How has the mask been inextricable from the technologies and infrastructures of counting, including the Enlightenment ideal of governmental rationality through counting votes in elections to political offices? What has the mask to do with differential mobility – the freedom or restriction to travel and move about? How does the mask operate from the U.S. but within global governmentalities such as the World Health

Organization or international flights? How has the exercise of *resistance* occurred through an ethico-politics of wearing the mask and/or refusing it? Within a history of Liberal objects, how does the COVID mask perpetuate or depart from the adoption (or the refusal) of protective masks in earlier pandemics governed through Modern Liberal institutions such as clinics and public schools or such as the Liberal city as a laboratory for governing the problem of individual freedoms and mobility? How or to what extent has the U.S. history of Liberal governance, particularly with respect to public hygiene as social security and biopower, shaped the current model and problem of citizenship and civic good? Rather than singularizing the mask as a Liberal object, how might we understand its governmental utility and instrumentality as part of 'actor-networks' – its relation to other things and objects, such as the self-testing and self-tracking applications, whose networking shapes and actualizes particular forms of agency in the pandemic? If the 'dusk mask' served as an everyday, household instrument of combat for the DHS's mobilization of a post-9/11 *citizen-soldier*, how has the COVID mask emerged within that history, becoming an affirmation of Foucault's thought (inverting Clausewitz's dictum) that politics, or security politics and current DHS policing, is war by other means? How does the mask fit into the current assemblage of 'weaponry', instruments, materials, and objects for 'combatting' COVID, deployed by citizens and professional security agents, possibly in a new 'civil' warfare?

From a 'War on Terror' to countering COVID-19 as a 'Weapon of mass destruction'

One way to address the last two questions in the prior section is to consider the concern raised by the DHS in July 2020 that enforcing face-mask regulations would complicate and possibly hinder the DHS's use of its current biometric, facial-recognition technology for protecting the Homeland by identifying and distinguishing citizens, non-citizens, criminals, illegal immigrants, and Terrorists. Thinking genealogically about the government of the COVID pandemic in the U.S. raises important, and still seldom discussed, questions not only about the changing political rationality of a 'homeland security' in virus government, but also about how the DHS has reinvented itself and rearticulated its purview so that its role in safeguarding citizens from and in a time of COVID intersected with its other objectives during the Trump presidency. Mask-wearing, which has been recommended though not highlighted or required as a safeguard by the DHS and its website, quickly complicated the department's self-described mission as enforcer of the Trump administration's multi-pronged immigration policy which has been bent on severely restricting the movement into U.S. territory of what it considered to be 'foreign elements' and on limiting drastically prior avenues for citizenship and visas. In 2018, when there was an outbreak of mumps in the detention centres that the DHS (through agents of its Customs and Border Protection and its Immigration and Customs Enforcement) oversaw for immigrants held along the southern U.S. border, Trump and his senior policy advisor, Stephen Miller, regularly equated immigrants with the viral spread of disease. In July 2020, the DHS website (without evidence) listed border protection as one of its primary roles and achievements in controlling COVID in the U.S., as Trump and many Republican legislators continued to refer to COVID as the 'China virus' and to claim that the virus originated due to failures of China's government to restrict sick passengers or due to a deliberate attempt to destabilize the U.S. by purposefully launching the virus as a weapon of mass destruction. In December 2018, Trump signed the Countering Weapons of Mass Destruction Act which authorized the creation of a CWMD agency within the DHS, and by May 2020 the CWMD began to lead the DHS's (and the U.S. federal) response to COVID (DHS 'Weekly Update', 18 May 2020), thus formalizing the department's folding of its policing of a residual War on Terror into its three-year aggressive policing campaign to restrict immigration, into its oversight of border-wall construction, and into the militarized policing technologies and objects of virus government. Lacking a permanent, vetted Director, the DHS's Interim Director, Chad Wolf, appeared in July 2020 on the DHS's COVID information website in a video mostly thanking ICE and CBP agents, and attempting to correct a 'public misunderstanding' about their operations, but having little to say about the DHS's virus response. By the summer of 2020, the Ready.gov website inserted Pandemic Readiness into its menu of kits and checklists for protecting one's family and household from the virus, with the hashtag #AloneTogether – a motto for virus government in the U.S. during the pandemic. These are the institutional rationalities and rationalizations about calibrating the control of a virus as a Weapon of Mass Destruction, and in a country where the front line of defense is a technological regime of self-testing, self-tracking, and self-responsibilization, wherein the COVID mask (ironically a *dusk* mask for our epoch) has thus become the primary counter-weapon and flimsiest protection against a virus objectified and governmentalized as 'a weapon of mass destruction'. When Foucault states that 'Modern man is an animal whose politics', and I would add whose technologies of freedom and government, 'places his existence as a living being into question', one should surely ask how that existence has become a politics/warfare of virus government, and whether through a new biopolitical regime we have entered a new Modernity, or the end of Liberalism as political modernity.

Disclosure statement

No potential conflict of interest was reported by the author(s).

Further information

This Special Issue article has been comprehensively reviewed by the Special Issue editors, Associate Professor Ted Striphas and Professor John Nguyet Erni.

References

Agamben, G., 1998. *Homo sacer: sovereign power & bare life*. Stanford, CA: Stanford University Press.

Federal Emergency Management Agency. 2004. *Are You Ready? An In-depth Guide to Citizen Preparedness*. https://www.fema.gov/pdf/areyouready/areyouready_full.pdf.

Foucault, M., 1990. *History of sexuality*, Vol. 1. New York: Vintaqe.

Foucault, M., 1998. *Ethics: subjectivity & truth*. New York: New Press.

Foucault, M., 2003. *"Society must Be defended": lectures at the college de France—1975-76*, trans. David Macey. New York: Picador.

Hay, J., 2007. The many responsibilities of the new citizen-soldier. *Communication & critical/Cultural studies*, 4 (2), 216–220.

Hay, J., 2006. Designing homes to be the first line of defense. *Cultural studies*, 20 (4/5), 349–377.

Hay, J., 2010. Television as everyday network of government. In: G. Kien and M. Levina, ed. *Post-global network & everyday life*. New York: Peter Lang, 149–176.

Hay, J., 2011. 'Popular culture' in a critique of the new political reason. *Cultural studies*, 25 (4/5), 659–684.

Hay, J. and Andrejevic, M., 2006. Homeland Insecurities: introduction. *Cultural studies*, 20 (4/5), 331–348.

Hearn, A., 2010. Structuring feeling: Web 2.0, ranking & rating, & the digital 'reputation'. *Economy. ephemera*, 10 (3/4), 421–438.

Humphries, L., 2018. *The Qualified self*. Cambridge, MA: MIT Press.

Lemke, T., 2015. New materialisms: foucault & the 'government of things'. *Theory, culture, & society*, 32 (4), 3–25.

Lupton, D., 2016. *The Quantified self*. Cambridge, UK: Polity Press.

Neff, G., and Nafus, D., 2016. *Self-tracking*. Cambridge, MA: MIT Press.

Otter, C., 2007. Making Liberal objects: British techno-social relations, 1800-1900. *Cultural studies*, 21 (4/5), 570–590.

Ouellette, L. and Hay, J., 2008. *Better living through Reality TV*. London: Wiley-Blackwell.

Rose, N., 1999. *Powers of freedom: reframing political thought*. London: Cambridge University Press.

Bio or Zoe?: dilemmas of biopolitics and data governmentality during COVID-19

Yeran Kim

ABSTRACT

Heralding the self-brand of 'K-prevention' (nuanced with nationalistic pride in line with K-wave, K-pop, etc.), Korea has operated within two methods of articulation against COVID-19. One method involves granting the population relative freedom within the actual, physical realm, while the other method involves strengthening data surveillance within the virtual realm. This articulation of the actual and the virtual, and of freedom and surveillance, is at the core of Korea's biopolitical governmentality, which is currently intertwined not only with an infectious virus, but also with data technology. I would like to suggest a slight silver lining with respect to the possibility of overcoming this dilemma: a dilemma that involves physical survival under data colonialism on the one hand, and freedom from data colonialism on the other – both elements complicated by the potential risk of transmission. This may be a starting point toward digital democracy in the age of pandemics: social equality for life instead of augmenting the thanapolitical database; respect toward vulnerable singularities instead of deceitful exclusion; and sensitivity toward redressing embedded inequality instead of reinforcing stigmatization. We must, in other words, reinvent an ethics of vulnerability and a politics of dependency as guiding principles for living together in pandemic times.

Introduction

COVID-19 is a corporeal, affective, social, economic, and political pandemic. At the least related to the reality in which the pandemic has significantly undermined human beings' fundamental norms regarding how to separate and connect with one another. COVID-19 has almost entirely ruptured the explicit or implicit distinction between the individual and the society. Instead of the old wisdom that states, 'If we are to live, we must unify', in Korean society nowadays, a new wisdom has emerged: 'If together, we all die. If we are to live, we must be alone'. This trendy neologism of the 'new normal' may be summarized as the bifocal procedure of *physically* isolating those who used to live together and of *virtually* connecting with those who need to have their privacy protected. The societal problem of connection and isolation is closely associated with the biopolitical matters of life and death in the current specificity of the pandemic.

South Korea has featured a peculiar mode of controlling the COVID-19 crisis, and (as I would like to argue) one of the main factors in preventing infection involves a hyper-tightened 'data governmentality' over the biopolitical matters of life and death. Korea was initially blamed for being a country where, after China, COVID-19 was rampant; however, Korea was gradually seen as having had considerable success in containing the infection. For example, relatively fewer cumulative cases were reported in comparison with other countries, with a total of 45,442 patients and 612 deaths as of December 16, 2020. Heralding the self-brand of 'K-prevention' (nuanced with nationalistic pride in line with K-wave, K-pop, etc.), Korea has operationalized a prevention policy using two methods of articulation: one method grants the population relative freedom of movement and economic activities within the physical realm, while the other method strengthens data surveillance within the virtual realm. This articulation of the actual and the virtual (and of freedom and surveillance) intersects with matters of life and death. The assemblage of biopolitics (Foucault 2003) and data governmentality has resulted in a novel controlling system in the pandemic. This is so not only in relation to health and safety with regard to COVID-19, but also to citizens' subjectivation to data governmentality: the power of granting people health and safety (or life) by submitting one's truth ('When and where are you, and with whom? And even in what temperature?') to the totalizing system of checking, tracing, identifying, and accumulating a massive scale of populational data. In the pages that follow, I will analyse the current system for controlling COVID-19 in Korea, specifically as the articulation of biopolitics and data governmentality. Next, dilemmas are formulated in the clash between *zoe,* as the biological terms, and *bio,* as the socio-political terms, under which operate the system for controlling COVID-19. Finally, an ethico-politics of vulnerability is developed. Based on a 'relational understanding of vulnerability', it is argued, we should accept and pursue 'interdependency as a condition of equality' and the possibility of non-violent coexistence (Butler 2016, 2020).

Data governmentality in everyday life in Seoul

My life in Seoul, the capital city of South Korea, has been significantly transformed since the COVID-19 outbreak in January 2020. Somewhat like other countries in Asia, South Korea has adopted a peculiar mode of controlling COVID-19. In contrast to most western countries, where total lockdown measures were initially taken, citizens in South Korea have generally been allowed to do daily outdoor activities. At the level of daily life, all shops and restaurants (including entertainment and places of leisure) have remained open, while public and private transportation still operate. Particular spots have been closed for certain periods of time when a visitor tested positive for COVID-19, but they were permitted to reopen in a couple of days after preventive treatment. Schools and universities were delayed for some weeks, starting in the spring semester of 2020; nevertheless, they eventually managed to run their classes alternatively online or offline while maintaining the necessary hygiene rules and facilities.

In terms of work, companies and public institutions have kept their employees working from home by operating in shifts. Though self-employed shops and services (including cafes, restaurants and sports centres) are the main groups that have been seriously affected by the pandemic, they have still been permitted to open as usual, with a partial restraint to stay open until 9 PM just during the peak COVID-19 period. Spatial elements have also been reshaped; for example, handles and buttons in buildings have been covered with antibiotic materials, and numerous campaign stickers and placards requesting people to maintain personal rules of prevention are frequently found in the streets.

Of course, human faces have become the principal target to protect from the coronavirus. In contrast to people in most western societies, Koreans have been passionate about facial masks and have been willing to wear them every time and place since the initial stage of the outbreak of COVID-19. A so-called 'great mask war' erupted during the early stage of the COVID-19 outbreak when a large number of citizens desperately rushed to buy facial masks. This happened when facial masks were sold out in the markets across the nation, and if any remained, the prices skyrocketed. The great mask war calmed down only when the government promulgated a 'public mask' scheme, a so-called 'five-day rotation face mask distribution system' making it mandatory for pharmacies to sell only one mask per person on fixed days, according to one's birth year. More specifically, highly advanced screening devices called 'untact AI sensors' (the exact meaning of which hardly anyone knows) have been set up in public spaces; thus, bare faces without masks are automatically flagged, and people without masks are prohibited from entry into buildings. Consequently, physical human faces have been defaced with respect to the danger of pandemic transmission. At the same time, their virtual identities have been recognized, assembled, and controlled through expansive and seemingly inexorable datafication.

At the cost of maintaining a relatively ordinary and free daily life, Korean society has built up an extraordinary surveillance environment. People who have tested positive for COVID-19 are given a numbered ID, such as 'a certain city district + serial patient number', which announces their every movement online. Moreover, those testing positive for COVID-19 are required to download apps onto their smartphones that check in real time whether they are following self-isolation rules. Information regarding their use of credit cards and GPS (embedded in their smartphones) is also aggressively utilised to track patients' previous movements. In fact, it has become a common joke among Koreans that we are less afraid of the coronavirus than we are of revealing every detail of our private lives.

Smartphone alarms keep ringing due to the increasing accumulation of coronavirus-related data at any moment. Messages mostly come from the Korea Centres for Disease Control and Prevention (KCDC) and local governments, informing residents about new COVID-19 infection cases and their trajectories. Citizens are required to indicate their residence and mobile number almost everywhere, either in writing or by using QR codes, in order to enter public places (e.g. cinemas, bars, clubs, etc.). Thanks to all the records and data mentioned above, people who are identified as having been in the same place with COVID-19 patients receive phone calls requesting that they get tested immediately. The monitoring networks operate not only in suspended places, but across the nation. When traveling across the city and passing through several districts, I find that my smartphone has become a kind of storage space for automated messages that (thanks to GPS) each local government spreads among anonymous citizens staying – even momentarily – within their jurisdictions. Thus, a huge data system has been synchronized with the spatialized human/non-human assemblage at every moment.

Specific groups of people, such as those who came from abroad or who contacted patients, are managed in distinctive ways that are mediated and augmented by advanced surveillance technologies. They are obliged to self-isolate and are legally forced to set up applications on their smartphones. One application, called the Self-Isolation App, was developed and distributed by the Ministry of the Interior and Safety (7 March 2020). The utilities of apps are plural for purposes of both protecting potential patients' health and managing the safety of the entire population. First, regarding individual health, the app should necessarily be attached to the user at all times: alarms automatically and simultaneously ring twice a day, both for users and local government officers, requiring users to check their temperature and symptoms and report them to the officers via the app to make certain that everybody is 'normal' .Next, with respect to managing the whole population, the app is used to control the movement of the people under supervision. When someone who is supposed to self-isolate deviates from the boundary of the allowed isolation space (normally his/her home), as identified by the position of the app on smartphones, governmental officers are authorized to call the police and search for the person who has violated established rules. They can also coerce him/her to return to the self-isolation space immediately, and if this individual refuses to follow the order, he/she is fined. Some people may attempt to leave their phones in their self-isolation place and go out. If such a mischievous act is revealed, this is also punishable by law.

The Korean app-based system of self-isolation and supervision can contrasted with some western models: in terms of technological operation, the German model, based on the Corona-Warn-App, is not intended for governmental tracking of individuals' locations, but rather for checking the proximity among anonymous people for purposes of preventing healthy people from unintendedly contacting patients. This method is premised on the notion that the citizens are free to take care of their health and safety in mutual relations. In comparison, the Korean model is grounded in a paradigm under which individual citizens are imminently subject to the government, a paradigm that authorizes police and other government officials to identify, and track locations and movements: not only of individuals but, potentially, the entire population. Moreover, the German model is based on the liberal framework in which a decision to adopt the app depends on the individual subject's own choice to do so. On the other hand, the Korean model makes it a legal obligation for certain groups of citizens, even those not confirmed to have COVID-19, to accept and follow the rules of the app. If the rules of the app are neglected or resisted, these citizens are punished under the law.

The assemblage of human bodies, digital technologies, laws, policies, and physical spaces (let alone the coronavirus) coalesces in the nation's control system against the pandemic. The unique rhetoric of K-protection emblematizes Korea's 'firstness' in introducing certain digital technologies as protections against COVID-19 transmission. Such measures are aimed to maximize the degree of maintaining normal everyday life, including the freedom of mobility, openness of public spaces, and liveliness in daily social interactions – but under the condition of everyone being 'ambient' and interconnected to ubiquitously-operative data technologies. For instance, it was publicized by the Central Disaster Management Headquarters and Central Disease Control Headquarters that a 'Residential Treatment Centre' was introduced in Korea (*first* in the world) as the core element of K-protection. This centre is intended to care for COVID-19 patients with no or mild symptoms in order to contain local transmission (14 May 2020). Such a strong nationalistic tone culminated in the government announcement of K-protection achievements (20 January 2021) on the one-year anniversary of COVID-19 in Korea. It was declared that Korea had invented a unique model to counterattack the pandemic over the past one year, made up of 'mobile screening stations' to facilitate prompt COVID-19 tests; QR codes (KI-PASS) to implement tracking and testing, both for the protection of privacy and to secure precise information; and the aforementioned residential treatment centres. It was reiterated that the principle of K-protection is 'democracy, transparency and openness', of which 'we all deserve to be proud'. The number of cases in Korea is 136.45 out of 100,000, the third lowest position following New Zealand and Australia, while the death rate is 2.31 out of 100,000, second to New Zealand. These records are especially remarkable, according to the government's assessment, considering that Korea has never ordered a national lockdown. Not surprisingly, the relatively good record of protection against COVID-19 has been accompanied with a rosy picture of the national economy, with the expectation that the economic growth rate of Korea was expected to be −1.1% in 2020, which falls in the best grade among Organisation for Economic Co-operation and Development (OECD) member countries.[1]

The infinitesimal and grand processes of surveillance are, where the pandemic is concerned, constitutive of the regime of data governmentality, which compels citizens to be 'docile' bodies (Foucault 1977). It is inevitable that most Korean citizens cannot help but answer 'Yes' (and hopefully 'No' to COVID-19) to the biopolitical mode of 'interpellation' (Althusser 1970) under the current pandemic situation. One is subject to data governmentality, spontaneously and perhaps willingly, for the sake of survival. There may be less casual damage in terms of privacy or temporary technological errors. However, as increasingly advanced technologies are adopted, data governmentality becomes more and more omnipotent and naturalized as a perfectly innocent entity, to the extent that the citizens, accustomed to the surveillant environment, no longer seem to doubt them. One of the most obvious examples is the QR code, considered to be the core technology of the KI-PASS. This measure was legalized and referred to as the Personal Information Protection Act, Act on the Protection, Use, etc. of Location Information, Infectious Disease Control and Prevention Act (Ministry of Health and Welfare), or as a legal system that has been significantly developed over recent decades to overcome serious infectious diseases (e.g. SARS and MERS). The KI-PASS has made it a legal obligation for everyone who enters public places to scan his/her own QR code and confirm his/her personal identity and current location. Regarding the privacy protection policy of the QR code, the personal identity information is channelled to the QR-providing companies (e.g. Internet portal service companies such as NAVER or Social Networking companies such as KAKAOTALK), while the location information is provided to the Korea Social Security Information Service. Thus, by separating the two sorts of information, one's privacy (matched information of identity and location) is untraceable and protected. In addition, both kinds of information are deleted after 4 weeks from the time of collection unless any COVID-19 cases occur in the related location. As the apparently advanced digital devices have spread to every corner of Korea, citizens have gradually accepted, internalized, and conducted themselves in line with this system of data governmentality.

Biopolitical and data-governmental powers sometimes conflict and nego-tiate with each other. Furthermore, they sometimes erupt in alternative direc-tions of social change with respect to pre- or post-COVID-19 political issues. For instance, visitors to gay clubs were tested anonymously when mass con-tamination broke out in those settings (10 May 2020). The unusual privacy protection of maintaining anonymity in testing was adopted in order to contain coronavirus transmission, particularly among sexual minorities, who are highly sensitive to privacy protection in the strongly conservative Korean society. Indeed, a common response from sexual minority groups was the concern that the outbreak of COVID-19 at gay clubs might be abused as grounds to legitimate homophobic attitudes ('They are so dirty, and COVID-19 is payback for their behaviour'). The issue of legitimating the Prohibition of Discrimination Act has been in the air since 2007 in Korean society, due mainly to conservative disagreement in approving equality, regardless of one's sexual identity and orientation. In these circumstances, it seemed obvious that, if individuals are identified as having contracted COVID-19 at gay clubs, they would be outed. As a result, they might even be fired from their workplace and alienated from society (Nah 2020). It is not surprising that the expression 'Dying alone from COVID-19 is better than being outed' became the prevailing mindset of sexual minorities after the COVID-19 outbreak at gay clubs (Yoon 2020). Sexual minority groups immediately founded the 'Corona Sexual Minorities Emergency Act Group' (12 May 2020) after the outbreak of COVID-19 at gay clubs and called for 'safety without discrimination'. This group requested that the government enact anonymous testing for COVID-19. This exceptional rule of an anon-ymous system for those who had visited these related places was decided by the government two days later (14 May 2020). This decision was the result of a biopolitical necessity (to contain disease transmission) overriding a homophobic ideology oppressive toward minorities, as well as the wilful force of data governmentality (if temporarily) to trace and identify and collect the individual subject's truth to establish a grand scale of population data.[2]

Fractures in controlling systems

An irony regarding the assemblage of biopolitical power and data govern-mentality is that this controlling system requires a certain alienation and dis-crimination, despite its universal (but fictional) claim of saving lives in the nation. Korea's controlling system during the pandemic is characterized by three related aspects: totalization, exclusion, and stigmatization.

The first element of controlling the population in the pandemic world is 'totalization'. Everyone, regardless of his/her social categories (e.g. age, gender, class, and ethnicity), may be exposed to the potential risk of

COVID-19. Once everyone is subject to a universal surveillance system, he/she is assembled into a massive data system, with the objective of achieving national immunity.

The second element concerns 'exclusion', which has rendered marginalized groups invisible and ignored, even in the midst of the pandemic. The unusually high number of COVID-19 deaths associated with BAME (Black Asian minority ethnic) groups is very often pointed out in critical approaches to the pandemic. For instance, the disproportionate rate of BAME deaths in western society is attributable to economic, cultural, and social factors such as (1) jobs, (2) household and working conditions, (3) residential areas, (4) cultural differences, (5) ideological segregation (racism), and (6) class (e.g. Jones 2020). In a similar vein, Reich (2020) identifies four emergent classes during the COVID-19 crisis: 'the remotes', 'the essentials', 'the unpaid', and 'the forgotten'.

Nevertheless, Korean society has paid very little attention to these already-existing and newly emerging social realities of inequality. Instead, everyone is simply too busy to track every individual movement with myopic, surveillant gazes. Thus, the critical question of how the so-called 'normal life' has 'failed' the poor has so far been dismissed; the poor have only now been recognized during these 'abnormal' times when 'cruelties [are] deliberately targeting' them to the extent of 'being deadly' (Harris 2020a, 2020b, The Guardian 2020). Those who have suffered from social, economic, and cultural poverty up until now have been figuratively picked up with tweezers and examined under a magnifying glass during this pandemic, in the process standing out as both vulnerable and dangerous subgroups.

Thus, the last category involves 'stigmatization'. COVID-19 patients are segmented and often 'branded' (Clough 2018) based on their social, economic, and cultural capital. A series of branding efforts have taken place, first toward foreigners (mostly Chinese), followed by 'inferior' individuals who have insufficient cultural and economic capital, and who are considered weak and incapable of self-control, such as religious groups, manual workers, decadent and irresponsible indulgers, elderly people, and prisoners. Mental hospitals, prisons, and churches were identified as 'super-spreaders' of COVID-19, and individuals from such venues were blamed for their unreasonable, immoral, and aggressive propensities in terms of threatening others ('good people') with death (Lyou 2021). Apart from these 'abnormal' people, the majority of 'normal' COVID-19 patients – mostly 'proper' middle-class citizens (Campbell 2011) – have been absolved of blame and given sympathy as victims of 'silent transmission'.

Distance but (Still) dependency

The Korean approach to the pandemic crisis might have saved many lives (in a biological sense); however, it has colonized human lives through data surveillance (in a virtual sense). In order to save lives in the biological sense, citizens rationalize that we must incur the 'cost' of being colonized by data (Couldry and Mejias 2019). Consequently, 'bio', understood as the socio-political formation of life under data colonialism, clashes with 'zoe', understood as the biological fact of living (Agamben 1998). A dilemma in which we are situated is that *bio* (which should have been respected as the critical criterion of socio-political autonomy and freedom) is recklessly neglected in pandemic-related data colonialism in favour of *zoe*.

It is no surprise that the power of digital surveillance, or *shareveillance,* is pervasive in the contemporary network society, in which the communitarian moral of 'sharing' is reformulated into a hegemonic mode of controlling networked populations (Birchall 2016). However, it may be difficult to agree upon a critique of *shareveillance* without hesitation in this pandemic situation. This is partly due to our feelings of anxiety and guilt regarding my claim for freedom from data surveillance. With respect to the pandemic, any 'obfuscation' of personal data (Birchall 2016) runs the risk of affecting others' health and safety. Moreover, some people would also argue – with good reason – that people are dying due to a lack of information. Consequently, our dilemma is situated in the reality in which we are supposed to abandon individual autonomy and freedom concerning data privacy for the sake of biological survival (Agamben 2020, Nancy 2020).

A matrix consisting of four couplets may be proposed as an analytical framework by which to account for the dilemma of (or tension between) biopolitics and data governmentality:

(1) **'Life x Isolation'** is conducted in self-isolation in the pandemic. This has been the most common form of enduring the pandemic in civil society.
(2) **'Life x Connection'** operates in the system of *shareveillance* across the digital network.

Unsurprisingly, 1 and 2 are complementary, articulated as physical isolation and a data network.

(3) **'Death x Isolation'** is embodied mainly by 'key workers' (delivery, public transportation, prevention service, care work), all of whom must travel across empty cities among self-isolated people during the lockdown, despite the risks of disease and death to themselves.
(4) **'Death x Connection'** is emblematized by those who gather in response to their desire to transgress the 'new normal' of self-isolation, many of

whom are doomed to become ill from herd infection. Manual workers (e.g. customer call centre workers), gay clubbers, or worshippers have been singled out for this category in Korean society.

We may then ask ourselves if the only options we have are biological safety (giving up data autonomy) or risking infection (free from data surveillance). Both options may sound humiliating and miserable. This is why we must realize our double-trapped reality of vulnerability in order to create an alternative ethics of vulnerability. How do we protect our valuable, and yet vulnerable, lives in the milieu of the virus-pervasive and data-saturated present?

Following Judith Butler, the recognition, affirmation, and practice of relations of 'dependency' shape an ethics of 'vulnerability'. I, you, we, and they cannot but co-exist merely because of our common sharing of vulnerability, argues Butler (2020). Thus, it is because of our political and existential ethics that we seek to 'safeguard', equally, others' lives in addition to our own. The COVID-19 crisis has made us recognize that we are not only digitally connected; more importantly, we are physically co-present, affectively compassionate, socially cooperative, and politically collective across life and death In 'Interrelationality'. Thus, we must go beyond the instrumentalist approach to connectivity, which is embedded in the total dominance of data power. Instead, we must reinvent an ethics of vulnerability in the shared process of 'our persistence', an ethics that should be 'relational, fragile, sometimes conflictual and unbearable, sometimes ecstatic and joyous' (Butler 2020, p. 64). A politics of 'interdependency' forms the basis of co-livable lives in the double-trapped lifeworld of vulnerability to biopolitical power and data governmentality.

Concluding remarks

Can we imagine even a slight silver lining – a means by which to possibly overcome the dilemma of physical survival under data colonialism (or freedom from data colonialism) with the potential risk of infectious illness? While the catchphrase 'social distancing' dominates the common discourse, the truth (which has become more obvious in the COVID-19 crisis) is that, ironically enough, the life and death of human beings is essentially connected and collective in society.

A practical solution may be that if information is necessary for survival, deliberate decisions and consensus must be made in terms of the kinds of data to be collected and utilized; the types of methodologies in terms of who will have access, and who will analyse and use the data; and what the particular aims are of such data collection. This may be a starting point toward digital democracy in the age of pandemics. More fundamentally, we may have to further develop the ethico-politics of life and death in to pandemic times. This is necessarily initiated from the critical reflection of biopolitics and data governmentality at such a precarious border between life and death: that is, social equality for life instead of augmenting the thanapolitical database; respect toward equally valuable and vulnerable singularities instead of deceitful exclusion; and reflexive sensitivity toward discrimination, instead of reinforcing stigmatization. And perhaps a politics of vulnerability will emerge in the course of this transition, a politics to help guide us to, in, and through a post-coronavirus era. A politics of vulnerability pursues 'connectivity *across and beyond* death' (overcoming the four dilemmas discussed earlier) in order to seek justice with respect to breathing equally and freely. Through reciprocal breathing, air flow, and eventually the world may change.

Notes

1. According to the government's account, Korea's situation of the national economy is in contrast to those of other countries. For instance, the average growth of OECD member countries is −.4.2%, while other powerful countries are much lower, such as Britain (−11.2%), Japan (−.5.3%), and the USA (−3.7%).
2. Anonymous testing was expanded to the general public during the third strain of COVID-19 in winter 2020. This was due to a dramatic increase in COVID-19 cases, and it has become the most urgent biopolitical task to find non-symptomatic COVID-19 patients.

Disclosure statement

No potential conflict of interest was reported by the author(s).

Further information

This Special Issue article has been comprehensively reviewed by the Special Issue editors, Associate Professor Ted Striphas and Professor John Nguyet Erni.

References

Agamben, G., 1998. *Homo sacer: sovereign power and bare life*. Stanford, CA: Stanford University Press.
Agamben, G. 2020. The invention of an epidemic. *European Journal of Psychoanalysis* (26. February 2020). Available from: https://www.journal-psychoanalysis.eu/coronavirus-and-philosophers/ [Accessed 19 July 2020)]

Althusser, L., 1970. *Lenin and philosophy and other essays*. New York: Monthly Review Press.

Birchall, C., 2016. Shareveillance: subjectivity between open and closed data. *Big data & society*, 3 (2), https://journals.sagepub.com/doi/full/10.1177/2053951716663965.

Butler, J., 2016. Rethinking vulnerability and resistance. In: J. Butler, Z. Gambetti, and L Sabsay, ed. *Vulnerability in resistance*. Durham, NC: Duke University Press, 12–27.

Butler, J., 2020. *The force of non-violence*. London: Verso.

Campbell, T., 2011. *Improper life: technology and biopolitics from heidegger to agamben*. Minneapolis, MN: University of Minnesota Press.

Clough, P., 2018. *The user unconscious: On affect, media, and measure*. Minneapolis, MN: University of Minnesota Press.

Couldry, N. and Mejias, U., 2019. *The costs of connection: How data is colonizing human life and appropriating it for capitalism*. Stanford, CA: Stanford University Press.

Foucault, M., 1977. *Discipline and punish: The birth of the prison*. New York: Random House.

Foucault, M., 2003. *"Society must be defended": Lectures at the Collège de France, 1975-1976*. London: Picador.

Harris, J. 2020a. 'Normal' life failed us. The coronavirus crisis gives us the chance to rethink a new economy. The Guardian (17 May 2020). Available from: https://www.theguardian.com/commentisfree/2020/may/17/normal-life-failed-coronavirus-rethink-economy-labour party [Accessed 19 July 2020].

Harris, J. 2020b. There's another pandemic stalking Britain: Hunger. *The Guardian* (28 June 2020). https://www.theguardian.com/commentisfree/2020/jun/28/pandemic-britain-hunger-boris-johnson [Accessed 19 July 2020].

Jones, O. 2020. The real message behind 'stay alert': It'll be your fault if coronavirus spreads. *The Guardian* (14 May 2020). Available from: https://www.theguardian.com/commentisfree/2020/may/14/stay-alert-coronavirus-blame [Accessed 18 July 2020].

Lyou, H. 2021. Korean Christian 'worship battle'? What are the reasons of frequent outbreaks of COVID-19 at churches? HanKook Ilbo. Available from: 한국 기독교 '신앙 배틀' 문화 탓? 교회 집단 감염 왜 자꾸 터지나 (hankookilbo.com) [Accessed 31 January 2021].

Nah, Y. 2020. How would the Corona situation be different with Prevention of Discrimination Act? Hankyere Sinmun (23. May. 2020). Available from: 차별금지법 있었다면, 코로나19 상황은 어떻게 달라졌을까: 사회일반: 사회: 뉴스: 한겨레 (hani.co.kr) [Accessed 31 January 2021].

Nancy, J.L. 2020. Viral exception. *European Journal of Psychoanalysis* (27. February 2020)   https://www.journal-psychoanalysis.eu/coronavirus-and-philosophers/ [Accessed 19 July 2020].

Reich, R. 2020. COVID-19 pandemic shines a light on a new kind of class divide and its inequalities. *The Guardian* (26 April 2020). Available from: https://www.theguardian.com/commentisfree/2020/apr/25/COVID-19-pandemic-shines-a-light-on-a-new-kind-of-class-divide-and-its-inequalities [Accessed 18 July 2020].

The Guardian. 2020. Editorial: The Guardian view on coronavirus harms: Pandemic shows inequities are deadly. Available from: https://www.theguardian.com/commentisfree/2020/jun/14/the-guardian-view-on-coronavirus-harms-pandemic-shows-inequities-are-deadly [Accessed 18 July 2020].

Yoon, I. 2020. Corona-19: Itaewon infection spreading to homophobia (In Korean). BBC Korea. Available from: https://www.bbc.com/korean/features-52803935 [Accessed 18 July 2020].

Predicting COVID-19: wearable technology and the politics of solutionism

James N. Gilmore

ABSTRACT

The COVID-19 crisis has helped facilitate and amplify a set of articulations between technology, public health, and culture. Among these connections is the idea that wearable technologies – with their attendant claims to know more and know better about the relationship between human bodies and daily life – are able to predict the onset of COVID-19 symptoms and, in doing so, to help mitigate its spread. This article considers this imaginary through a case study of the Oura 'smart ring' and Oura's partnership with medical researchers and the National Basketball Association. Through a close, critical reading of popular press reports, I examine how Oura is imagined as a productive articulation between technology and public health capable of compensating for the failure of the United States government to implement adequate COVID-19 testing. This analysis demonstrates one way cultural studies scholars might interrogate and map the politics of this unfolding conjuncture – that is, to understand how a series of public failings is offloaded to private companies in an effort to develop quick solutions that only further entrench existing crises.

'Can a wearable detect Covid-19 before symptoms appear?' So went the headline of an April 2020 feature published in the technology and science magazine, *Wired* (Goode 2020). Though mostly comprising a glowing profile of researchers trying to use sensors embedded in wearable technology to 'help track the onset of infections or illness' (Goode 2020), the latter half of this article answers its leading question with a resounding: *probably not.* Despite little in the way of completed studies or peer-reviewed research, the promise of wearables to predict disease symptoms flourished throughout the spring and summer of 2020. In June 2020, the National Basketball Association (NBA) announced it would be convening an abbreviated season inside a manufactured 'bubble' in Orlando, Florida (Chariana 2020). Apart from constant COVID-19 testing, the NBA also announced the purchase of over 2,000 'smart rings' produced by the company, Oura. Oura Rings, though available since about 2017, became a flashpoint in the articulations between technology and public health during the pandemic. Some researchers are employing the Ring in attempts to continuously track whether a wearer is developing fever-like symptoms – and, in turn, developing COVID-19 (Smarr *et al.* 2020). In news reporting and commentary, the mere existence of this research has led to the repeated assertion that Oura Rings can predict COVID-19 symptoms in individuals (Fowler 2020).

This predictive claim reveals some of the stakes in how academic research is translated during crises – a process that can allow emergent technologies to figure as magical solutions to complex problems. In this article, I am concerned with the cultural politics of purported solutions to COVID-19 testing, or at the very least of measures that are imagined to create feelings of security among people compelled to navigate the crisis and its many modalities. In particular, the Oura example demonstrates how wearable technologies are discursively constructed as determinist, that is, as capable of generating change and solutions in and of themselves (Peters 2017). Solutionism, as one variant of determinism, refers to the belief that technical devices can (and should) be offered as a means to address, or even resolve, complex social problems (Morozov 2013).

Solutionism entails the rapid application of a perceived fix to a pressing crisis. Instead of focusing on contextual issues and systemic responses, problem solving is reduced to a set of tools and techniques. As Ajjawi and Eva (2021) have characterized it in relation to medical education throughout the COVID-19 pandemic, 'there is increasing pressure to accept simple solutions, to dive headlong into strategy before understanding the problem' (p. 2). Milan (2020) has further clarified that solutionism offers a feeling of certainty during times of 'global uncertainty' (p. 1), like the COVID-19 pandemic. This is something close to what Binde (2000) calls 'emergency time', 'an immediate protective reflex rather than a sober quest for long-term solutions' (p. 52). Henry Giroux (2002) has contrasted emergency time with Castoriadis's 'public time' (1991), the latter of which offers more space for reflection, education, and planning as individuals consider the role of government in addressing matters of concern. While Giroux examined this tension in the context of responses to the September 11, 2001 terrorist attacks, it is also relevant to the conjunctural crises of COVID-19, in that the need to respond (and respond as quickly as possible) in order to mitigate community spread, hospitalization, and death makes objects marketed as solutions seem particularly valuable.

These so-called solutions are not only considered valuable because of the tendency toward emergency time in a public health crisis. In his work on Google, Siva Vaidhyanathan (2011) has used the phrase 'public failings' (p. 6) to describe how Google enters into daily life relatively unimpeded because it claims to respond to – if not to solve – problems that government entities have been unable to properly address. Wearable devices like Oura functioned much the same way here: because of the relative lack of availability of rapid and effective testing in the United States during the initial months of the pandemic, such technologies could be positioned as attractive – if not necessary and viable – alternatives (Schneider 2020). Oura compensates for a lack of access to testing; its promoters promise a relatively affordable, at-home, always-on way to monitor and track a variety of metrics, which can in turn help an individual to predict the onset of COVID-19.

In my ongoing research on the ways in which wearable technologies gain legitimacy and exercise authority at the level of the everyday (Gilmore 2016, 2017, 2019, 2020), I have repeatedly stressed how the promoters of wearable technologies reproduce imaginaries about the transformation of everyday life via what some have called 'datafication' (Mayer-Schönberger and Cukier 2014), or the conversion of habit and routine into (largely quantified) data sets to be analyzed, standardized, and used to model and even predict populational behaviour. Imaginaries describe how values and meanings are formed socially, discursively, and culturally (Taylor 2004, Balsamo 2011, Markham 2021).

Oura's imagined solution to the problem of predicting COVID-19 symptoms in individuals is, in many ways, a familiar story about how emergent technologies are used to signal supposedly innovative means of solving intractable problems. The COVID-19 pandemic has accelerated a variety of articulations, bringing aspects of technology, public health, and culture, among many other elements, into complex assemblages. Oura is one part of a larger problematic, I argue, where datafication becomes a primary logic by means of which solutions are proposed and legitimated. In tracing some of the translations between scientific research and news reports, I demonstrate one way imaginaries are produced through the discursive articulations between technoculture and public health, allowing purported solutions to be formulated in absence of evidence. These solutions stem from a faith in, if not a desperation toward, technology in the moment of COVID-19. Wearables like Oura do not solve the ongoing crisis around the status of knowledge in society, which Grossberg (2018a) has characterized as (in part) 'the increasing politicization of knowledge – of assumptions about what is true, what one knows, or even how one goes about knowing' (p. 152). Rather, Oura propagates such crises: its promoters, and the replication of their promotional language in news outlets, embrace particular assumptions about how one goes about knowing one's wellness, readiness, and potential susceptibility to COVID-19. As tools for making particular claims about the articulation between technoculture and public health, they add confusion about which tests are reliable, about which technologies provide supposedly accurate reports of bodily function, and about how to create appropriate means of mitigating viral spread.

Imagining Oura as predictive tool

'Prediction' has been a persistent trope in critical inquiry into machine learning (Mackenzie 2015), policing (Brayne 2020), recommendation systems (Cohn 2019), social welfare (Eubanks 2018), criminality (Fussell 2020), and surveillance (Andrejevic 2019). Oura Rings construct biometrics using the band's sensors – including heart rate variability and body temperature – and employ machine learning software to build correlations for predicting one's wellness in the form of 'scores'. Like many wearable technologies – e.g. Fitbit, Apple Watch, and other trackers – Oura quantifies elements of lived experience; it attempts to make legible seemingly ineffable qualities of our bodies so as to render them not just knowable, but also trackable (Neff and Nafus 2016). Oura's 'Readiness Score', available on an accompanying smartphone application, monitors 'signals from your body and picks up on daily habits to determine how well-rested you are' (Oura 2020a). Like weather forecasts trying to predict the likelihood of severe rain and changing conditions, Oura is part of a growing ensemble of products trying to produce forecasts for human bodies.

Oura's website aggrandizes the device's accuracy as a tracking tool: 'While Oura is not a medical device, its capabilities are near perfect when compared to advanced medical technologies', including claims of a 98.4 percent reliability rating (Oura 2020b). The sales pitch to be *near perfect* is qualified significantly in the 'Precautions' section of the device's Terms and Conditions document: 'Oura Services are not intended to diagnose ... any disease or medical condition' (Oura 2018). The advertising here – as *so close* to a medical technology that it might as well be one – amplifies Oura's claims about the ring's capacity for prediction.

Much of Oura's status as a predictor for individual COVID-19 symptoms came, in mid-2020, both from anecdotal evidence of Oura users and from preliminary results of a study based at West Virginia University (WVU)'s Rockefeller Neuroscience Institute (RNI). The WVU researchers, who are formally partnered with Oura, developed a separate smartphone app that 'goes beyond physical symptoms and body temperature tracking through a holistic integrated neuroscience approach – measuring daily changes in physiological, psychological, cognitive, and behavioral biometrics' (Rockefeller Neuroscience Institute 2020). The app reportedly allows 'the data analytic team ... to predict the onset of physical symptoms *before they occur*' (emphasis in original). In order to do this, passive data collected from multiple wearables (including heart rate variability and body temperature) are integrated with user-submitted data (survey questions about fatigue, attention, memory, exposure to COVID-19, sense of smell, and other factors) in a smartphone app. These data are then combined and analyzed in the RNI Cloud to forecast the likelihood of individuals having contracted the virus, as well as model outbreaks and recovery periods across participants.

While Oura is part of this 'holistic and integrated neuroscience platform' (Anon 2020), it is, importantly, only one component. A press release from May 28, 2020, which was heavily cited in the subsequent reporting, claimed 'the RNI has created a digital platform that can detect COVID-19 related symptoms up to three days before they show up'; but, again, there are no publicly available findings for researchers to actually assess this claim, as the studies are still ongoing and as of January 2021, the project's website gives no indication its studies or datasets have been formally peer reviewed and published (WVU Medicine 2020). While an unrelated study of Oura's capacity to detect temperature fluctuations (and, thus, fever) was published in December 2020 (Smarr *et al.* 2020), it was very careful to hedge its results, suggesting (quite obviously) 'people are different, and so are physiological systems' (p. 7). While some researchers have centred Oura in their studies, in other words, they are relatively careful to indicate Oura in-and-of-itself cannot offer much of a solution.

Nevertheless, reporting on the WVU press release was immediately taken out of context. Take an *Engadget* headline from June 1: 'Researchers say Oura rings can predict COVID-19 symptoms three days early'. The first paragraph of this story contradicts, if clarifies, this claim: 'The researchers claim their *digital platform* can detect COVID-19 related symptoms' (Fisher 2020, emphasis mine). After the NBA announced its partnership with Oura, the *New York Post* similarly reported that the Ring itself and Oura's algorithms – rather than WVU's proprietary platform – could predict COVID-19 symptoms (Previte 2020). Some outlets, such as *Tech Crunch*, did note that the Oura data was one part of a larger platform experiment (Etherington 2020). But in side-stepping the complexities of the NRI's platform, most reporters simplified the study and reduced the platform largely to the Oura Ring, period. Oura takes on the qualities of a solution to the problem of knowing whether or not one has contracted COVID-19. This imaginary seemed so attractive to some observers precisely because it responds to particular political problems; notably, the broader failure of public health in the U.S. and also its failure to suitably plan for COVID-19 (and, by extension, possible future pandemics) (Maxmen and Tollefson 2020). In this, Oura acts as a proxy for long-term planning, preparation, and public mindedness.

Oura's partnership with the NBA helped legitimize the company and solidify a perception that the Ring is capable of responding to a public health crisis (Abbate 2020). Popular technology blog *CNet*, in discussing Oura's integration with the NBA, suggested 'The RNI said the Oura ring enables them to' predict symptoms–again without acknowledging how the RNI's platform is working with a variety of data from multiple sources (Reichert 2020). Even articles critical of Oura's capacity to provide a solution have reproduced the claim that the Ring itself detects illness (Mak 2020), while others bury an acknowledgement of Oura's limitations near the end of effusive praise

(Pickman 2020). There is, in other words, an observable pattern of translation that either inflates or simplifies what, exactly, Oura does and is being used to do. This translation demonstrates the emergence of an imaginary around Oura Ring: one that, despite minimal reviewable findings, has led major news outlets and sports leagues to position Oura as a compensatory technology, one whose purpose is to solve the failings of public health testing in the United States by allowing economically advantaged individuals to predict, supposedly, the onset of COVID-19. Seen in this way, the inflation and simplification in news reporting becomes a desperation toward technology, a way to try and cultivate a sense of security in the face of the United States' generally botched response to the COVID-19 pandemic.

Solving the crisis

If conjunctural analysis entails, in part, mapping the key problematics of a given conjuncture (Slack and Wise 2015, p. 218), then the emergence of imagined technocultural solutions to public health crises represents a particular problematic for mapping COVID-19. Here, technology developers promise to accomplish what a federal government could not: to provide accessible, understandable ways of monitoring one's body for disease on a constant basis. Such a promise – even if it were to work – locates the solution to COVID-19 squarely on the individual's responsibility to constantly track their own body for illness. It does not address broader crises of funding, administration, logistics, and knowledge that have continued to politicize and exacerbate the spread of COVID-19 in the United States. In evading these related crises, the politics of solutionism further dismantles faith in the capacity for such public institutions to help care for people. Companies like Oura provide the implementation of sensor-based datafication as a proxy for institutional reform, partnering directly or indirectly with research universities, sports leagues, and the press to legitimize the (largely unproven) capacities of such technology and, indeed, to do so without waiting for the time-consuming process of completing, writing, reviewing, and publishing research studies. Again, emergency time trumps public time.

The crisis of COVID-19 is in many ways a technocultural one as much as it is a health crisis, in that the pandemic affects how we conceptualize and practice our ways of life, and how technologies figure in the practice of daily life. The imaginaries surrounding wearable technology generally, and Oura particularly, are explicitly technocultural interventions in ostensibly political dimensions of health, safety, logistics, and other such affairs. We are asked to bring these artifacts into our habits, to value the data they can generate as useful and necessary, and to live with them bound to our appendages in order to improve – or, at least, to know more about – our body's wellness.

There are at least two interrelated paths that cultural studies might continue to follow in its pursuit to make sense of what's going on amidst this articulation of technoculture and public health. The first has to do with legitimation and authority: Claims to solve a crisis are in part about the way in which particular forms of power become expressed and taken-for-granted. If datafication has reached something close to social authority, then this demonstrates how these solutions can be so readily accepted and reproduced amongst journalists and commentators. It also explains why devices like Oura seem like viable means of predicting one's potential COVID-19 diagnosis. This viability only happens because of the second intertwined path: that the ongoing public failing of government in the United States has created a vacuum of authority and expertise, where private companies can offer means to respond to emergency time without consideration of public time. Particularly in the United States, the chaos of the Trump administration (Grossberg 2018b) and its hollowing out of faith in public institutions contribute to the characterization of the United States federal government as failing to care for citizens (e.g. Packer 2020).

Finally, purported solutions are not only evidence that a crisis is ongoing, and hence that ever-more solutions may be required to bring the crisis to an end. The proposed solutions themselves participate in, exacerbate, and are perhaps even imminent to other contextual crises. The embrace of Oura Ring as a potential solution to the public failure of COVID-19 testing is itself participating in contextual, still-unfolding concerns about what it will mean for devices like wearable computers to become delegates of human knowledge and well-being. Solutionism does not simply offer quick, often technical, solutions for complicated problems, it also encourages its adherents to consider crises as linear or contained, rather than as unfurling assemblages. Thinking COVID-19 as a series of crises entails, at least in part, seeing how proposed solutions to some elements of the pandemic further entrench other crises in related domains.

Disclosure statement

No potential conflict of interest was reported by the author(s).

Further information

This Special Issue article has been comprehensively reviewed by the Special Issue editors, Associate Professor Ted Striphas and Professor John Nguyet Erni.

References

Abbate, E. 2020. Here's how the NBA's coronavirus-fighting ring might help. *GQ*, 17 June. Available from: https://www.gq.com/story/oura-ring-nba [accessed 6 July 2020].

Ajjawi, R. and Eva, K.W., 2021. The problem with solutions. *Medical education*, 55, 2–3.

Andrejevic, M., 2019. *Automated media*. New York: Routledge.

Anon, 2020. WVU Rockefeller Neuroscience Institute says it can predict COVID-19 related symptoms up to three days in advance. *The Intelligencer: Wheeling News-Register*, 28 May. Available from: https://www.theintelligencer.net/news/top-headlines/2020/05/wvu-rockefeller-neuroscience-institute-says-it-can-predict-covid-19-related-symptoms-up-to-three-days-in-advance/ [accessed 6 July 2020].

Balsamo, A., 2011. *Designing culture: the technological imagination at work*. Durham: Duke University Press.

Binde, J., 2000. Toward an ethics of the future. *Public culture*, 12 (1), 51–72.

Brayne, S., 2020. *Predict and surveil: data, discretion, and the future of policing*. Oxford: Oxford University Press.

Castoriadis, C., 1991. *Philosophy, politics, autonomy*. New York: Oxford University Press.

Chariana, S., 2020. Inside the NBA Bubble: Details from NBPA memo obtained by The Athletic. *The Athletic*, 16 June. Available from: https://theathletic.com/1876737/2020/06/16/inside-the-nba-bubble-details-from-nbpa-memo-obtained-by-the-athletic/ [accessed 5 July 2020].

Cohn, J., 2019. *The burden of choice: recommendations, subversion, and algorithmic culture*. New Brunswick: Rutgers University Press.

Etherington, D., 2020. Researchers use biometrics, including data from the Oura Ring, to predict COVID-19 symptoms in advance. *Tech Crunch*, 28 May. Available from: https://techcrunch.com/2020/05/28/researchers-use-biometrics-including-data-from-the-oura-ring-to-predict-covid-19-symptoms-in-advance/ [accessed 6 July 2020].

Eubanks, V., 2018. *Automating inequality: how high-tech tools profile, police, and punish the poor*. New York: St. Martin's Press.

Fisher, C., 2020. Researchers say Oura rings can predict COVID-19 symptoms three days early. *Engadget*, 1 June. Available from: https://www.engadget.com/west-virginia-university-oura-ring-covid-19-symptoms-003239603.html [accessed 6 July 2020].

Fowler, G.A., 2020. Wearable tech can spot coronavirus symptoms before you even realize you're sick. *The Washington Post*, 28 May. Available from: https://www.washingtonpost.com/technology/2020/05/28/wearable-coronavirus-detect/ [accessed 5 July 2020].

Fussell, S., 2020. An algorithm that 'predicts' criminality based on a face sparks a furor. *Wired*, 24 June. Available from: https://www.wired.com/story/algorithm-predicts-criminality-based-face-sparks-furor/ [accessed 6 July, 2020].

Gilmore, J.N., 2016. Everywear: wearable fitness technologies and the quantified self. *New media & society*, 18 (11), 2524–2539.

Gilmore, J.N., 2017. From ticks and tocks to budges and nudges: The smartwatch and the haptics of informatic culture. *Television & new media*, 18 (3), 189–202.

Gilmore, J.N., 2019. Design for everyone: Apple AirPods and the mediation of accessibility. *Critical studies in media communication*, 36 (5), 482–494.

Gilmore, J.N., 2020. Securing the kids: geofencing and child wearables. *Convergence: the international journal of research into new media technologies*, 26, 1333–1346. https://doi.org/10.1177/1354856519882317

Giroux, H.A., 2002. The politics of emergency time versus public time: Terrorism and the culture of fear. *Culture Machine*. https://culturemachine.net/interzone/the-politics-of-emergency-versus-public-time-giroux/ [accessed 30 December 2020].

Goode, L., 2020. Can a wearable detect Covid-19 before symptoms appear? *Wired*, 14 April. Available from: https://www.wired.com/story/wearable-covid-19-symptoms-research/ [accessed 5 July, 2020].

Grossberg, L., 2018a. Tilting at windmills: a cycnical assemblage of the crises of knowledge. *Cultural studies*, 32 (2), 149–193.

Grossberg, L., 2018b. *Under the cover of chaos: Trump and the battle for the American right*. London: Pluto Press.

Mackenzie, A., 2015. The production of prediction: what does machine learning want? *European journal of cultural studies*, 18(4-5), 429–445.

Mak, A., 2020. What the NBA's $300 COVID-detecting rings can actually accomplish. *Slate*, 22 June. Available from: https://slate.com/technology/2020/06/nba-coronavirus-oura-ring-orlando.html [accessed 6 July 2020].

Markham, A., 2021. The limits of the imaginary: challenges to intervening in future speculations of memory, data, and algorithms. *New media & society*, 23, 382–405. https://doi.org/10.1177/1461444820929322

Maxmen, A. and Tollefson, J., 2020. Two decades of pandemic war games failed to account for Donald Trump. *Nature*, 584, 26–29.

Mayer-Schönberger, V. and Cukier, K., 2014. *Big data: A revolution that will transform how we live, work, and think*. London: John Murray.

Milan, S., 2020. Techno-solutionism and the standard human in the making of the COVID-19 pandemic. *Big Data & Society*, July-December, 1–7.

Morozov, E., 2013. *To save everything, click here: The folly of technological solutionism*. New York: Public Affairs.

Neff, G. and Nafus, D., 2016. *Self-tracking*. Cambridge: The MIT Press.

Oura, 2018. Terms of use. *Oura Ring*. Available from: https://ouraring.com/terms-and-conditions [accessed 6 July 2020].

Oura, 2020a. Readiness: Your complete guide. *Oura Ring*. Available from: https://ouraring.com/readiness-score [accessed 6 July 2020].

Oura, 2020b. The Oura difference. *Oura Ring*. Available from: https://ouraring.com/the-oura-difference [accessed 6 July 2020].

Packer, J., 2020. How to destroy a government. *The Atlantic*, April. Available from: https://www.theatlantic.com/magazine/archive/2020/04/how-to-destroy-a-government/606793/ [accessed 30 December 2020].

Peters, J.D., 2017. 'You mean my whole fallacy is wrong': On technological determinism. *Representations*, 140, 10–26.

Pickman, B., 2020. The story behind the Ring that is key to the NBA's restart. *Sports Illustrated*, 1 July. Available from: https://www.si.com/nba/2020/07/01/oura-ring-nba-restart-orlando-coronavirus [accessed 6 July 2020].

Previte, S., 2020. NBA to use 'smart rings,' big data to fight coronavirus in Disney bubble. *New York Post*, 19 June. Retrieved from: https://nypost.com/2020/06/19/nba-to-use-smart-rings-to-detect-coronavirus-within-bubble/ [accessed 6 July 2020].

Reichert, C., 2020. NBA players could wear smart ring to track COVID-19 symptoms as season resumes. *CNet*, 22 June. Retrieved from: https://www.cnet.com/news/nba-players-could-wear-a-smart-ring-to-track-covid-19-symptoms-as-season-resumes-at-disney-world/ [accessed 6 July 2020].

Rockefeller Neuroscience Institute, 2020. Understanding the spread; protecting our health and economy. *WVU Rockefeller Neuroscience Institute*. Available from: https://wvumedicine.org/RNI/COVID19/ [accessed 6 July 2020].

Schneider, E.C., 2020. Failing the test—the tragic data gap undermining the U.S. pandemic response. *New England journal of medicine*, 383, 299–302.

Shear, M.D., *et al.*, 2020. The lost month: how a failure to test blinded the U.S. to Covid-19. *The New York Times*, 28 March. Available from: https://www.nytimes.com/2020/03/28/us/testing-coronavirus-pandemic.html [accessed 8 July 2020].

Slack, J.D. and Wise, J.M., 2015. *Culture and technology: a primer*. 2nd ed. New York: Peter Lang.

Smarr, B.L., et al. 2020. Feasibility of continuous fever monitoring using wearable devices. *Scientific reports*, 10. article number 21640.

Taylor, C., 2004. *Modern social imaginaries*. Durham: Duke University Press.

Vaidhyanathan, S., 2011. *The googlization of everything (and why we should worry)*. Berkeley: University of California Press.

WVU Medicine, 2020. WVU Rockefeller Neuroscience Institute announces capabilities to predict COVID-19 related symptoms up to three days in advance. *WVU Medicine*. Available from: https://wvumedicine.org/news/article/wvu-rockefeller-neuroscience-institute-announces-capability-to-predict-covid-19-related-symptoms-up-/ [accessed 6 July 2020].

Learning From Lana: Netflix's *Too Hot to Handle*, COVID-19, and the human–nonhuman entanglement in contemporary technoculture

Fan Yang

ABSTRACT

The Netflix popular reality series *Too Hot to Handle* (*THTH*), released during the coronavirus outbreak in 2019, requires all contestants to refrain from sexual activities of any kind in order to win a cash prize in the end. Mirroring the physical distancing mandate during the COVID-19 crisis, the show offers an opportunity to discern a set of interrelated human and nonhuman entanglements in contemporary technoculture that the outbreak has brought into sharper relief. This essay probes into the conditions of possibility for the popularity of *THTH* by placing an analytical focus on the role of Lana, a nonhuman sensor centrally featured in the show with a female voice typical of digital assistants. Lana, a cone-shaped device from 'Factory, China', is a surveillance robot embodying the operation of Netflix as part of the expanding regime of data colonialism, which extracts personal data for profit. Her nonhuman identity is evocative of China as at once a manufacturing locale for the material gadgets that make up the global digital economy and an authoritarian state that has deepened its censorship and surveillance practices during the COVID-19 outbreak. Instructing the contestants to care for their entrepreneurial selves while encroaching upon their autonomy, Lana invites us to rethink the common framing of China – a coveted market for Netflix – as the nonhuman Other of the liberal-democratic West. During a time when the nonhuman virus keeps humans apart while intensifying their reliance on nonhuman machines for communication, Lana promotes a kind of intimacy without proximity characteristic of the global infrastructures of connection. A symptomatic reading of *THTH*, which also conjures a vision of collectivity as a basis for surviving the pandemic, thus allows us to recognize the entanglement of the human and the nonhuman and to imagine new paths toward global social justice.

The Netflix reality series *Too Hot to Handle* (*THTH*) hit the top charts in the United States (#2), the United Kingdom (#1), and Canada (#2) upon its release on April 17, 2020 (O'Brien 2020). As Judy Berman (2020) writes in the *Time* magazine, the producers of this 'unabashedly trashy' show could not have predicted that it'd become so 'weirdly relevant in the time of coro-navirus', as 'the participants face a low-stakes version of the ethical drama playing out across nations trying to flatten the curve'. Like many of its dating reality TV predecessors, *THTH* is premised on an experiment. That is, all contestants must refrain from sexual activities of any kind – including kissing and self-gratification – in order to develop 'deeper and more mean-ingful connections' with those to whom they are attracted (Newton 2020a). Violations are penalized in the form of deductions from the $100,000 prize money, with winner(s) to be determined at the end.

At first sight, the popularity of *THTH* amid an unfolding global pandemic seems self-explanatory. The show follows in the footsteps of *The Circle* and *Love is Blind*, two other reality series released by Netflix since the beginning of 2020[1] whose mandate of physical separation has made them 'seem like touching, hilarious portraits of all our lives right now' (Reklis 2020). Nonethe-less, in an era of Netflix's expanding global influence, it is worthwhile to subject this 'remarkably prescient artifact for the lockdown age'(Garland 2020) to a symptomatic reading.

Just as the coronavirus sometimes produces asymptomatic carriers, cul-tural artifacts like *THTH* demand a mode of critical engagement that, as Louis Althusser (1970) tells us, works to unveil what they do not immediately manifest. Indeed, probing the reality that creates the conditions of possibility for the popularity of *THTH* reveals a set of interrelated entanglements that the COVID-19 crisis has brought into sharper relief. As the nonhuman virus keeps humans from touching one another while intensifying the reliance of their connection on nonhuman machines, recognizing these intricate human-non-human entanglements becomes crucial for imagining new forms of collectiv-ity and politics.

The premise of *THTH* is not unlike many of its gamified counterparts in the dating shows genre, whose origins may be traceable to the production of *The Dating Game* in 1965 or *Temptation Island* in 2001 (Feuer 2018). Compared to many of its contemporary rivals that follow a heteronormative 'romantic love to marriage' trajectory, *THTH* seems quite unabashed about sex as a common, if not legitimate, goal of human encounter.[2] The first verbal exchange and onscreen monologues among the contestants in Episode One, for instance, highlight their clear preference for casual hook-ups to long-term commit-ment, lending legitimacy to the voiceover host's description of them as 'the horniest, commitment-phobic swipsters' (Newton 2020a). This apparent defiance of the dating-for-marriage show convention notwithstanding, the contestants learn, upon their arrival on the beautiful island in Mexico (unnamed throughout the show), that they cannot engage in sex, not even self-gratification.

The self-described 'first sex-less dating show' of course, remains full of sexual innuendos and heated moments thanks to the rebelliousness of numerous contestants; after all, they were chosen via Instagram based on the criteria of being 'sexy, sex-ed up, and charismatic' (*Too Hot To Handle Revealed - The Secrets of How They Film The Show 2020*). Yet for many contestants and viewers alike, the sexiest presence on screen is not a human but takes the form of a cone-shaped device. A 'virtual guide' of this 'no bone zone' is how the comedian-narrator Desiree Burch first introduces her, prior to the arrival of all contestants (Newton 2020a).

With a sleek design aesthetic reminiscent of Apple products, the robot is easily mistaken for an air freshener or a sex toy. In a voice resembling that of Siri's and Alexa's – reflecting 'the merging of woman, machine, and work … with the advent of the 'digital assistant'' (Hester 2016) – she reveals early on that 'Lana' is her name. Netflix announced later that the producers have intentionally chosen the name for how it is spelled backwards (*Too Hot To Handle Revealed - The Secrets of How They Film The Show 2020*). Lana's accent is British,[3] and her tone, cool and rational, even distant. 'Flirting is not a function I am programmed for' is her response to one of the contestants' attempt to get more intimate (Newton 2020b).

Placed at various spots of the resort, including the bedroom and the bathroom, Lana is presented – by the producers who write her role and lines into the script – as the ultimate surveillance machine. For the first twelve hours of the contestants' stay, Lana is said to be 'secretly gathering personal data before she lays down the sex ban' (Newton 2020b), though it is never clear what kinds of data she has collected. Throughout the show, Lana always lights up unannounced to deliver messages and give orders to the contestants. She is believed to be scrutinizing behaviours and assessing intimacies 'in order to help them towards better relationships' (Newton 2020a). She grants couples dates and rewards them with brief rule-lifted moments during which they can kiss or touch without penalty, but only when she deems the connection genuine.[4] She even offers an itemized 'bill' of prize deductions on the mornings following those rule-breaking nights.

Because of Lana's power – or more precisely, the power that the *THTH* writers have given her – it is little wonder that 'The Too Hot To Handle Revealed – The Secrets of How They Film', a video released on Youtube by Netflix UK & Ireland, calls Lana 'the real star' of the show. Based on tweets collected on Buzzfeed, Lana is also very popular among fans of *THTH*. One tweet demands Netflix to 'put Lana in more shows'; another declares: 'GOAL of 2020 – to be as sarcastic and witty as Lana the cockblocking cone' (Yapalater 2020).

Such a fascination with a technology's on-screen presence is certainly not brand new. In making Lana a visible figure, the producers of *THTH* have arguably channelled the creators of *Black Mirror*, the dystopian Channel 4-turned-Netflix series that centrally features one (futuristic) technology in each episode.[5] 'Hated in the Nation' from Season Three of *Black Mirror*, for example, visibly displays a technology called Autonomous Drone Insects (ADI). When hacked, these bee-like machines can turn into killing armies that target online users of a viral hashtag, thus putting a visceral spin on the term 'virality'. The airing of *THTH* during the pandemic, likewise, latches on to these complicated feelings toward the power of the nonhuman, be it biological or technological. 'Too hot to handle is real life rn [right now] and Lana is the corona virus', says one tweet (Byrne 2020). Just as the coronavirus is a nonhuman agent that has made humans vulnerable, thereby exerting control over their behaviour, Lana the nonhuman machine is able to limit humans' capacity to engage in bodily interactions with one another.

Netflix has arguably opted to capitalize on this fear and fascination with the nonhuman during the COVID-19 crisis. Another heavily marketed and hugely popular documentary series, *Tiger King*, for example, depicts the human obsession with the nonhuman entity that is the big cat. The show became a hit at the onset of the US lockdown and has been seen by 64 million viewers (Rushe and Lee 2020). Calling it the 'first media event of the lockdown', Jeff Scheible (n.d.) suggests that the show has 'in many ways … domesticated' the perceived wildlife origin of the coronavirus in a Wuhan wet market. An 'accidental allegory', *Tiger King* 'coincides with the strange moment in which it, like COVID-19, went viral' (Scheible 2020, p. 1). Its virality also evokes the ways in which 'Netflix itself acts as a deadly contagion', as 'the streaming service has in many senses algorithmically "infected" our viewing practices and the entertainment industry alike, leaving studios struggling to find their footing and forced to reform their business models' (Scheible 2020, p. 3).

Just as the nonhuman animals caged in *Tiger King* have come to remind quarantined, Netflix-binging viewers of their own confinement, Lana in *THTH* has also taken on awe-inspiring characteristics of the coronavirus and in turn the 'viral' power of Netflix itself. On May 5, 2020, in an obvious attempt to promote *THTH*, Netflix released a horror-film parody titled 'Lana Knows What You Did' on Youtube. Clips from the show and Lana's voiceover are interspersed with dark screens with blood-stained titles in white such as 'She's Always Watching', 'Always listening', 'She knows what you did', and 'Test Your Temptation'. In the end, 'A Netflix Horror Series' appears, with the word 'horror' replaced by 'reality' seconds later. A contestant's exclamation 'Oh my God!' is followed by Lana declaring: 'I'm taking it all in' (*Lana Knows What You Did* 2020). If the heightened sense of horror in this clip accentuates the association between Lana and the coronavirus, the *THTH* parody has also made clear that Lana is quite self-referential of Netflix as a company. Like Lana, Netflix is always watching you watch it. It gathers all-encompassing user data to inform its production, programming, and recommendations (Harris 2012) – not unlike the virus, which adapts and mutates in constant interactions with the host environment (Dupré and

Guttinger 2016). Variously termed 'surveillance capitalism' (Zuboff 2019), 'platform capitalism' (Srnicek 2016), or 'data colonialism' (Couldry and Mejias 2019), Netflix's operation characterizes a distinctive mode of economic value creation that is predicated on the extraction of behavioural data.

Importantly, as Sarah Arnold (2018, p. 49) points out, 'Netflix posits the use of data mining systems as beneficial for the consumer and suggests that such systems allow the company to better understand and respond to audience tastes'. This 'marketing ideology of personalization', as Nick Couldry and Ulises A. Mejias (Couldry and Mejias 2019, p. 16) argue, 'makes ... tracking and surveillance attractive'. It is, therefore, quite reasonable for the audience to perceive Lana – an embodiment of Netflix's reliance on Artificial Intelligence – as 'sexy'.

Just like the enigmatic Lana who never tells us how she does her job, Netflix has until recently been reluctant to reveal the specificities of the viewing data collected (Laporte 2014). Its lack of transparency allows the company to frequently declare shows on the platform as 'the most watched' without the backing of actual numbers. In part thanks to its veiled 'sexiness' and the 'deeper connection' encouraged between Netflix and its users, the company has accrued 15.77 million new subscribers since the global pandemic began, more than doubling its predicted numbers (Rushe and Lee 2020). Its stock value has also risen quite remarkably since March 16, when the outbreak sent much of the (developed) world into isolation mode. The linkage between Lana and the coronavirus thus takes on a new shade; Netflix, working like Lana and quietly permeating human lives like the virus, is no doubt a beneficiary of the pandemic.

Yet Lana's identity has another intriguing layer. In the first episode, when the contestants' hometowns are displayed on screen to accompany their first appearances (e.g. 'British Columbia, Canada' for Francesca), we learn that Lana is from 'Factory, China'. Of course, 'factory' is not exactly a geographical location. But its invocation brings immediately to mind the well-told story of the globalized production of electronics. China, the manufacturing powerhouse often dubbed 'the world's factory', is an all-too-familiar locale in that story. Once 'China' is noted, no more geographical specificity would appear to be necessary; 'factory' the abstract concept would suffice. One can even argue that Lana's gendered voice simultaneously evokes and erases the labour of the female workers who toil on the assembly lines in China producing the material gadgets that make up the global digital economy (e.g. Pun 2005, Qiu 2017).

China, an expanding media market, has also had an intricate relationship with Netflix. Reed Hastings (2016), the CEO and cofounder of Netflix, during his keynote at the 2016 Consumer Electronics Show (CES) in Las Vegas, informed the audience: 'The Netflix service has gone live in nearly every country of the world but China – where we also hope to be in the future'.

By 2019, it has appeared that the chance of launching Netflix in China is looking slimmer due to the extant success of homegrown platforms like iQiyi – with which Netflix has once partnered – and the tremendous state censorship to which the platform must subject itself (Kharpal 2019).

Naming 'factory, China' as the birthplace for Lana can thus be read as one way in which Netflix is coming to terms with its 'loss' of the Chinese market, by representing China as a place for merely making, not *creating*, technologies or contents. But this mention becomes more significant when China was also emphasized, most (in)famously by the former President of the United States, as the place of origin of the coronavirus. The narrative of 'Coronavirus: Made in China' surfacing in both official and vernacular settings (Riechmann 2020) has had a pervasive effect in spreading the perception that not only was the coronavirus most likely manufactured in China (Schaeffer 2020), it is the censorship of the Chinese state – an anti-human (-rights) practice – that has created a false initial impression of the severity of the virus, thus causing the spread of COVID-19 globally (Smith 2020).

The nonhuman, then, appears to not only connect Lana and Netflix to the coronavirus, but also to China as well. The 'anti-human' framing of China is indeed operative in shaping the narrative of state control and surveillance during the COVID-19 crisis. This may be seen in the reportage of the Chinese government's order to lock down Wuhan (Kuo 2020a) and the subsequent rollout of symptom monitoring and contact tracing (through the Health Code on the app Alipay, for example) (Kuo 2020b). Highlighting the inhumane level of China's repressive state apparatus – often through the voices of human rights activists interviewed by the journalists – offers an easy explanation for the low number of reported cases daily out of China. This, in combination with the critique of China's state censorship, also helps to lessen the embarrassment of staggering numbers emerging in places like the United States since March 2020. Arguably, such rising Sinophobia has contributed in no small part to the recently growing number of racist attacks on people of Chinese/East Asian descent in the West, whose dehumanizing tendency is part of a long history of the Yellow Peril discourse (Billé 2018).

However, as David Eng *et al.* (2011, p. 2), editors of a special issue in *Social Text*, caution us, neither 'China' nor 'the human' should be taken for granted as 'a pre-given object of knowledge'. There is much need to destabilize China as a 'paradigmatic site of the inhuman, the subhuman, and the humanly unthinkable' vis-à-vis 'the universal human' construed by the West (Eng *et al.* 2011, p. 5). Instead of pitting China as an authoritarian Other against Western democracies, it is important to recognize here that 'China, the censor' may not be so different from 'Lana, the sensor'. While the former restricts the movement of information and the latter limits the proximity and interaction of bodies, both rely on the sensing and tracking of data generated by citizens/users, presumably to make or serve them better.

Akin to Netflix's recommendation system marketed to enhance the viewers' experience of media, Lana is not only bent on detecting and tracking the contestants' feelings and actions but also takes as her ostensible goal to promote their sense and care of the self. At a time when major components of what some call 'the experience economy', from fitness to travel, are restricted, Lana has put together a series of 'New Age-y' workshops (Berman 2020) designed to cultivate the contestants' self-awareness and self-respect. However, the emphasis of such 'experiential learning' on inner personal growth invariably comes into tension with Lana's (and Netflix's) ability to encroach upon the 'boundedness that constitutes a self *as a self*', or what Couldry and Mejias (2019, p. 156) call the 'minimal integrity' of the self.

For Couldry and Mejias, the invasion of the space of the self constitutes the major costs of internet-based human connection, as individual autonomy is increasingly subject to the control of external power, whether it is that of the state, like China, or corporations, like Netflix. Under this regime of data colonialism, the continuous dispossession of human life has rendered 'the orders of "liberal" democracies and "authoritarian" societies ... increasingly indistinguishable' (Couldry and Mejias 2019, p. 20). In this light, the tongue-in-cheek joke of 'Lana (Factory, China)' serves as an invitation to more carefully consider the deep technocultural entanglement of – rather than ideological opposition between – China and the West.

The boundary between the human and the nonhuman – be it Lana or China – is thus a blurred one at best. Indeed, the kind of 'intimacy without proximity' (Metcalf 2008) that Lana promotes among the *THTH* contestants is a practice long embraced by the global infrastructures of connection. The lack of physical contact depicted in *The Circle*, *Love is Blind*, and *THTH*, as Colin Horgan (2020) suggests, is more reminiscent of 'life pre – and post-pandemic', for these shows have merely dramatized the 'basic idea ... that people these days often default to distanced communication over personal interaction'. The key, however, is that 'these shows are fantasizing about an extreme we currently inhabit' (Horgan 2020). The contestants on screen get to 'go home' to reality after the shows. By contrast, our reality of social distancing, which extends the already intensely mediated interpersonal communication prior to the pandemic, is one from which we can no longer escape (Horgan 2020).

It is tempting to speculate, as many have done, that China's stringent surveillance system under the 'state of exception' that is COVID-19 will become the norm not just in China but the world at large (Kuo 2020b). Meanwhile, a seemingly halted global economy – as indicated by massive unemployment, among other things – has not thwarted the growth of a financial market dominated by key players in surveillance capitalism, sometimes dubbed the 'FAANG Stocks', encompassing Facebook, Amazon, Apple, Netflix, and Google. In highlighting the dominating role of Lana, the technological nonhuman, *THTH* indeed appears to provide no less than an 'allegory for the sad and frustrating predicament plaguing our pandemic-stricken world' (Berman 2020). After all, it is communication technologies that also allow the privileged to be sheltered at and working from home, deepening the longstanding divide (Patton 2020) between the 'knowledge workers' and 'essential workers'; the latter, often consisting of populations long subject to dehumanizing racism, have no choice but to put their bodies at risk to sustain the lives of the former.

Nevertheless, it is equally worthwhile to reflect on another lesson taught by Lana. As mentioned, *THTH*'s contestants are chosen from Instagram. This process of selection arguably reverses the standard 'reality-to-influencer trajectory' taken for granted in other shows of similar premise and 'is now obvious to everyone watching, as well as those participating' (Horgan 2020). In essence, Lana has instructed these fully entrepreneurialized neoliberal 'selves' to form deeper bounds with others, as 'the success of the community relies on the compliance of every individual' (Berman 2020).

To be sure, this gamified premise of *THTH* references a dominant myth of data colonialism, that 'today's infrastructures of connection and data extraction fulfil human beings' collective potential in some transcendent way' (Couldry and Mejias 2019, p. 17). But under the conditions of COVID-19, this collective potential deserves more rethinking. The kind of intimate sociality that Lana calls for among humans, so frequently dependent on all those nonhuman devices and infrastructures 'made in China' (including masks), now arguably also forms a basis for surviving the pandemic, if not the climate crisis for which it is said to be 'a dress rehearsal' (Latour 2020).

A conjunctural analysis of the deepening COVID-19 crisis through the lens of *THTH* is understandably open-ended. In fact, Netflix has already begun advertising *Too Hot To Handle: Brazil*, tantalizingly suggesting different perspectives that may emerge from the Global South. Learning from Lana the nonhuman does not necessarily mean a disavowal of human agency, just like cultural studies and human rights can be critically examined through each other (Erni 2018) without reducing the latter to a Sinophobic trope. During and after the US Presidential Election in 2020, the talk of decoupling between China and America – the so-called superpowers and past and present epicentres of the pandemic – continues to escalate. Meanwhile, despite the effects of the Trump-era trade war, stay-at-home holiday shoppers in the US have re-distributed their disposable income from spending on (now restricted) travels and dining to the purchase of more Chinese-made goods (Swanson 2020). In this context, Lana from 'Factory, China' serves as a helpful reminder that acknowledging – by way of critically unfolding – the multiple and serial entanglements of the human and the nonhuman in the realm of popular culture is an urgent and necessary step for imagining new paths toward global social justice.

Notes

1. In *The Circle*, released on January 1, 2020, eight contestants are isolated in separate apartments and compete for social-media popularity. Only those eliminated are granted an opportunity to visit one other contestant in person. In *Love is Blind*, released on February 13, 2020, ten couples are placed in isolated pods to talk to their dates strictly through verbal communication for ten days and are not allowed to meet their romantic partners until a marriage proposal is made.
2. Arguably, such popular series as *The Bachelor* franchise on ABC, its newer competitor *Married at First Sight* on Lifetime, and Netflix's more adventurous *Love is Bind* all simultaneously uphold marriage as a sanctified ideal while undermining this sacredness by rendering the search for love a playful game.
3. All of the contestants come from English-speaking countries, including the United Kingdom, Ireland, the United States, Canada, and Australia. The choice of British accent appears quite reasonable given its relation to Britain's colonial history and the air of superiority with which it is often associated.
4. Mid-way through the series, a watch-like device akin to self-monitoring tools like the Apple Watch is given to the contestants to convey Lana's approval with a green light.
5. A similar technological presence is also discernible in *The Circle*, where the large TV screens placed in contestants' rooms periodically display a ring – an obvious logo for the fictitious social media platform named 'The Circle' - that sends out alerts and invites participants to chat, rate others, and play games.

Disclosure statement

No potential conflict of interest was reported by the author(s).

Further information

This Special Issue article has been comprehensively reviewed by the Special Issue editors, Associate Professor Ted Striphas and Professor John Nguyet Erni.

References

Althusser, L., 1970. *Reading capital*. Translated by B. Brewster. London: New Left Books.
Arnold, S., 2018. Netflix and the myth of choice/participation/autonomy. In: K. McDonald, and D Smith-Rowsey, ed. *The Netflix effect: technology and entertainment*

in the 21st century. Reprint ed. New York London Oxford New Delhi Sydney: Bloomsbury Academic, 49–62.

Berman, J. 2020. Netflix's too Hot to Handle is a trashy dating show. It's also strangely relevant. *Time*, 16 April. Available from: https://time.com/5820865/too-hot-to-handle-netflix-review/ [Accessed 18 July 2020].

Billé, F., 2018. Introduction. In: S. Urbansky, and F Billé, ed. *Yellow perils: China narratives in the contemporary world*. Honolulu: University of Hawaii Press, 1–34.

Byrne, A. 2020. Too Hot to Handle is real life rn and Lana is the corona virus. *Twitter*, 19 April. Available from: https://twitter.com/ainebyrne97/status/1251986571210952705? ref_url=https%3a%2f%2fwww.buzzfeed.com%2flyapalater%2ftoo-hot-to-handle-lana-the-robot-voice [Accessed 24 June 2020].

Couldry, N., and Mejias, U.A., 2019. *The costs of connection: how data Is colonizing human life and appropriating It for capitalism*. 1st ed. Stanford, California: Stanford University Press.

Dupré, J., and Guttinger, S., 2016. Viruses as living processes. *Studies in history and Philosophy of biological and biomedical sciences*, 59, 109–116. doi:10.1016/j.shpsc. 2016.02.010.

Eng, D.L., Ruskola, T., and Shen, S., 2011. Introduction: China and the human. *Social text*, 29 (4 109), 1–27. doi:10.1215/01642472-1416073.

Erni, J.N., 2018. *Law and cultural studies: a critical rearticulation of human rights*. London; New York: Routledge.

Feuer, J., 2018. The making of the bachelor nation: reality TV and layered identification. *Critical quarterly*, 60 (4), 46–61. doi:10.1111/criq.12440.

Garland, L.O., Emma. 2020. "Too Hot to Handle" is the sistine chapel of horny reality shows. *Vice*, 21 April. Available from: https://www.vice.com/en_us/article/y3m8jw/ netflix-too-hot-to-handle-review [Accessed 10 May 2020].

Harris, D. 2012. *Netflix analyzes a lot of data about your viewing habits, Gigaom*. Available from: https://gigaom.com/2012/06/14/netflix-analyzes-a-lot-of-data-about-your-viewing-habits/ [Accessed 14 June 2017].

Hester, H. 2016. Technically female: women, machines, and hyperemployment. *Salvage*, 8 August. Available from: https://salvage.zone/in-print/technically-female-women-machines-and-hyperemployment/ [Accessed 20 July 2020].

Horgan, C. 2020. *Reality TV Is no longer a form of escapism, medium*. Available from: https://gen.medium.com/reality-tv-is-no-longer-a-form-of-escapism-35400d3bc29c [Accessed 23 June 2020].

Kharpal, A. 2019. *Netflix has a China strategy — but it doesn't involve launching there soon, CNBC*. Available from: https://www.cnbc.com/2019/05/10/netflix-has-a-china-strategy-it-doesnt-involve-launching-there-soon.html [Accessed 3 July 2020].

Kuo, L. 2020a. Coronavirus: panic and anger in Wuhan as China orders city into lockdown. *The Guardian*, 23 January. Available from: https://www.theguardian.com/world/2020/jan/23/coronavirus-panic-and-anger-in-wuhan-as-china-orders-city-into-lockdown [Accessed 21 July 2020].

Kuo, L. 2020b. "The new normal": China's excessive coronavirus public monitoring could be here to stay. *The Guardian*, 9 March. Available from: https://www. theguardian.com/world/2020/mar/09/the-new-normal-chinas-excessive-coronavirus-public-monitoring-could-be-here-to-stay [Accessed 21 July 2020].

Lana Knows What You Did. 2020. Available from: https://www.youtube.com/watch?v= S-b2eEBN1TU&feature=youtu.be [Accessed 24 June 2020].

Laporte, N. 2014. Netflix: The red menace. *Fast Company*, 17 January. Available from: https://www.fastcompany.com/3024158/netflix-the-red-menace.

Latour, B. 2020. Is this a dress rehearsal? *In the Moment*, 26 March. Available from: https://critinq.wordpress.com/2020/03/26/is-this-a-dress-rehearsal/ [Accessed 29 March 2020].

Metcalf, J., 2008. Intimacy without proximity: encountering grizzlies as a companion species. *Environmental philosophy*, 5 (2), 99–128.

Newton, P. 2020a. Too Hot to Handle. Episode 1. Netflix.

Newton, P. 2020b. Too Hot to Handle. Episode 2. Netflix.

O'Brien, J. 2020. *Too Hot to Handle skyrockets to top of Netflix charts in US, UK & Canada, screenrant.* Available from: https://screenrant.com/too-hot-handle-top-netflix-charts-us-uk-canada/ [Accessed 18 July 2020].

Patton, E.A., 2020. *Easy living: the rise of the home office.* New Brunswick: Rutgers University Press.

Pun, N., 2005. *Made in China: women factory workers in a global workplace.* Durham, [NC] Hong Kong: Duke University Press; Hong Kong University Press.

Qiu, J.L., 2017. *Goodbye iSlave: a manifesto for digital abolition.* Urbana, Chicago: University of Illinois Press.

Reed Hastings, Netflix - Keynote 2016. 2016. Las Vegas. Available from: https://www.youtube.com/watch?v=I5R3E6jsICA [Accessed 1 August 2019].

Reklis, K., 2020. Reality TV for the socially distanced. *Christian century*, 137 (9), 44–45.

Riechmann, D. 2020. *Trump officials emphasize that coronavirus 'Made in China', US News & World Report.* Available from: https://www.usnews.com/news/politics/articles/2020-03-12/trump-officials-emphasize-that-coronavirus-made-in-china [Accessed 31 March 2020].

Rushe, D., and Lee, B. 2020. Netflix doubles expected tally of new subscribers amid Covid-19 lockdown. *The Guardian*, 21 April. Available from: https://www.theguardian.com/media/2020/apr/21/netflix-new-subscribers-covid-19-lockdown [Accessed 10 May 2020].

Schaeffer, K. 2020. Nearly three-in-ten Americans believe COVID-19 was made in a lab. *Pew Research Center*, 8 April. Available from: https://www.pewresearch.org/fact-tank/2020/04/08/nearly-three-in-ten-americans-believe-covid-19-was-made-in-a-lab/ [Accessed 30 July 2020].

Scheible, J. n.d. Aca-Media. (Talking Television in a Pandemic). Available from: http://www.aca-media.org/pandemic-tv [Accessed 30 July 2020].

Scheible, J., 2020. Tiger king as accidental allegory. *Communication, culture and critique*, 13 (4), 1–3.

Smith, M. 2020. Blame the Chinese Communist Party for the coronavirus crisis. *USA TODAY*, 5 April. Available from: https://www.usatoday.com/story/opinion/2020/04/05/blame-chinese-communist-party-coronavirus-crisis-column/2940486001/ [Accessed 5 April 2020].

Srnicek, N., 2016. *Platform capitalism.* Cambridge, UK; Malden, MA: Polity.

Swanson, A. 2020. China trade deal details protections for american firms. *The New York Times*, 14 January. Available from: https://www.nytimes.com/2020/01/14/business/economy/trump-china-trade-deal.html [Accessed 17 January 2020].

Too Hot To Handle Revealed - The Secrets of How They Film The Show. 2020. Available from: https://www.youtube.com/watch?v=z023yB9_oaE&feature=youtu.be [Accessed 29 June 2020].

Yapalater, L. 2020. *I'm obsessed with lana, the robot voice from 'Too Hot To Handle', BuzzFeed.* Available from: https://www.buzzfeed.com/lyapalater/too-hot-to-handle-lana-the-robot-voice [Accessed 9 May 2020].

Zuboff, S., 2019. *The age of surveillance capitalism: The fight for a human future at the new frontier of power.* 1st ed. New York: PublicAffairs.

COVID bread-porn: social stratification through displays of self-management

Ravindra N. Mohabeer

ABSTRACT

Much has been and will continue to be made of 'official responses' to the COVID-19 pandemic, particularly around the varying success of prescribed isolation practices and how well (or not) people, taken in aggregate, complied with them. This paper examines a more spontaneous response to COVID-19 isolation: bread-porn. Taken literally, bread-porn is the competitive display of gratuitous pictures of home-baked bread across social media (particularly in the 'west'), shared by people isolated at home. On the surface, such pictures perfunctorily depict bread; yet, it is argued that these pictures are more nuanced than that, and that the bread itself is almost immaterial. 'COVID bread-porn' was a jockeying for social standing and represented one of many unique, if temporary, forms of do-it-yourself (DIY) cultural currency while people were less able to access other extant systems of representational social stratification. The paper discusses the value and significance of the suffix 'porn' with respect to struggles to understand the extremities of new systems of value, by linking how temporary COVID culture fit into the flow of the cultural changes that preceded it. The paper argues that the world faced the COVID pandemic at a tumultuous time marked by liminality between historically 'physical' and emerging 'cerebral' cultural practices in many societies (i.e. the move from manufacturing to 'knowledge' economies). Thus, it situates bread-porn as an attempt to 'win' at isolation by demonstrating prowess with available domestic resources, and highlights the productive tension of bread-porn that extends and potentially resists the social imperatives of pandemic self-management.

At the start of the COVID-19 pandemic, many people faced a deep and sudden strangeness, hemmed in, inside a global patchwork of previously unimaginable social isolation and stay-at-home orders. This pronounced cultural ebb in the usual global and local flows occasioned new material priorities, words, techniques of interaction, and relations between people and institutions, each other, and ourselves. We recalibrated our sense of social hierarchies where consciousness and celebration of professions like medical care, teaching, service work, and other often under-glorified sectors occupied by invisible labourers (Sharma 2009) necessitated a collective pause to contemplate how ordinary things were ever previously accomplished. Many households, caught unprepared, were forced to evaluate how they could get by, having to make do with whatever was on hand to realize everything from work, to school, to the meeting of basic needs. It can be argued that all people in all societies faced at least some form of momentary adaptation that might be thought of as transient COVID culture(s).

Social responses to the COVID-19 pandemic have tended to focus on undertakings at the scale of institutions, nations, and regions. While assessment of these official tactics is imperative, so too is thinking about the seemingly mundane things that people did and continue to do during COVID-19 isolation, and considering what those actions might imply. This paper reflects on one such phenomenon, 'COVID bread-porn', by considering it within a constellation of self-management techniques put on display by people who, as a matter of class standing, may not have regularly spent much time thinking or sharing about them before.

As if lost in a daze, COVID isolation meant that people whose previously busy lives were delineated by other external markers of achievement, were suddenly displaced into an almost foreign domesticity, needing to find a way to feel normal. Left with questions like, 'when will I be able to go back to work? Send my kids to school? Travel for vacation?', candid displays of home-baked bread offered a tool to 'find other ways to have a say in [their] lives' (Levin 2020). The explicit nature of these displays, it can be argued, was often pornographic in tone. But why? Throughout COVID-19, fresh, home-baked bread, along with the outputs of other self-management activities, have frequently found their way into curiously porned domains in some (privileged) social circles. To be sure, the labouring classes who make bread for a living were not likely at the centre of bread-porn, or other self-management porn. Rather than bread-porn being a celebration of bread and traditional bread-makers, it represents an important marker of other, more spontaneous, COVID distinctions.

The term 'porn' as it is used here as a suffix has both visceral and social significance. The word carries weight and draws attention. Yet, when one experiences a barrage of home-bound people publicly circulating intimate pictures of their baked goods across social media, there is something about it that justifies the addition of the suffix, *porn*. It evokes implicit feelings about what *porn* is, what it should be, and what it should do. The suffix form appends the term *porn* to new locales, ushering it well beyond any expected focus on fleshiness or sex, toward new territories of obsession: in the case of COVID-related bread-porn, toward a productive homeliness. Yet, outside of the work of Hester (2014) in the field of porn studies, the dearth of literature that critically theorizes the rhetorical dexterity of *porn* as a suffix is notable.

What does the term 'bread-porn' attached to the COVID-19 pandemic signify, if not sex? Bread-porn is not the use of bread for traditional porn, but instead is bread depicted pornographically. While the idea of bread-porn here is used as a central example, it is meant as a stand-in for other forms of highly conspicuous displays of quarantine self-management, used as attempts to re-produce what Clifford (2020) describes as a sense of community, and, YPulse (2020) notes, as a way to satiate a need for comfort, normalcy, and order within that community. Making sense of what the suffix of *porn* means in this context, in the time of the COVID-19 pandemic in particular, offers value. That is, COVID bread-porn encapsulates the idea that bread baking as a form of self-management is presented pornographically to create a loose and indefinite acceptance of its stylized display as a way of asserting one's social position in an upside-down social world.

COVID bread-porn is a temporary attempt to demonstrate social prowess using the resources one has on hand. It assumes that the act of putting home baked bread, and other forms of relatively ordinary and personal self-care, on public display across social media for the consumption of our ambient social relations (Lin *et al.* 2016) is about sharing our ability to 'win' at isolation, as we muddle our way through pandemic turmoil. What the *bread* part is in 'bread-porn' should be materially obvious, carrying with it particular cultural meaning. The *porn* part follows former US Supreme Court Justice Potter Stewart's famous saying, 'I know it when I see it' (cited in Williams 1989, p. 5).

This paper, then, considers what happens when the two words come together as 'bread-porn' during the time of COVID-19. It also examines how this type of display, in some social circles, manifests class belonging, social identity, and acts of competitive self-management at a time of decreased physical sociality and increased uncertainty. This type of belonging, though purportedly ubiquitous, is highly selective, generally situated amongst those whose lives were forced to be paused by the pandemic, shifted to working from home, bereft of the opportunity to work 'in the outside world'. Equally, bread-porn as a gratuitous display denies the risks faced by essential workers who continued to go to factories to make mass-produced bread for a living. Unable to work from home, their risk of COVID exposures were more uncontrollable and acute. Their bread, not typically the stuff of COVID bread-porn, remained objectively mundane. This difference makes the social stratifications of COVID bread-porn all the more curious.

Why bread?

Bread-porn refers to pictures of homemade bread shared on social media platforms, and bears a strange resemblance, both aesthetically and substantively, to sexually explicit imagery. But rather than being about bread per se, bread-porn is, within the context of COVID, a competition. Following Trigg's

(2001) reading of Thorstein Veblen's notion of 'conspicuous consumption', one could argue that the *bread* of bread-porn is not only the display of 'tra-ditional [i.e. economic] value' but represents a tool for communicating social standing at a time of limited access to other tools that would normally assert the same. The physical act of baking bread, important as it may be as a symbol of survival, here is also something of a double entendre. The edibility of bread is less important to bread-porn than the display of that bread in a constant game of social one-upmanship that 'feeds' social media algorithms, the purpose of which is to leverage cultural capital and satisfy changeable norms in an effort to prove oneself the best at managing social-isolation in a time of global pandemic. While COVID bread *making* signifies survival and the meeting of basic needs, bread-*porn* acts as an embodiment of cul-tural capital. It uses what Bourdieu (1984/2006) describes as a conflation of the necessary and the aesthetic to create this significance. Its value is judged not singularly by how good one's bread looks, since even the display of 'bread fails' is not uncommon. On a deeper level, bread-porn reflects the underlying negotiation of representational acquiescence to that which is deemed necessary as a marker of distinction in pandemic times.

To appreciate the scope of 'COVID bread-porn', one need only search *bread* and other homemaking hashtags on Instagram and other social media platforms (see Hutchinson 2020, compared to Koman 2018). While a bread-porn community has existed on the Internet platform Reddit since 2011, COVID commandeered, expanded, and migrated the concept to other settings, and with ulterior purposes. In its new homes, you will find scores of images carefully curated by people with time on their hands during COVID isolation, presenting their new-found bread-making profi-ciency. While Ahmad (2020) might suggest that these breads embody how people conveyed to others that they had adapted to a collective trauma, thinking about this sharing as 'bread-porn' takes these stories of bread-making to represent a different, if related, layer of culture.

Writing for academic colleagues new to crisis, Ahmad (2020) captures lessons learned from experience. She instructively outlines three stages of dealing with COVID isolation as a crisis, directing energies to, first, support others and meet immediate needs, then, slow down and observe, and, even-tually, accept uncertainty toward developing a 'new normal'. In this process, Ahmad advises to ignore the urge toward 'productivity porn', opting instead for the management of everyday material and social needs. This does not mean that we must abandon who we *were*, but that we must adjust *how we are* during the crisis. People do not easily give up hard won social stand-ing, even if they are forced into a foreign experience that requires fundamen-tal re-tooling. COVID bread-porn acts as a union of meaningful substitutes for pre-pandemic activities that might symbolize survival, and learning, while also demonstrating one's ability to maintain and assert an enviable lifestyle.

Why porn?

Articulating something as *porn* signifies it as an idealized extreme that reflects a sort of sublime achievement. Thus, COVID bread-porn displays an idealized version of being the best at being stable in a time of great tumult. As people individually must struggle to stabilize the uncertainties of 'new-to-them normal' things, becoming good at the hyper-ordinary generates a familiar and comparative measure of self-management and control, shifting the assessment of comfort-making practices from being that of just meeting needs to that of also being able to assert social standing by meeting those needs first, or best.

What makes COVID bread-porn *porn* is the nature of displaying ritual experience, and the explicit *studium* of vicarious hyper-perfect fantastical exemplifications of excellence at control that make the ordinary extraordinary. As Levin (2020) notes, 'we cook out of necessity, but we bake to celebrate special times'. It may be odd to consider this pandemic 'special' in the same way one might consider a birthday as such, but perhaps it is fair to consider it 'special' as in the sense of being exceptional. In this exceptional time, Clifford (2020) claims that bread-porn's purpose is to 'share and connect', though YPulse (2020) and Munro (2020) suggest that it is not done neutrally or altruistically. Bread-porn is the 'the ultimate humblebrag' (Munro 2020), a way of posturing for status without seeming to be overtly garish. This competition applies specifically to those who have the time to devote their energies to crafting an image as a means to 'share and connect', more so than to those who rely on bread-making to earn a living.

Showing off your bread across social media demonstrates control in the face of real and perceived food shortages, which is to say nothing of the loss of control over what is going on in the surrounding world. Thinking about life after COVID, the marketing web-publication YPulse (2020) says that 'while at-home bread baking is at its peak [during COVID], and flour and yeast shortages will end, young consumers will likely continue to cook the things that bring them comfort'. Under these circumstances, self-sufficiency is an ultimate achievement. For some people, this means that those who master bread-making, win at COVID isolation. Of course, this proposition is very western, classist, gendered, and culturally specific. Making some variation of bread every day is not new to many. Yet, COVID bread-porn is shared in some settings as if 'new', or at least 'newly discovered', almost as by colonists claiming ownership and definition of an existing place by asserting their own rules to make the space their own. To consider the display of bread pornographically, then, is to consider how its gratuitous display acts as a referent to temporarily avow one's place in an emergent, potentially temporary, social order unfolding with respect to a world in chaos. This is particularly true for those for whom making bread is out of the ordinary and could be appropriated as a physically accessible arena in which to display mastery when denied access to other, more known, physical spaces.

Bread-porn winners and losers

Bread-porn, like all porn, does not require you to engage in its production to help create its value. Consuming bread-porn is a complicit value-making act. It strips the affective obligations between subject and viewer since one knows in advance that, as Linda Williams (1989) describes it, 'the money shot' is on the way regardless of whether you can achieve it on your own, or not. In this way, you do not have to be a (good) baker to play the game of COVID bread-porn. Consuming it acknowledges and elevates its social import. Using the framework provided by Hester (2014), this dynamic suggests an alternate value for the term *porn*. It needs to 'no longer [be] discussed as if it is a single thing to be either condemned or defended, but it is, instead, viewed as being as mutable and multifaceted as any other regime of representation' (Hester 2014, p. 2). This framework can help us to understand an alternate purpose for sharing so many sensual pictures of bread during the COVID-19 pandemic. They helped some people replace systems of social differentiation that went 'offline', displaced by social isolation, but not forgotten or unwanted.

Bread-porn demonstrates the assertion of ordinary dominion by people within society at large, rather than professional skill deployed by specialists. Anyone who has the time can potentially be a bread pornographer, maybe not even by being good at baking and sharing bread as much as by being good at sharing pictures of bread, explicitly. Bread-porn thus offers a consideration of the spontaneous cultural emergence of ordinary practices of social stratification that surface in response to COVID-19 when other extant systems of display and differentiation are restricted. Bread-porn, again, used as a stand-in for other forms of self-management during COVID-19, emerges as a way of chronicling daily activities hierarchically; it is an effort to jockey for position in a game whose stake is to take 'ownership' of daily life in isolation.

To be fair, it is entirely possible that 'bread-porn' might not be a 'real' thing as much as a fantasy of community asserted through the artifice of hashtags which are then aggregated across digital platforms. By lacking lexicographic certainty, bread-porn is necessarily user- and algorithmically generated, always already emerging, and devoid of centrally governed boundaries. This explains how bread-porn could be so easily co-opted into a modified system of stratification, rather than being a point of similarity in a specialist r/breadporn community of enthusiasts on Reddit. In COVID times, the essence of bread-porn and its purpose is consummately subjective yet deeply bounded by anecdotal and fleeting knowability, making it prime for spontaneous exchange as a value system. It does not take much training or effort to spot differences between displays of an object being celebrated, and pornographic glorification for the sake of display itself. For ordinary home bakers, the bread displayed in COVID bread-porn should not be thought of as belonging strictly to the category of food but also, more broadly, to social currency.

In the case of COVID bread-porn, the 'rediscovering' of basic skills (and hence the privilege of never having had to learn them in the first place) becomes a marker of one's standing in an emergent, socially isolated social hierarchy among the 'work-from-home' classes, rather than the physical labouring classes. We, thus, take away the providence of the labour-identity group 'bakers' and replace it with a more ubiquitous cultural display-value of baking as a tool of social stratification and self-righteous self-management. Ironically, the sharing of bread-porn might do little to ameliorate class and gender distinctions, or the actual sharing of bread in times of hardship, where baking for subsistence or from within a prescribed gendered role may not be elevated in value at all. Bread-porn-making does not signal that we intend to use bread-making to develop an artisanal political consciousness, but it could. Right now, all that bread-porn says is that during COVID-19, those with the privilege of time, and sense of a loss of known systems of control, seek the cultural capital that displaying baked goods pornographically can offer as a part of a competition with others who are similarly positioned. Bread-porn, during COVID, allows social media users to leverage baking in such a way that it becomes less of a craft than a social tool and, indeed, to do so without ever really caring about bread at all.

Conclusion

Bread-porn asks us to consider our fascination with the limits of culture(s), how far they can expand, and also to accept our prurient desire to witness the 'ultimate' manifestation of ability in contest with others.

It is hard to say if the ubiquity of competitive at-home bread baking (or instances of engaging in other self-sustaining, do-it-yourself activities shared on social media that rose to prominence during COVID-19) will persist. Post-COVID, our 'new normal(s)', may well include vestigial elements of COVID behaviour like competitive bread-porn, since, as YPulse (2020) reminds us, the 'desire for comfort and connection in the kitchen will not end anytime soon'.

It is clear, though, that the sharing of these activities across social media during the pandemic reflects a jostling for community and status, specifically as a stand-in for other means of social participation that were suddenly inaccessible. Bread-porn emerges from COVID culture(s) to parallel other forms of social stratification that were, owing to the pandemic, less readily available. It provisionally relocates the traditional boundaries of socially valued behaviour to different social places, without necessarily elevating consciousness or appreciation of the classes to which that behaviour is more traditionally associated. Bread-porn embodies how relatively privileged people in their everyday pandemic lives have tried to assert their place in society using a temporary representational currency, devoid of any obligation to acknowledge the typically utilitarian status they ascribe to most breads, and the social standing often placed on the people who normally mass produce bread for a living.

The pornographic display of these accomplishments as personal 'artisanal' achievement is particularly instructive. Indeed, the suffix 'porn' brings into focus aspects of a culture that are extraordinary and, when titillating, often, quasi-taboo, while also laying bare underlying social relations. It could also reveal some self-awareness through the use of the moniker 'bread-porn', signalling a type of rejoinder to 'productivity porn'. In the case of COVID breadporn specifically, when controlling bread ostensibly becomes social status, displaying it conspicuously and intimately reflects a much wider and deeper dynamic. It implies, as Hester (2014) argues, *porn* as a framework for considering how every culture, COVID culture(s) included, has aspects that can be displayed in a totemic manner and can thus be understood systematically and contextually. In the context of COVID culture, the suffix of *porn* helps us to think about how the display (and not making) of bread reflects how the politics of presence can be adapted spontaneously as needed to proclaim social standing at will.

Disclosure statement

No potential conflict of interest was reported by the author(s).

Further information

This Special Issue article has been comprehensively reviewed by the Special Issue editors, Associate Professor Ted Striphas and Professor John Nguyet Erni.

Funding

This project has received funding support from a VIU Publish Grant.

References

Ahmad, A.S., 2020. Why you should ignore all that coronavirus-inspired productivity pressure. *Chronicle for Higher Education*, 27 March. Available from: https://www.chronicle.com/article/Why-You-Should-Ignore-All-That/248366.

Bourdieu, P., 1884/2006. "Introduction; the aristocracy of culture" from Pierre Bourdieu, "introduction" and "the aristocracy of culture." *In: Distinction: A social critique of the judgement of taste*, 1–3, 5–7, and 11–13. Translated by Richard Nice. Cambridge: Harvard University Press, 1984, in Durham, M. and Kellner, D. eds. *Media and cultural studies keyworks*, Revised Edition. Blackwell Publishing.

Clifford, C., 2020. Coronavirus: why everyone is baking their way through the pandemic. 28 March. Available from: https://www.cnbc.com/2020/03/27/coronavirus-why-everyone-is-baking-their-way-through-the-pandemic.html.

Hester, H., 2014. *Beyond explicit: pornography and the displacement of sex*. Albany: State University of New York Press.

Hutchinson, A., 2020. Pinterest outlines rising trends amid COVID-19 lockdowns. 17 April. Available from: https://www.socialmediatoday.com/news/pinterest-outlines-rising-trends-amid-covid-19-lockdowns/576233/.

Koman, T., 2018. The only guide you need to Instagram food hashtags: think before you #nom. 10 December. Available from: https://www.delish.com/food-news/a25456620/food-hashtags-instagram-guide/.

Levin, S., 2020. The hashtag connecting home bakers in isolation. 23 March. Available from: https://www.sbs.com.au/food/article/2020/03/23/hashtag-connecting-home-bakers-isolation.

Lin, R., Levordashka, A., and Utz, S., 2016. Ambient intimacy on Twitter. *Cyberpsychology*, 10 (1). doi:10.5817/CP2016-1-6.

Munro, C., 2020. How hobbies have become the ultimate humblebrag. 8 April. Available from: https://www.refinery29.com/en-us/hobbies-during-quarantine-social-media-trend.

Sharma, S., 2009. Baring life and lifestyle in the non-place. *Cultural studies*, 23 (1), 129–148. doi:10.1080/09502380802016246.

Trigg, A.B., 2001. Veblen, Bourdieu, and conspicuous consumption. *Journal of economic issues*, 35 (1), 99–115. Available from: https://www.jstor.org/stable/4227638.

Williams, L., 1989. *Hard core: power, pleasure, and the frenzy of the visible*. Berkeley: University of California Press.

YPulse. 2020. These food & Bev trends are a hit during quarantine – here's what they say about what comes next. 23 April. Available from: https://www.ypulse.com/article/2020/04/23/these-food-bev-trends-are-a-hit-during-quarantine-heres-what-they-say-about-what-comes-next/.

Parodies for a pandemic: coronavirus songs, creativity and lockdown

Jon Stratton

ABSTRACT
One of the common responses to the coronavirus pandemic and the lockdowns that have been a feature of almost all countries has been the making of what have come to be called parodies. These are songs with new lyrics set to the tunes of established and well-known popular songs. The new lyrics describe life during the pandemic, the experience of isolation during lockdown, the importance of wearing masks and washing hands, the importance of social distancing when one is out. The pandemic parodies are a comment, sometimes jocular sometimes more anguished, on the new normal. They are posted on social media sites, mostly YouTube but also other sites such as TikTok, and invite comments from their audience about everything from the quality of the recording to the accuracy of the lyrics in reflecting people's lives during this time. Some of these parodies are by semi-professional singers, others by amateurs. Most of the parodists are white males and most of the songs parodied are from the 1970s and 1980s, part of the cultural capital of Generation X. This article argues that calling these songs parodies invites misunderstanding. They function more like the ballads of the eighteenth and nineteenth centuries when new lyrics would be written to be sung to well-known tunes. Often these lyrics would be commentaries on significant public or political events. This article argues that the pandemic parodies function similarly only now rather than the new lyrics being sold in the streets by hawkers, the songs are available on the web. At a time when the popular music industry is undergoing a fundamental transformation as a consequence of the impact of new technologies such as streaming, these pandemic parodies suggest another transformation in the production and consumption of popular music.

Immediately prior to, and during, the lockdown that took place across many countries in an attempt to slow and perhaps halt the spread of the novel coronavirus many people turned to music as a way of expressing themselves. In this article I discuss what have come to be described as coronavirus parodies. These songs are called parodies because they lift off from the tunes of preexisting, well-known songs giving them new lyrics which express people's experiences during the lockdown, sometimes also their anxieties, and sometimes they offer advice as to how to manage behaviour in order to avoid catching the virus. This article also examines who was making these parodies, mostly Generation X white males often, but by no means always, with some creative background as professional, or amateur, singers, as entertainers or as actors. The internet, and especially Web 2.0, has transformed the nature of the audience, no longer the either passive or active recipients of the creative products distributed by the mass media, audience members can now themselves create and place their creations on the web, on platforms like YouTube. Here is where we find the coronavirus parodies. Finally, this article argues that it is a mistake to call these songs parodies. They are better understood in the tradition of folk songs, broadly understood, where new lyrics would be created, and sometimes sold, to be sung to already existing well-known tunes.

As the novel coronavirus spread across the world most countries instituted some form of lockdown, an isolation of the population to prevent as much social interaction as possible. This was in line with World Health Organization (WHO) guidelines for managing a pandemic. The purpose of the lockdown was to slow and restrict the spread of infection. The lockdown was more extreme in some countries than others and also, confusingly, went by different names in different jurisdictions. Lockdown, quarantine, isolation, shelter at home, and more, were all used, sometimes in the same jurisdiction where they could mean different degrees of social separation required, for example, for returning travellers as compared to the resident population. Nevertheless what all the terms had in common was some amount of personal isolation either on one's own or with close family at the residence where one lived. Large numbers of people lost their jobs, going within the space of a week from having a liveable income to poverty. In addition, if one was allowed to venture out there were further things to remember; keep a social distance from other people, cough and sneeze into your elbow, and, above all, wash your hands regularly for at least twenty seconds or, as we were informed, as long as it took to sing Happy Birthday twice. For most people this new regime was related to a constant sense of anxiety.

Performing on the internet

During this time the internet offered a cheap and easily accessible means of distraction, of communication, and a site for sharing. TikTok, which used to be primarily the province of teenage girls has been transformed. In the British experience:

> Before the coronavirus pandemic TikTok was predominantly favoured by British teenagers, who posted prank videos of the latest trending dance routine on it.

But since the lockdown, TikTok has become a seething leviathan of user-generated content, chewing down our boredom, our fatigue and our fear and spitting
them back at us in 15-second chunks, to be digested ad infinitum (Kale 2020).

The term for this form of involvement is participatory culture. The concept
was first elaborated by Henry Jenkins *et al.* (2006). Christian Fuchs (2014,
p. 52) explains that participatory culture designates, 'the involvement of
users, audiences, consumers and fans in the creation of culture and
content.' TikTok presentations are a specific genre the form of which is determined by the fifteen seconds (in the first half of 2020 increased to sixty
seconds) the platform offers for the length of content. It turned out to be
the ideal distraction for adults as well as teens confined to their homes
without an end-date.

Commenting on what he calls the post-television audience, Michael Strangelove (2010, p. 158) explains:

Amateur online video has changed who can see what (almost everyone) and
what gets represented (almost everything). It has deepened our involvement
in the universals of shared culture and heightened our awareness of the particu-
lars of local culture and difference. It has also changed our status as audiences
and consumers. ... Audiences are watching and interpreting YouTube videos
not just as passive viewers but as active commentators and as producers of
their own videos.

YouTube is also one of the platforms identified by Fuchs as enabling participatory culture. YouTube videos are normally limited to fifteen minutes but it
is possible to extend the length to two hours. The fifteen seconds offered by
TikTok and the endless scrolling system, coupled with the ease with which
the short videos can be produced, makes it an intensely involving platform.
YouTube is, to use Marshall McLuhan's term, a cooler medium and allows
the audience of its videos to leave comments which are displayed below
the video.[1] Leaving comments is also possible with TikTok but the comments
page is not continually visible as with YouTube, rather it needs to be called up
using a button. The standard length for YouTube videos makes it an ideal
platform for music. Indeed, YouTube hosts huge numbers of tracks, often
recorded live but also offerings of recordings sometimes posted legitimately
by record companies but often placed on the site by enthusiasts making
available rare, and not so rare, tracks from their own collections. Nevertheless,
while YouTube is the main platform for coronavirus songs, short songs have
also been posted on TikTok. For example, vicki-dinos sings Quarantine to the
tune of Dolly Parton's Jolene about how she has been in her house 'too dang
long' and is sick of trying to spell quarantine.

The coronavirus songs are perhaps best described as examples of participatory culture. These songs are identified as parodies. They take the tunes,
and sometimes even the instrumental backing, of existing and well-known

songs and add new lyrics related to the experience of the pandemic, for example the predicament of isolation. Sometimes they function as public service announcements explaining to listeners how to behave to keep safe. Often the performers are artists: the English soul singer Jamiroquai has repurposed the musical backing of David Bowie's 'Let's Dance' for 'Locked Down', while Americans Chris Mann and Sarah Golden have both competed on *The Voice* and both have made albums in their own right. Dana Jay Bein, who wrote the lyrics for the popular parody of Queen's 'Bohemian Rhapsody', 'Coronavirus Rhapsody', works as a stand-up comedian and Adrian Grimes, whose version using Bein's lyrics is the most viewed on YouTube, perhaps because his voice bears a strong similarity to Freddie Mercury's, is the singer in a rock and roll covers band called the Solution. Grimes' version with Bein's lyrics has over five million four hundred thousand views (at the time of writing in October, 2020. All subsequent figures in this article are from this date also). There are a number of other versions using Bein's lyrics, such as that by Raul Irabien, an actor and singer, which has nearly four million views.

However, there are other contributors to the genre who are not trained or professional singers. Gregory Finsley, who is a member of a Queen tribute group called Queen Nation, sings a coronavirus version of the Police song 'Don't Stand So Close To Me' with Masha McSorley who, her website tells us, plays wineries, pubs, weddings, fairs and similar events (Masha McSorley). Their harmonization is earnest but inexpert yet they have almost 13,000 views and comments that recognize and respect the worth of their posting. For example, Lavonne Frierson comments 'horrible / I love it, I hope you two go viral!' and Pedro Guedes endorses this view: 'This is honesty (sic) so embarrassing. I feel sorry for them. This will be going viral shortly. Great job!'[2] What protects the attempts by people like Finsley and McSorley is the web's tolerance. Nick Douglas (2014, p. 315) has developed the idea of what he calls the Ugly Aesthetic:

> The ugliness of the amateur internet doesn't destroy its credibility because it's a byproduct of the medium's advantages (speed and lack of gatekeepers), and even its visual accidents are prized by its most avid users and creators. As opposed to media like TV or print, where the amateurish is marginalized and audience attention is centred on mainstream blockbusters, the internet is built to give outsized attention to the amateurish, the accidental, the surprise hit. Creators with no traditional skill or talent often become online celebrities for their work, and creators with skill or talent often suppress their abilities or manufacture amateurish conditions to better achieve the Internet Ugly aesthetic.

The comments on Finsley and McSorley's video mostly eschew the quality of the performance and concentrate on the lyrics. Laura Estey, for example, writes: 'Lyrics are the best of the parodies of this song that I have seen.'[3] The web offers a space where anybody can transform from audience to performer and, although sometimes criticized, will likely find somebody who enjoys the performance. At the same time we need to recognize that everybody on the web is not treated equally. Power relations discriminate against minorities. In the United States and other parts of the western world this includes those identified as non-white and those identified as non-heterosexual and non-binary.

A similar acceptance is given to Claire and Mel Vatz who provide a coronavirus version of Simon and Garfunkel's 'Homeward Bound' as 'We're All Home Bound – the Corona Virus Song'. Claire Vatz is a speech pathologist and Mel Vatz is an attorney. The song has over three quarters of a million views. One of the things that is unusual about the Vatzes is their age. They are clearly baby boomers and they are remaking a song from their youth. 'Homeward Bound' was released in 1966 on the album *Parsley, Sage, Rosemary and Thyme*. As a single it reached number five on the American Billboard chart. Some comments reflect the age of the listeners and their enjoyment at hearing a song from their past remade in the present time of disturbance and anxiety. Elaine Wilt, for example: 'Love this! You made us feel we aren't the only seniors with a great sense of hope. We will survive this! Thank you for making our day!' Catwoman writes: 'Wonderful! We all remember the original. Who would have thought we would be living this rewrite. BRILLIANT!!! Thank you.'[4] The 'we' here signals a particular community. Not everybody remembers the original, and it is not a part of the cultural capital, to use Pierre Bourdieu's term (1987 [1979]), of many Generation Xers. Catwoman's 'we' is the baby boomer generation, one little represented in the songs reworked as coronavirus parodies.

Who makes coronavirus songs?

Most of the parodists are Generation Xers, while most of the songs parodied are from the 1970s and 1980s. Thus, to give some examples: My Sharona, by the Knack, was released in 1979, Bohemian Rhapsody, by Queen, in 1975, I Want To Know What Love Is, by Foreigner, in 1984, Kokomo, by the Beach Boys, in 1988, I Want To Break Free, again by Queen, in 1984 and Staying Alive, by the Bee Gees, came out in 1977. These are the songs that the singers likely grew up listening to – the songs their parents played on the home sound systems and that they would have heard playing on mainstream radio stations. They are a part of the pop-cultural capital of Generation X. There are very few songs from the 1960s. It would seem that either those who decide on the songs to parody aren't familiar with those songs or they think their likely listeners will not know them.

As some of the comments I have already quoted indicate, the parody songs lift off from, and reinforce, a sense of community among those who make the parodies and those who listen to them. It is worth briefly elaborating what is meant here by community. We can go back to Howard Rheingold's foundational definition that he offered in his 1993 book, *The Virtual Community*. He described virtual communities as 'social aggregations that emerge from the Net when enough people carry on … public discussions long enough, with sufficient human feeling, to form webs of personal relationships in cyberspace' (Rheingold 1993, p. 5). In a discussion of marketing, John Hagel III and Arthur Armstrong (1997, p. 1) refine this definition, writing about virtual communities as, 'groups of people with common interests and needs who come together online. Most are drawn by the opportunity to share a sense of community with like-minded strangers, regardless of where they live.' Web 2.0 and the development of social media has made virtual social interaction, and therefore community, much easier. At a time of anxiety and uncertainty, and especially when people are forced to isolate, this feeling of being a member of a community, one built on a sense that we are all striving through this dreadful situation together, is very comforting.

What songs there are that have been repurposed from the 1960s are those that have realized a classic status. Thus, the Kiffness does a version of the Beatles' Yesterday and Terry Young has a version of the Beatles' I Wanna Hold Your Hand which he calls I've Got To Wash My Hands. Neil Diamond himself performs a version of his 1969 hit, Sweet Caroline, in which he changes the chorus to 'Hands washing hands.' In the video Diamond is wearing a black pullover, has on a cap, and is playing an acoustic guitar in front of a wood fire. The video begins with a large dog nuzzling the camera. The scene is made to seem cosy though the room, very probably his lounge room, is expensively decorated. We have here another form of the Ugly Aesthetic in which the rich entertainer, with the best of intentions, seeks to enable his audience to identify with him and be reassured by his performance while seemingly being unaware of the wealth divide between himself and the majority of that audience.

The majority of performers of coronavirus songs are American, and are white and male. One exception to the predominance of males is Stephanie Forryan, who calls herself One Woman Band. She has reworked 'My Sharona' and has over 96,000 views. There are few African Americans. Jinx Da Rebel remakes Akon's 'Locked Up' with the same title equating being locked down at home with being in jail and LL Bars remakes Bruno Mars' '24K Magic' as 'COVID-19K'. Neither has many views, Jink Da Rebel's Locked Up has just over three thousand views and LL Bars' remake has under thirty views. Even the high production quality track by SExT, the multiracial Sex Education by Theater group, a remake of Shaggy's 'It Wasn't Me' called 'It Wasn't Me (A Quarantine Parody)' only has just under thirteen and a half thousand views. The first point to make here is that these parodies are of twenty-first century songs: 'Locked Up' was released in 2003, '24K Magic' is from 2016 and 'It Wasn't Me' was released in 2000. There is no generational cultural capital being mined here. There is little sense of a shared sense of community in adversity, perhaps because, as a racialised community, African Americans already share other forms of oppression. This is made clear in the two versions of 'Locked Up', the one about being in prison, which got to number eight on the Billboard chart, the other about being forced to stay at home. Being locked down can be substituted easily for being locked up. The lack of views of the African-American parodies suggests a lack of interest by the dominant, white population.

In the context of race and power it is worth noting that while there seem to be no African-American coronavirus parodies of songs identified with the white musical tradition, there are versions of African-American tracks by white artists. Strangelove (2010, p. 161) writes that:

> The power that active audiences have to make their own meanings has been called appropriation power. As audience members we are constantly altering the original, or *intended*, meanings of texts (a movie, book, film, and so forth). ... YouTube is filled with millions of acts of appropriation that are often incorrectly seen as copyright infractions by entertainment corporations. [italics in the original]

Strangelove's point is that as audience members we actively interact with cultural texts giving them meanings unintended by the creators of those texts. Web 2.0 gives the audience the power to take this further. Members of the audience for cultural texts are able to appropriate and remake part or all of those texts themselves. This gives great power to audience members. However, appropriation takes place in the context of social power. Chris Mann, who has made a number of coronavirus parody songs, has remade Lil Nas X's 'Old Town Road' as a song about the loss of child care, 'Day Care Closed', and the Holderness Family, who also have made many parody songs, have parodied Michael Jackson's 'Billy Jean' as 'Quarantine (Is Not Quite Over)'. There is here a sense of white entitlement, that all popular music regardless of its origin, is available to be parodied. We might remember Amiri Baraka's position, in *Black Music*, published in 1968 when he was known as LeRoi Jones, that: 'They take from us all the way up the line. ... what is the difference between Beatles, Stones, etc., and Minstrelsy' (p. 235). Power tends to be invisible to those who have it.

The lack of parodies of white songs by black artists calls into question the claim that all music is available to everybody. We should be reminded here of the pressures on African-American artists not to play rock music. Maureen Mahon (2004, p. 6) tells us that, 'by the late 1980s when [black rock group] Living Colour released their first album, *Vivid*, African-American musicians had been relegated to rhythm and blues, dance, and rap music.' The whiteness of rock music, and the cultural power of white Americans, has made white popular music less available for African-Americans to parody, and of less interest. At the same time, one of the relatively few parodies by women is Sarah Golden's remake of MC Hammer's 'U Can't Touch This', the original having climbed to number eight on the Billboard chart and number one on Billboard's Hot Black Singles chart in 1990. Like 'Billy Jean' and 'Old Town Road' the crossover success of 'U Can't Touch This' provided an opportunity for white parody.

Outside of the United States there are coronavirus parody songs by performers in Hong Kong, Singapore, the United Kingdom, Canada and South Africa, among other countries. In Hong Kong, the singer Kathy Mak parodied the Natalie Imbruglia hit Torn, in Singapore the entertainer Alvin Oon parodied Simon and Garfunkel's 'Sound of Silence' with 'Fight The Virus', and the actors Edward Choy and Jo Tan parodied Dexys Midnight Runners' hit 'Come On Eileen' with 'COVID-19'. In the UK there was The Singing Dentist, a dentist of Iranian heritage who had put a number of parodies on YouTube this time remaking Vanilla Ice's 'Ice Ice Baby' as 'Virus … Baby'. What all these parodies have in common is that they are of well-known songs from either the UK or the United States and they emanate from predominantly white popular culture. 'Ice Ice Baby' was notoriously not only by a white American artist, in 1989 it was also the most successful rap track up to that time topping the Billboard Hot 100. Unlike the American tracks which group around the 1970s and 1980s, these tracks are drawn from a wider temporal field though still before 2000: Torn was a hit in 1997, The Sound Of Silence in 1964, Come On Eileen in 1982. Again we have the sense of a sedimented, shared cultural capital, a cultural capital which, we might say, is a function of Anglo-American cultural imperialism. The broader spread could be put down to a lack of generational differentiation as the knowledge of the tracks is more significant than the eras from which they come.

Parody and popular music

I have called the versions of the original tracks with new lyrics *parodies* because this is the generally accepted term. The performers themselves identify their work as parodies and journalistic comment likewise refers to them as such. For example, Greg Callaghan (2020) in *The Sydney Morning Herald* writes that: 'Parody songs are striking a chord when it comes to spreading coronavirus information.' Lanre Bakare (2020) in *The Guardian* headlines his article: 'Coronavirus Rhapsody: isolation is catalyst for slew of parody songs.' Here I will argue that these confections are not parodies but, rather, function more like folk songs before the advent of recording systems when lyrics would be sold with advice as to which well-known tune the lyrics should be sung. Jean Burgess has developed the idea of 'vernacular creativity'. She argues that such creativity should not be thought of as in opposition to the mass media but rather it should include 'as *part* of the contemporary vernacular the experience of commercial popular culture' (Burgess 2006, p. 207). She continues: 'Above all, the term signifies what Chris Atton [in *Alternative Media*, 2002, p.77] calls "the capacity to reduce cultural distance" between the conditions of cultural production and the everyday experiences from which they are derived and to which they return' (Burgess 2006, p. 207.). Vernacular creativity is a way to understand the productive work that performers are doing when they give new lyrics to well-known songs.

Traditionally, parody has tended to be thought of negatively, as a dull revision of a preexisting work. As Linda Hutcheon (1985, pp. 3-4) explains:

> Parody has been called parasitic and derivative. [FR] Leavis's famous distaste, not to say contempt, for parody was based on his belief that it was the philistine enemy of creative genius and vital originality. ... What is clear from these sorts of attacks is the continuing strength of a Romantic aesthetic that values genius, originality, and individuality.

The English literary critic FR Leavis laid the foundation for modern literary judgement in the 1930s and 1940s. Parody was criticized because it depended on another, prior text for its existence. Hutcheon (1985, p. 6) argues that parody is a characteristic form of the modern era and, even more, a foundational practice of postmodernity: 'what is remarkable in modern parody is its range of intent – from the ironic and playful to the scornful and ridiculing.' Parody has become an increasingly accepted form of expression.

The prevalence of parody is acknowledged in recent copyright law. The most significant case is still the Supreme Court's judgement in 1994s Luther Campbell *et al.* v Acuff-Rose Music, Inc. To complicate matters, because of its use of a prior text parody has become closely associated with sampling. In 1989, on their album *As Clean as They Wanna Be*, 2 Live Crew, led by Luther Campbell, released a reworking of Roy Orbison's 'Pretty Woman'. 2 Live Crew's version had new lyrics which made plain the coarse sexual desire that could be read as underlaying Orbison's original yearning romanticism. At the same time, making plain the track's intimate relationship with the original, 2 Live Crew sampled the guitar, bass and drums from the Orbison's track. Acuff-Rose Music, who owned the publishing rights to the song, sued. In the Supreme Court in 1992 they lost on the ground of fair use with the court recognizing the 2 Live Crew version as a parody. David Sanjek (2006, p. 180) explains that:

> Even when the transformative work amounts to 'criticism with a vengeance', in the words of Judge David A. Nelson, the addition of the new material to the public dialogue provides the necessary salve to ameliorate whatever alteration or alleged injury it has inflicted upon the original act of expression.

Parody is a typifying form of vernacular creativity when that involves, as it does on platforms like TikTok and YouTube, the reworking in some way by an active audience member of a given popular culture text disseminated through commercial media. It remains within established social systems of power.

Returning to an earlier point, Sanjek notes that Acuff-Rose appeared to have no trouble allowing the Orbison track to be used in the film *Pretty Woman* and another Orbison track to be used in David Lynch's film *Blue Velvet*. The suggestion here is how copyright can be employed to patrol the racial appropriation of songs. As Anjali Vats (2020, p. 10) notes, discussing the relationship between copyright and white culture, and here implicitly referencing the romantic idea of genius:

> True imagination, which emerged in the United States in the 1700s, is anchored by a binary of originality/unoriginality. That binary is legible in the racialized 'transformativeness' around sampling in the 1990s and the (neo)colonial management of the public domain in the 2000s.

In what Vats calls Euro-American creatorship the privileging of originality has meant that parody has been denigrated.[5]

However, let us take a step back for a moment and think about parody in popular music. Here, its primary purpose has been for humour, often intending to undermine the apparent seriousness of popular songs. Sometimes answer songs, songs that claim to respond to positions taken in other songs, have been grouped with parodies (Cooper 1987, pp. 57–77). However, while these tracks are dependent on the prior song they are not parodies. They develop the original song in a new direction. Thus, for example, after Elvis Presley released 'Are You Lonesome Tonight' in 1960, Dodie Stevens released 'Yes, I'm Lonesome Tonight'. As Hutcheon (1985, p. 6) defines parody: 'Parody … is a form of imitation, but imitation characterized by ironic inversion, not always at the expense of the parodied text.' Answer songs do not typically imitate the prior text. Rather they give that text depth by establishing a relationship. They offer the opportunity for a further riposte which, as it happens, rarely if ever comes.

Starting in the early 1950s Stan Freberg made numerous parody records including, in 1952, a parody of Johnnie Ray's 'Cry' called 'Try' and in 1956 of Elvis Presley's 'Heartbreak Hotel' where Freberg exaggerates Presley's accent and the echo on his voice gets out of control. Freberg was unsympathetic to rock and roll. His parody of 'Heartbreak Hotel' was humorous but, in Hutcheon's term, ridiculing. Freberg's singing is overwhelmed by the echo while, at one point, he mentions that he has ripped his jeans. The song's structure falls apart as Freberg asks amid the echo for it to be turned off. We are supposed to laugh with Freberg at Presley and the musical dynamics of the original song's recording.

There is a sub-genre of popular music parody which helps us to under-stand the coronavirus songs. In the 1940s through to the 1960s there were American Jewish parodists who took well-known songs and gave them new lyrics. The two most relevant here are Mickey Katz and Allan Sherman. Katz was a clarinetist with his own orchestra. He would write new lyrics to established songs which would speak to a migrant Ashkenazi audience illuminating their experience in America. He often included Yiddish phrases which added to the familiarity and humour, and increased the feeling of community for his listeners. For example, in 1950 Katz rewrote Frankie Lane's 'Mule Train' as 'Yiddish Mule Train' where the driver uses what is now a donkey to take salami to the Jews of Miami and lox and bagels to those in Las Vegas (Kun 2005, pp. 86-112). Katz's most successful parody was his 1955 rewriting of 'The Legend Of Davy Crockett' as the Jewish Duvid Crockett who was brought up on the Lower East Side's Delancey Street in New York. Katz respected the original songs and revised them for a migrant community that was taking on American culture but wanted to continue to feel comfortable with the culture with which they had grown up.

Katz was followed as a parodist in the 1960s by Allan Sherman. Sherman's rewritings were aimed at the next generation of Jews, more established in America and less at home with Yiddish but who still saw themselves as a com-munity apart. On his first album, *My Son the Folk Singer*, released in 1962, Sherman rewrote 'The Streets Of Laredo' as 'The Streets of Miami' and 'The Battle Hymn Of The Republic' became 'The Ballad Of Harry Lewis', a tailor. Writing about Sherman, and referring to the blurb on the cover of *My Son the Folk Singer*, Jeffrey Shandler (2017, p. 115) comments,

> it implies that the act of parody is itself a distinctively Jewish idiom. Jewishness is thus defined as a self-conscious difference in relation to the sensibilities of others, a distinction with which Jews are familiar and against which they take measure of themselves. The skewing of folk songs through this parodic sensibil-ity constitutes a performance of Jewishness.

Neither Katz nor Sherman were ridiculing the songs they parodied. Indeed, quite the reverse. They were taking mostly American songs that had become a part of their Jewish audience's cultural capital and reworking them from a migrant, Jewish perspective. The distance between the original lyrics of the songs and their parodic revisionings can be thought of as the cul-tural distance, and the corresponding sense of identity, of the Jewish audi-ence from the mainstream of American society.

The most immediate comparison with the coronavirus songs from the per-spective of parody are the parodies of Weird Al Yankovic. Yankovic has been parodying popular music since the early 1980s. In his book on Yankovic, Nathan Rabin (2012, p. 22) writes that:

… as an adult he would disassemble the songs of his favorite artists and recon-struct them in his own image for his pastiches. He would determine just what made a Devo song a Devo song or a Talking Heads song a Talking Heads song then reassemble the parts into a new creation.

While humour is fundamental to Yankovic's parodies, his intent is not to diminish the original. Rather, the humour of the parody is a function of the inimitability of the song, that is, the particularity of the original song is what gives Yankovic's parody its quality.

It so happens that Yankovic's first released parody was of the Knack's 'My Sharona', a track which has served as the basis for a number of coronavirus songs. Yankovic's parody is titled 'My Bologna'. The lyrics tell of the singer's enjoyment of the sausage. Yankovic's focus is on the original work. His intent is to create a new, amusing version of that work which depends on the original for its humour. 'My Bologna' is funny because of the musical and lyrical distance from the original. Food is a common theme in Yankovic's parodies. Simon Reynolds (2016) remarks that:

> One of his trademark moves is the food-substitution trick: 'My Bologna' (based on 'My Sharona'), 'I Love Rocky Road' (based on 'I Love Rock 'n' Roll'), and of course 'Eat It', his parody of Michael Jackson's 'Beat It'. … There seems to be something about food that makes it inherently un-rock 'n' roll (think about it: it only ever figures in songs as a metaphor for something else, usually sex).

If you don't know the original, 'My Bologna' simply sounds pointless and stupid. The basis of Yankovic's humour is bathos. In this case the bathos can be found in the difference between the topic of the original song and the topic of Yankovic's parody. Don Fieger, the lyricist and singer with the Knack wrote 'My Sharona' about his desire for a young woman named Sharona Alperin. However, as the popularity of the song suggests, it can be read more generally as an expression of young male desire. Yankovic's lyrics are about his craving for sausage. The humour of the parody lies in the transposition of a liking for Bologna, for food, with a desire for a girl. The difference between these two desires, reinforced by Yankovic's very un-rock 'n' roll use of an accordion, is what creates bathos.[6]

The coronavirus parodies

The humour of the coronavirus songs comes primarily from the lyrics as a com-mentary on people's experience and if related to the original song uses that song to make a point about the present circumstance. So, the 'My Corona' songs make points in their lyrics about the experience of managing the threat of the virus. In Chris Mann's 'My Corona', he sings: 'Gotta make a grocery run, well that sounds fun / Why 'm I out here risking my life, corona? / Where's a goddam parking space / Shit, I touched my face / Wait, I think I finally caught my corona.' These lyrics don't relate to the original song at all except for the known tune of the lyrics and the rhyme of corona with Sharona. This is unlike 'My Bologna' which derives its humour from the bathetic relation to the original song. Rather, Mann's lyrics express the anxiety of going out during the lockdown and the fear of catching the coronavirus. In My Corona Home, Joe Pumper uses the tune of the Beach Boys track, 'Kokomo'. He keeps the same first verse which lists various Caribbean islands thought of as exotic such as Aruba, Bermuda and Jamaica ending with 'why don't we go' and then departs abruptly from this fantasy: 'Cause we can't, we're in / Quarantine in our own corona homes / That's where you have to go to stay away from it all / Dinner's from a can, after-noons coloring with crayons / It's been thirteen seconds since I last went to wash my hands / In my corona home.' The idea of a desirable holiday is contrasted with the mundanity of life in lockdown. The singer doesn't even have a properly cooked meal, it can be assumed because he can't get to the shops to buy the ingredients, and in his afternoons he is reduced to a childlike state, using crayons and colouring-in books. The reference to having washed his hands so recently suggests that he washes them even more frequently than is asked for in the guidelines. Many of the song lyrics reference hand washing. Finsley and McSoorley sing 'Wash hands, sanitiser, did you just touch your eyes … No soap in the bathroom, I think I'm gonna die.' Often this concern with hand washing can be read as an expression of anxiety. The virus cannot be seen without a microscope so we don't know if we have picked it up from some surface and we therefore also don't know if we have washed our hands enough.

The Holderness Family, in 'I Want To Know What Day It Is', sung to the tune of Foreigner's 'I Want To Know What Love Is', describe the experience of being locked down in isolation: 'I have no concept of time / Is it May or October / I took the trash cans out at 9.00 / But the collection it was over / She said TGIF because she thought that it was Friday / But there are still two days left / And Wednesday is a dry day.' The lyrics speak to the experience of a loss of temporal organization. When there is no division between work and leisure, and when every day is essentially the same because you are almost always at home, people lose track of time. This is the experience of everyday life in modernity portrayed by Henri Lefebvre. Philip Wander (2017 [1984], pp. vii–viii) provides this summation:

'Everyday life' refers to dull routine, the ongoing go-to-work, pay-the-bills, homeward trudge of daily existence. … In this sphere of nonwork relations we live out our lives with our acquisitions, compulsions, and fears.

Commentators on the Holderness song on YouTube remark that it feels like *Groundhog Day*, a reference to the film of that name where the protagonist finds himself forced to live the same day every day. In another comment Juliann Davis writes: 'This would be totally funny except it's a documentary of my life.' In the Vatz rewrite of 'Homeward Bound', they sing:

I'm getting used to sleeping late / Should clean the house but it can wait / I try to work from my PC/ But soon the fridge is calling me / I eat some snacks, turn on tv / Without Netflix what would life be?

Here is another version of living in lockdown with which people identify. Here is the feeling of aimlessness without the focus of work, the resort to food and the importance of Netflix, the streaming service which in 2018, the latest year for which figures are available, offered over 5,500 films and television series which can be watched as fodder for distraction. Lockdown intensifies the experience of everyday life in late modernity described by Lefebvre. This is the dull banality of the quotidian. The lyrics to both the Holderness family and the Vatz songs, as in the lyrics to many other coronavirus songs, are detailed and easily relatable to in a world where we all have very similar experiences as a consequence of governments following the WHO guidelines.

Running through many of the lyrics is a popular culture vernacular. In the Vatz lyrics we have references to a PC and to Netflix. In the Holderness Family's lyrics we have TGIF, known generally now as short for Thank God It's Friday where the video shows a woman pouring herself a glass of wine until she realizes that it's only Wednesday, which is a dry day. In the Finsley and McSoorley lyrics of 'Don't Stand So Close To Me' there is a reference to 'that Dean Koontz book.' This book is a thriller called *The Eyes of Darkness*. Published in 1981, it references a virus made in a laboratory which in the first edition is in Gorki, Russia, but in the 1989 edition Koontz has changed the city to Wuhan, which is where the novel coronavirus is supposed to have originated. Koontz's virus has a hundred percent mortality rate. Circulating on the web is a claim to Koontz's prescience and the suggestion that he has an insight into the virus being human in origin rather than having naturally evolved. In the Kiffness' remake of ABBA's 'Dancing Queen' as 'The Quaranqueen', he sings in the persona of Colleen who can't go out on Friday night. Instead she watches the Netflix documentary series, *The Tiger King*. This is a key popular culture reference for 2020. The Kiffness gives his/Colleen's take on the Joe Exotic and Carole Baskin dispute described in the show in which circumstantial evidence suggests that Baskin may have murdered her husband and fed him to her tigers. The proliferation of these popular culture references in the coronavirus song lyrics can be understood in the terms of vernacular creativity and shared popular cultural capital. They develop from, and help create, a sense of community.

Repurposing melodies

The lyrics of coronavirus parodies point away from the original songs. For this reason these songs do not function like traditional parodies. Their humour does not derive from their specific relation to the original songs though, sometimes, the lyrics do reference the original song. This is especially apparent in titles like 'My Corona' and 'Corona Rhapsody'. The songs use of new lyrics to well-known tunes has a history in folk songs. In their discussion of the ways songs can be used in social movements Rob Rosenthal and Richard Flacks (2010, p. 10) write that,

> songs are easily adapted and changed to fit circumstances. What is sometimes called the 'folk process' involves the ongoing tendency for songs transmitted orally to be reworked accidentally or on purpose. Listeners mishear words or tunes. Musical elements may get adapted to particular traditions with respect to tonality, tempo, or rhythm. A familiar melody may be put to new lyrics, which are readily learnt and sung because of the familiarity of the tune.

In the coronavirus songs we are seeing the process of reworking taking place with recorded songs as they are actively engaged with by listeners who find other uses for the tunes.

This is not a new development. E. David Gregory (2006, p. 23) tells us that,

> not all sixteenth- and seventeenth century broadsides were political, topical, sensational, or salacious in content. In fact some were Puritan exhortations to piety and morality. Many were intended simply as entertainment and often consisted of new lyrics put to old and well-known melodies.

Putting new lyrics to established melodies has been a common practice for many centuries. The melody enables the lyrics to become familiar more quickly and also aids in the remembering of the new lyrics. Printing enabled lyrics to be distributed easily before the technology allowed tunes to be printed, and even then people needed to be able to read music in order to learn new tunes. Before recorded music people would buy lyrics sold on broadsheets. Ian Pettway (2016) explains:

> Ballad buyers would hear the song at the point of sale, as ballad mongers stood in the street, singing their wares. Occasionally more than one tune was indicated, which suggests a rather liberal attitude to the melody. It was, after all, the words that ballad-mongers were selling, with the tune as a vehicle for them.

Today those songs that have sedimented as cultural capital are being given new lyrics offered for free to those who want to hear them, and maybe even sing them themselves.

For a century recorded music was sold on records, and later on cassettes and later still on CDs. It was a mass medium. As long ago as 1983 Pekka Gronow (p. 53) wrote that: 'Common sense tells us that sound recording—that is, records and cassettes—is a mass medium just like newspapers, films or television.' Listeners, members of a dispersed mass audience, would often make up their own words to the songs they heard but these new lyrics would go no further than the bedroom or perhaps the local schoolyard (see Opie and Opie 1960, pp. 87-118). Web 2.0 has helped to change all this. Active audience members can now write, and sing, their own lyrics to established tunes and put them on platforms like YouTube, sometimes with an accompanying video. These songs are not parodies, though this is the term used. The commercial songs can be treated like folk songs. New lyrics can replace those that have seemingly been immutably linked with the tunes to which they have been sung. Strangelove (2010, p. 161) notes that: 'YouTube is filled with millions of acts of appropriation that are often incorrectly seen as copyright infractions by entertainment corporations.' We can note here a point that McLeod (2005, p. 83) makes in relation to the 2 Live Crew Supreme Court case discussed earlier: 'The Court voted unanimously that this wasn't an infringement; instead, it qualified as fair use, even though the record was sold commercially'. Copyright law is murky. Fair use is most easily identified where there is likely to be little or no financial gain. The coronavirus parodies discussed here have been created for the enjoyment of the makers and an audience which finds the parodies online. They have not been sold commercially. As such, it would seem, until a test case may prove otherwise, they exist outside the reach of companies anxious to preserve their ownership of songs for financial reasons.

Conclusion

Coronavirus songs are not parodies, they are a herald for a new musical future which, in an important way, takes us back to the past before tunes and lyrics were fused in recordings. However, this is not the past. The tunes are known because of the popularity of the original songs, because they are played on the radio and because people own recordings or more recently have downloaded them from streaming services. The vernacular creativity made possible by Web 2.0 is one of the ways that the music industry is being transformed. As Strangelove indicates, these kinds of appropriations cause a problem for a copyright system that has always limited the ways audiences can interact with songs.

   At the same time, the active audience offers new possibilities for the creation of virtual communities. While new communities may be formed, the appropriation and reworking of music existing in the recording mass medium is inherently subversive, disturbing not only the commercial structure of popular music but also expanding what music is available and the uses to which popular music can be put. This development overlaps with the DIY (Do It Yourself) movement. Ellis Jones (2019, p. 2) notes that, 'it is in the late 1970s, as part of the first wave of punk, that DIY gains its contemporary meaning as a specifically politicised approach to organizing popular music culture.' Just as punk was often considered to be critical of capitalism and the popular music industry which functions as a capitalist enterprise so DIY is frequently understood to be resistant to the hegemonic popular music industrial apparatus. Whether or not it is resistant, DIY artists are situated outside of that apparatus. DIY has been made possible by technological developments that have enabled people to set up recording studios in their homes and even their bedrooms. One version of DIY is known as bedroom pop. Broken Stereo (2020) explains:

> Gone are the days of paying producers, engineers and labels thousands and thousands of dollars to release a song. Now everything an artist needs is on the internet. You can write a song, record it in your bedroom and release it with an online label all in the same week.

The artists making the coronavirus parodies might come under the umbrella of DIY. They take advantage of the same technological innovations.

The proliferation of coronavirus songs is an outpouring that expresses people's experiences and anxieties during the pandemic. It is a way people have found to communicate with each other at a time when isolation and social distancing have forced most people into staying at home. For example, Chris Mann has reworked Adele's 'Hello', in which she sings about wanting to meet an ex-lover, to 'Hello (From The Inside)', where he tells us, 'It's me, I'm in California dreaming about going out to eat,' expressing the pain of being locked down. This has a video in which Mann has his face pressed agonizingly against a window as he looks out at a world he cannot visit. The track has garnered almost thirteen and a half million views. The idea of going out to eat provides bathetic humour, as with Yankovic's references to food, but also offers detail about the effect of the restrictions enforced by having to shelter in place and a seriousness about the possible impact of isolation. For some people the inability to go out to eat is not bathetic.

We must also recognize that appropriation functions in terms of power. The whiteness and maleness of the majority of the performers of these songs reflects the predominance of white males in the American entertainment industry, and it correspondingly reflects who has most access to the technology to produce the songs and, often, the videos with which they are uploaded. We can note that at this time, 2020, a digital audio work station like the Apple Logic Pro X costs around US$200 and an iMac to run it on is about US$2000. This also suggests a class argument in a country where race and class are profoundly imbricated. The kinds of appropriation discussed by Strangelove are limited to certain groups of people. Nevertheless, the coronavirus songs, like DIY more generally, indicate a future where the abilities to interact in these productive ways with popular music can become even more widespread and the meaning of the term popular music will take on a more accurate sense, a sense closer to, but of course very different from, what is understood as folk music.

Notes

1. I am using cool here in the way Marshall McLuhan used it. Matthew Crick, in *Power, surveillance and culture in YouTube's digital sphere* (2016, p. 69), argues that, 'a medium like YouTube would be considered a cool medium due to its all-encompassing highly interactive nature.'
2. These comments can be found underneath the video on YouTube at: https://www.youtube.com/watch?v=CjHf1ESsJCl.
3. This comment can be found at: https://www.youtube.com/watch?v=CjHf1ESsJCl.
4. Both these comments can be found at: https://www.youtube.com/watch?v=k0ci5EYb9qA.
5. This can be compared to the importance of repetition in African-American culture (see Rose 1994, pp. 87–107).
6. The accordion has been used in rock songs, for example, Talking Heads 'Road To Nowhere', the Rolling Stones 'Backstreet Girl' and the Who 'Squeezebox'.

Disclosure statement

No potential conflict of interest was reported by the author(s).

Further information

This Special Issue article has been comprehensively reviewed by the Special Issue editors, Associate Professor Ted Striphas and Professor John Nguyet Erni.

References

Atton, C., 2002. *Alternative Media*. London: Sage.
Bakare, L., 2020. Coronavirus rhapsody: isolation is catalyst for slew of parody songs [online]. *The Guardian*, 6 Apr. Available from: https://www.theguardian.com/world/2020/apr/05/coronavirus-rhapsody-isolation-catalyst-slew-of-parody-songs. [Accessed 22 Nov 2020].
Bourdieu, P., 1987 [1979]. *Distinction: a social critique of the judgement of taste*. Trans. R. Nice. Cambridge: Harvard University Press.

Broken Stereo. 2020. Bedroom pop and the rise of the DIY artist [online]. *Medium*, 24 Jan. Available from: https://medium.com/@brokenstereo/bedroom-pop-and-the-rise-of-the-diy-artist-1946e83bc7e0. [Accessed 22 Nov 2020].

Burgess, J., 2006. Hearing ordinary voices: cultural studies, vernacular creativity and digital storytelling. *Continuum: Journal of Media & Cultural Studies*, 20 (2), 201–214.

Callaghan, G., 2020. Parody songs are striking a chord when it comes to spreading coronavirus information [online]. *The Sydney Morning Herald*, 10 Mar. Available from: https://www.smh.com.au/culture/music/parody-songs-are-striking-a-chord-when-it-comes-to-spreading-coronavirus-information-20191231-p53nwr.html. [Accessed 22 November 2020].

Cooper, B.L. 1987. Response recordings as creative repetition: answer songs and pop parodies in contemporary American music. *Onetwothreefour: a Rock 'n' Roll Quarterly*, 4, 57–77.

Crick, M., 2016. *Power, surveillance and culture in YouTube's digital sphere*. Hershey, PA: IGI Global.

Douglas, N., 2014. It's supposed to look like shit: the internet ugly aesthetic. *Journal of Visual Culture*, 13 (3), 314–339.

Fuchs, C., 2014. *Social media: a critical introduction*. New York: SAGE Books.

Gregory, E.D., 2006. *Victorian songhunters: the recovery and editing of English vernacular ballads and folk lyrics, 1820–1883*. Lanham, MD: Scarecrow Press.

Gronow, P., 1983. The record industry: the growth of a mass medium. *Popular Music*, 3, 53–75.

Hagel III, J. and Armstrong, A.G., 1997. *Net gain: expanding markets through virtual communities*. Brighton, MA: Harvard Business Review Press.

Hutcheon, L., 1985. *A theory of parody: the teachings of twentieth-century art forms*. London: Methuen.

Jenkins, H., et al., 2006. *Confronting the challenges of participatory culture*. Cambridge: MIT Press.

Jones, L., 1968. *Black music*. London: MacGibbon & Kee.

Jones, E., 2019. DIY and popular music: mapping an ambivalent relationship across three historical case studies. *Popular Music and Society*, 1–19.

Kale, S., 2020. How coronavirus helped TikTok find its voice [online]. *The Guardian*, 26 Apr. Available from: https://www.theguardian.com/technology/2020/apr/26/how-coronavirus-helped-tiktok-find-its-voice. [Accessed 21 Nov 2020].

Kun, J., 2005. *Audiotopia: music, race and America*. Berkeley: University of California Press.

Mahon, M., 2004. *Right to rock: the Black coalition and the cultural politics of race*. Durham, NC: Duke University Press.

McLeod, K., 2005. *Freedom of expression: overzealous copyright bozos and other enemies of creativity*. New York: Doubleday.

McSorley, M., n/d. Website at: https://mashamcsorley.com/home [Accessed 21 Nov 2020].

Opie, I. and Opie, P., 1960. *The lore and language of schoolchildren*. Oxford: Clarendon Press.

Pettway, I., 2016. One song to the tune of another: early music common practice, 800 years before Humph [online]. *Early Music Muse*, 22 Nov. Available from: https://earlymusicmuse.com/one-song-to-the-tune-of-another/. [Accessed 22 November 2020].

Rabin, N., 2012. *Weird Al: the book*. New York: Abrams.

Reynolds, S., 2016. Killer riffs: a guide to parody in popular music [online]. *Pitchfork*, 19 Oct. Available from: https://pitchfork.com/features/lists-and-guides/9967-killer-riffs-a-guide-to-parody-in-popular-music/. [Accessed 22 Nov 2020].

Rheingold, H., 1993. *The virtual community: homesteading on the electronic frontier*. Reading, MA: Addison-Wesley Publishing Co.

Rose, T., 1994. *Black noise: rap music and black culture in contemporary America*. Hanover: University Press of New England.

Rosenthal, R. and Flacks, R., 2010. *Playing for change: music and musicianship in the service of social movements*. London: Routledge.

Sanjek, D., 2006. Ridiculing the 'white bread' original: The politics of parody and preservation of greatness in Luther Campbell a.k.a. Luke Skyywalker et al. v. Acuff-Rose Music, Inc. *Cultural Studies*, 20 (2-3), 262–281.

Shandler, J., 2017. "If Jewish people wrote all the songs": the anti-folklore of Allan Sherman. In: M. Renov, and V. Brook, eds. *From Shtetl to Hollywood: Jews and Hollywood*. West Lafayette, IN: Purdue University Press, 109–124.

Strangelove, M., 2010. *Watching YouTube: extraordinary videos by ordinary people*. Toronto: University of Toronto Press.

Vats, A., 2020. *The color of creatorship: intellectual property, race, and the making of Americans*. Redwood City, CA: Stanford University Press.

Wander, P., 2017 [1984]. Introduction. In: H. Lefebvre, ed. *Everyday life in the modern world*. Trans. S. Rabinovitch. London: Routledge, vii–xxiii.

Fashion in 'crisis': consumer activism and brand (ir)responsibility in lockdown

Rimi Khan ⓘ and Harriette Richards ⓘ

ABSTRACT

The Covid-19 pandemic precipitated an 'existential crisis' in the global fashion industry. The effects of the crisis on the retail sector resulted in many brands deferring or cancelling orders from supplier factories without paying workers, which had an instant and calamitous impact on the lives of garment workers in the global South. While activist organizations were quick to launch campaigns demanding that fashion brands #PayUp and take responsibility for their producers, these calls seemed futile in the face of fashion supply chains that have long been structured in ways that absolve brands of responsibility. The stories of worker exploitation and abuse in the garment industry that emerged during the pandemic were not discussed as effects of global capitalism, but rather were recast as evidence of a world suddenly in 'crisis.' In this article, we reflect on how the language of 'crisis' adopted in the early months of the pandemic produced particular modes and instruments of (ir)responsibility. We present an analysis of the effects of the pandemic on the global fashion industry, as well as the #PayUp and #WeWearAustralian campaigns, and argue that the exceptionalism underpinning the crisis discourse has both diffused and narrowed responsibility for garment worker exploitation, reiterating the very racialised inequalities that allow such exploitation to occur in the first place.

Introduction

In late March 2020, reports began circulating about the 'existential crisis' facing the fashion industry in the wake of Covid-19 (Industriall 2020). The pandemic was devastating fashion's global supply chains and threatening up to 60 million garment workers who risked job losses and destitution (BHRC 2020a). The Centre for Global Workers' Rights reported on 'three phases of crisis' that had resulted in the complete or partial shutdown of thousands of garment factories in Bangladesh, one of the world's largest apparel exporters (Anner 2020, p.1). First, lockdown restrictions in China in late 2019 meant delays in raw material imports to Bangladesh and increased shipment costs. Second, as similar restrictions spread to the rest of the world, fashion brands and retailers were forced to close their doors and, faced with major losses, began deferring payments for already-produced orders from supplier factories. Finally, in mid-March, as the scale and gravity of the pandemic became clear, brands started to 'abruptly cancel' both future orders and orders in progress (Anner 2020, p.5). These cancelled payments had dire consequences for supplier companies and their employees. In Bangladesh alone an estimated 2.3 million garment workers have been laid off or temporarily suspended (BHRC 2020b). By November 2020, a reported US $16.7 billion of unpaid orders have resulted in over US $5.8 billion of unpaid wages for garment workers worldwide (BHRC 2020a). While the plight of garment workers has long been the focus of labour rights campaigners, the pandemic has galvanized a new wave of digital activism propelled by the language of crisis. This article reflects on how this discourse of crisis produces particular spaces and instruments of (ir)responsibility. We argue that the exceptionalism underpinning the crisis discourse both diffuses and narrows responsibility for garment worker exploitation, and reiterates the racialised inequalities that allow such exploitation to occur in the first place.

In 2013 the Rana Plaza building collapse in Bangladesh that killed at least 1134 workers also became a signifier of 'crisis' in the industry. The tragedy was used by labour rights activists to develop instruments that could better regulate factory safety and hold fashion brands to account. At the same time, the event offered an opportunity for brands to *disavow* themselves of responsibility. A common response was for brands to deny knowledge that their clothes were manufactured in the Rana Plaza factories, citing the complexity of industry supply chains over which they had little oversight or control (Le Baron et al. 2017). In this way, moments of crisis call for accountability while obscuring the underlying relations of irresponsibility that lead to these events.

News of the fashion industry's current 'crisis' came at a time when many around the world were already confronting a deluge of data detailing infections, deaths, jobs lost, and days in isolation. We have come to understand the Covid-19 pandemic via this 'avalanche of numbers', a term coined to describe the quantification of human sickness in the nineteenth century, and which offers an uncomfortably apt metaphor for the current moment in which we are being buried by numbers (Hacking 1982). Statistics about the numbers of garment workers in Bangladesh whose livelihoods are at risk form a small part of the much wider reckoning taking place as economies go into recession around the world. During Covid-19, news of Bangladesh's garment workers is simply more bad news. However, these reports about the garment industry reflect a multiplication of the Covid-19 crisis, where the biopolitics of disease becomes linked to other forms of economic calculation and cultural speculation. In the case of the garment industry, stories of worker exploitation are being reframed as ostensibly unforeseeable side-effects of the pandemic. Fashion markets that have routinely relied on worker abuse and global inequality are recasting these phenomena as evidence of a world suddenly in 'crisis'. In what follows we discuss how these proclamations of crisis produce particular modes of responsibility. Crises can create spaces for action or intervention, but they also attribute and conceal responsibility in specific ways.

Exceptionality and irresponsibility in crisis

Constructivist accounts of crisis reveal the various kinds of historical imagination through which events come to be framed as extraordinary or unexpected (Samman 2015, Patrona 2018). By tracing the etymology of the term Samman (2015) examines the contradictory temporalities of crisis. 'Crisis' is widely used to imply a break or rupture from the past, obscuring historical continuities and entanglements. However, crises are often mediated or interpreted in relation to prior, related crises, which posit relations of affiliation with other historical moments. The Rana Plaza disaster, for example, has been regularly compared with the Triangle Shirtwaist Factory fire that took place in New York in 1911, in which 146 garment workers died (Bain 2018). The comparison emphasizes the enduring problem of poor labour conditions in the fashion industry, at the same time as it articulates a geography and trajectory of global 'progress' that relies on a contrast between the 'first' and 'third' worlds (Saha 2019). In this way, narratives of crises are fraught with historical ambiguity. Crisis moments can be read as 'symptoms of systemic failure' in ways that also 'absolve that same system from blame' (Samman 2015, p. 977). The current fashion industry crisis invokes a similar temporal ambiguity – brands have long depended on the opacity of supply chains to exonerate themselves of responsibility for worker welfare but are now attributing this problem to the unprecedented nature of the Covid-19 pandemic. Brands' sudden inability to pay their workers, framed as a 'rupture,' obscures the fact that the impoverishment and exploitation of workers in fashion supply chains is part of the industry's natural order.

A number of major brands have invoked the *force majeure* clause in their contracts to claim unforeseen and exceptional circumstances (Anner 2020). In April, the European retail giant Primark defended the non-payment of its apparel producers because the pandemic had presented them with 'unprecedented and frankly unimaginable times' (Kelly 2020). Following intense pressure from campaigners, the brand announced it would set up a wage fund to support garment workers. However, in November, the activist group Labour Behind the Label was still calling on Primark to pay all its suppliers, arguing that the wage fund did not cover major production countries including Turkey and China, and that Primark workers in Bangladesh,

Myanmar and Cambodia were continuing to protest mass dismissal, unpaid wages and reductions in pay (Lewis 2020). Brands using Covid-19 to excuse themselves of their contractual obligations uphold the pretence that these responsibilities were taken seriously in the first place. The fashion industry's disclosure of supply chain information may have increased in recent years,[1] yet its persistent lack of transparency means that many unethical fashion production practices remain invisible – providing both consumers and brands a sense of plausible deniability. While brands are alleging 'unprecedented impacts to their viability' (ILO 2020, p.1) such claims are difficult to reconcile with the scandalously large profits reported by many apparel companies, including brands who have reported profits *during* the pandemic (Debter 2019, BHRC 2020c).[2]

Dispersing responsibility

As reports surfaced about international fashion brands cancelling in-production orders and not paying for orders already produced, two distinct calls to action emerged via social media. The first was an appeal by labour rights and sustainable fashion advocates[3] for fashion brands to #PayUp and commit to paying for back orders. A petition on change.org, launched by Remake on 30 March 2020, emphasized the obligations of fashion consumers to support garment workers in Bangladesh who 'will go hungry and be forced onto the streets' if they are not paid (Change.org 2020).

Since launching in March, the campaign received support from models such as Cameron Russell, Arizona Muse and Amber Valletta and, by the time the petition closed in October it had received over 272,000 signatures. The campaign focused on the need for consumers to take responsibility for holding brands to account, stating on Instagram: 'We need you more than ever' (10 April 2020). To be removed from the list of brands who needed to #PayUp (tracked by the Worker Rights Consortium), brands had to commit to paying suppliers for all orders that were cancelled or paused as a result of the pandemic. By mid-July, significant public pressure led companies such as Gap and Levi's to join other fashion brands that had already committed to the pledge. The success of the campaign, in which the #PayUp hashtag has been used in over 793,000 Instagram posts to date, not only ensured that numerous brands committed to paying for their orders but also contributed to the launch of PayUp Fashion, an activist movement to reform labour rights in the fashion industry. This movement is continuing to call on brands such as Forever 21, Fashion Nova and URBN (Urban Outfitters, Free People, Anthropologie), all of whom remain silent on their order payment status.

The second campaign arose from concerns about the impact of lockdown restrictions on the viability of 'local' fashion brands and retailers. In Australia, activists implored fashion consumers to support local production, brands and designers through the #WeWearAustralian movement, driven by Australian fashion industry stalwart Richard Poulson. Heavy with concern, if not patriotic duty, campaigners proclaimed that the survival of the Australian fashion industry was 'up to us' – the consumers. In one of the many features publicizing the #WeWearAustralian campaign, owner of Australian womenswear brand Bondi Born, Dale McCarthy, made clear: 'If people stop shopping, the industry will disappear' (Jane 2020). The call to arms demanded that shoppers use their buying power to prop up local businesses; many local fashion brands and industry bodies declaring that the industry 'needs your support now, more than ever' (Ethical Clothing Australia 2020).

The effect of these campaigns is decidedly parochial: *don't* shop from global brands who haven't paid their workers, and *do* shop from local designers and brands. This global/local dichotomy offers a reductive picture of a complex industry reality. It ignores those local designers who manufacture offshore with no guarantee of compliance with fair labour standards, and it overlooks the unethical *local* production practices of some domestic brands. Moreover, it invokes a model of consumer responsibility that collapses class differences and assumes shoppers' capacity for boycotts, 'ethical consumption' and 'responsible choice' (Barnett *et al.* 2010, p.1). Critiques of 'ethical consumption' as an individualized, feminized response to structural problems of global capitalism are well rehearsed (Bartley et al. 2015, Horton 2018). Consumer responsibility is also drawn along racialised lines, in which rich white women save or empower brown garment workers, deemed unable to be responsible (Pham 2017, Khan 2019). These examples of 'hashtag activism' (Jackson et al. 2020) are the mediated forms of visibility and outrage through which we come to know the crisis in the fashion industry. And while they rely on the individualization of consumer action, the #PayUp and #WeWearAustralian campaigns also illustrate a widening of 'horizons of blame and responsibility' in ways that ultimately diffuse and detract from the culpability of corporations (Fitz-Henry 2012, p.184). When 'everyone' is responsible, no one is truly responsible, and responsibility is largely unenforceable.

These consumer movements ask individuals to respond to globalized relationships of commodity production by 'caring at a distance' (Goodman 2004). The question of how to cultivate such care is especially pertinent during the protracted period of quarantine and isolation triggered by the Covid-19 pandemic. As people retreat into local spaces and confront immediate threats to their physical and economic security, how can they be expected to attend to global interdependencies and obligations? In an emotional YouTube video published on 23 March, the President of the Bangladesh Garment Manufacturers and Exporters Association draws explicitly on the language of trust, partnership and care as she implores fashion brands to pay their apparel producers. 'Please do not give up on us,' she urges, 'we've been partners for so long … it's not a huge amount of money for you' (Haq 2020). She highlights the shared interests between global brands and suppliers in Bangladesh, remarking that in this potentially catastrophic time for the industry, 'the only thing we have is hope, trust and the spirit of collaboration.' Such statements reflect the contradictory geographies shaping Covid-19. On the one hand there are appeals for global solidarity and assertions that 'we are all in this together' (Gaztambide-Fernandez 2020, Guterres 2020). Equally vocal, however, is the chorus of commentators reminding us that 'we are not in this together,' and that, if anything, the pandemic has foregrounded structures of entrenched inequality (Fitzpatrick 2020, Guarnieri 2020). Such inequities make the need for collective responsibility and action more pressing, but they also highlight how poorly-positioned we are to mobilize in collective ways.

Narrowing responsibility

Fashion brands' responses to the current pandemic highlight how they evade responsibility by articulating and codifying it in narrow terms. In a global industry where many companies operate beyond government regulation, responsibility for labour conditions falls on companies themselves, or to their third-party auditors and consultants, and is expressed via statements of social responsibility and transparency. But transparency instruments can often reiterate colonial relations of visibility and power. Systems of factory auditing that offer assurances about labour standards for consumers in the global North arguably form part of a transparency 'industry' that serves Western interests, and have little connection to the needs and experiences of workers in these local places (de Maria 2008). The Business and Human Rights Resource Centre, for example, has launched a 'Covid-19 Action Tracker' that is evaluating the responses of 35 major fashion brands to the pandemic (BHRC 2020a). Brands are asked whether they have committed to pay their workers, and about the terms of their contracts with suppliers, but participation in the BHRC's survey is voluntary. In many cases participating brands have responded to the survey in generalities, stating that 'most of our contracts' aim to meet particular benchmarks, or by claiming that it is not possible to disclose details about contracts because such information is commercially sensitive (BHRC 2020a). These transparency instruments measure only what is allowed to be made visible in an otherwise opaque system of commodity production and private regulation.

Narrow instruments of accountability offer a way of *moving on* from crisis. In response to the current pandemic, brands have been declaring their support for the International Labour Organisation's *Call to Action*, a statement that commits brands to various kinds of 'action' but which also disperses responsibility to a variety of other actors, including governments and financial institutions, who might lend credit to supplier factories and extend social support to workers at risk of impoverishment (ILO 2020, p.2). The hollow nature of these 'actions' aside,[4] brands' endorsement of this document is itself promoted as evidence that the industry is addressing the crisis. Although a crisis potentially marks a period of struggle, contestation or transformation, the accountability instruments through which apparel companies respond to crisis permit business as usual. Similarly, the social movements which anchor brands' responsibilities to specific, isolated demands – to commit to #PayUp, for example – allow brands to then claim the crisis has been resolved. Such campaigns might effectively pressure brands to meet specific obligations, but they are not good at imagining a future beyond crisis.

Conclusion

Fashion supply chains have long been built on a foundation of opacity and invisibility, structured in ways that absolve brands of responsibility. While the effects of Covid-19 have brought a new wave of outrage, visibility and attention to these realities, a meaningful response to fashion's current crisis demands thinking beyond exceptionality. There is growing recognition that the climate crisis is a symptom of a much longer 'anthropocenic era' (Bhavnani 2019), and that the global refugee crisis is an expression of ongoing geopolitical conflicts and colonial violence (Allen et al. 2018). In fact, it could be argued that the racialised and unequal impacts of the pandemic on the fashion industry are inseparable from these other historical currents. The global protests that erupted after the killing of George Floyd saw an overlapping of the #PayUp and #BlackLivesMatter campaigns, in which labour rights campaigners stressed the garment industry's historical reliance on the exploitation of people of colour. Despite recent efforts to diversify fashion runways and imagery, the #BlackLivesMatter movement provoked some commentators to admit that 'racism in fashion runs to the very core of the industry' (Legesse 2020).[5]

While media attention in the early days of the pandemic focused on garment workers in the global South, as the months continued, reports emerged about the conditions of workers elsewhere. In the UK city of Leicester, Labour Behind the Label revealed that sick employees were ordered to continue working long hours in densely populated factories to keep up with demand from fashion brand Boohoo (Bland and Campbell 2020).[6] The 'slave-like' conditions of these factories, long an 'open secret,' had become the site of a Covid-19 'hotspot' and was suddenly of concern to the wider community (O'Connor 2020, Wright and Nillson 2020). Significantly, a large proportion of Leicester garment workers are of South Asian heritage. Exposing these conditions through the language of crisis has revealed and amplified existing practices of racialised exploitation, and complicated simplistic oppositions between the 'local' and 'global' in the fashion industry.

Early conjecture that Covid-19 had the potential to bring about the 'end of capitalism' now seems unpersuasive (Mason 2020). As the #WeWearAustralian campaign illustrates, the imperative to rebuild economies is itself being framed as a responsibility of consumer-citizenship. Far from abating consumer appetite, the pandemic has spurred significant e-commerce growth (Business of Fashion and McKinsey & Co., 2020) and has resulted in many brands recording profits (Davey 2020, BHRC 2020c), confirming speculation that there might be a 'bounce' in sales once the threat of the virus subsided (Uddin 2020). The discourse of crisis may energize those consumers and campaigners who become suddenly responsible, but such responsibilities are largely expressed in ways that do not imagine alternative kinds of cultural economy, and do not consider how workers themselves might be positioned as equal agents in longer-term processes of economic transformation.

Gibson-Graham (2008) have argued that the point of academic reflection on 'post-capitalist possibilities' is not to hypothesize about what a utopian future should look like but to make visible, and affirm, existing forms of ethical and economic experimentation that emphasize solidarity, hospitality and collectivity. In this way, academic commentary forms part of the performance of alternative economies and an 'ontological reframing' of economic problems (2008, p.1). Such an approach is especially productive for rethinking the fashion industry, not as an intractable and totalizing global system in which exploitation is inevitable, but as part of a complex 'global assemblage' that is constituted by diverse 'ethical regimes' (Ong and Collier 2005). Such assemblages are comprised of disjunctures *and* interdependencies between different economic orders and agents, including garment producers, entrepreneurs, consumers and activists in diverse places. Keeping these entanglements and continuities in view, rather than a politics of exceptionality, might help to rethink 'action' in terms of interconnected responsibilities.

Notes

1. Improved industry transparency since the Rana Plaza factory collapse has been a result of efforts by labour rights groups, consumer activism and the visibility brought to this issue by garment workers themselves. Regular protests by garment workers in Bangladesh have demanded greater accountability from fashion brands, including compensation for Rana Plaza victims and increased wages. Alongside these movements, activist groups such as Fashion Revolution, and labour rights organisations such as Clean Clothes Campaigns have been mobilising consumers and lobbying fashion brands to improve transparency.
2. In a recent survey by the Business Human Rights Centre (2020c), 29 out of 55 fashion brands reported profits since the onset of the pandemic.

3. Organisations included Labour Behind the Label, the Clean Clothes Campaign and Remake.
4. The actions include brands' commitment to 'engaging with financial institutions, governments and donors' without detailing the nature of this engagement, and to 'strongly support access to relief funds' without providing such support themselves (ILO 2020, p.2).
5. One high profile example is the resignation of Yael Aflalo, the founder and former-CEO of sustainable fashion brand, Reformation. Although the brand, like many others in 2020, embraced the BlackLivesMatter hashtag, the testimonies of black employees highlighted the ways in which racism was embedded in the brand's operations and ethos (Nesvig 2020).
6. Similar reports have emerged of Bangladeshi garment workers, including pregnant women (Politzer 2020), and garment workers in Los Angeles (Miller 2020) being forced to work despite the risks of Covid-19 within overcrowded factories.

Disclosure statement

No potential conflict of interest was reported by the author(s).

Further information

This Special Issue article has been comprehensively reviewed by the Special Issue editors, Associate Professor Ted Striphas and Professor John Nguyet Erni.

ORCID

Rimi Khan ⓘ http://orcid.org/0000-0001-5346-8115
Harriette Richards ⓘ http://orcid.org/0000-0001-6557-5495

References

Allen, W., et al., 2018. Who counts in crises? the new geopolitics of international migration and refugee governance. *Geopolitics*, 23 (1), 217–243.

Anner, M. 2020. Abandoned? The impact of Covid-19 on workers and businesses at the bottom of global garment supply chains. *Centre for Global Workers' Rights*. https://www.workersrights.org/wp-content/uploads/2020/03/Abandoned-Penn-State-WRC-Report-March-27-2020.pdf [Accessed 3 April 2020].

Bain, M. 2018. Two garment factory disasters a century apart show how globalization has sapped labor's power. *Quartz*, 25 April. https://qz.com/1255041/two-garment-factory-disasters-a-century-apart/ [Accessed 10 December 2020].

Barnett, C., et al., 2010. *Globalizing responsibility: The political rationalities of ethical consumption*. West Sussex: Wiley-Blackwell.

Bartley, T., et al., 2015. *Looking behind the label*. Bloomington: Indiana UP.

Bhavnani, K., 2019. *Climate futures: re-imagining global climate justice*. London: Zed Books.

Bland, A., and Campbell, D. 2020. Some Leicester factories stayed open and forced staff to come in, report warns. *The Guardian*, 30 June. https://www.theguardian.com/uk-news/2020/jun/30/some-leicester-factories-stayed-open-and-forced-staff-to-come-in [Accessed 16 July 2020].

Business and Human Rights Resource Centre. 2020a. COVID-19 action tracker. *Business and Human Rights Resource Centre*. https://covid19.business-humanrights.org/en/tracker/ [Accessed 21 June 2020].

Business and Human Rights Resource Centre. 2020b. COVID-19 action tracker: Bangladesh. *Business and Human Rights Resource Centre*, 10 December. https://www.business-humanrights.org/en/from-us/covid-19-action-tracker/bangladesh/ [Accessed 10 December 2020].

Business and Human Rights Resource Centre. 2020c. Major fashion brands record profits while vulnerable workers languish in poverty. *Business and Human Rights Resource Centre*, 11 November. https://www.business-humanrights.org/en/from-us/media-centre/major-fashion-brands-record-profits-while-vulnerable-workers-languish-in-poverty/ [Accessed 10 December].

Business of Fashion and McKinsey & Co. 2020. *The State of Fashion 2021*.

Change.org. 2020. #PayUp Petition. https://www.change.org/p/unless-gap-primark-c-a-payup-millions-of-garment-makers-will-go-hungry [Accessed 4 July 2020].

Davey, J. 2020. Asos sees quadrupling of profit on strong pandemic demand. *Business of Fashion*, 14 October. https://www.businessoffashion.com/articles/retail/asos-sees-quadrupling-of-profit-on-strong-pandemic-demand [Accessed 10 December 2020].

De Maria, B., 2008. Neo-colonialism through measurement: a critique of the corruption perception index. *Critical perspectives on international business*, 4 (2/3), 184–202.

Debter, L. 2019. The world's largest apparel companies 2019: Dior remains on top, Lululemon and Foot Locker gain ground. *Forbes*, 15 May. https://www.forbes.com/sites/laurendebter/2019/05/15/worlds-largest-apparel-companies-2019/#28315fcc390a [Accessed 25 July 2020].

Ethical Clothing Australia. 2020. #WEWEARAUSTRALIAN ... , Instagram, 22 April. https://www.instagram.com/p/B_RbWcVg2cN/ [Accessed 21 December 2020].

Fitz-Henry, E., 2012. Rethinking 'remoteness': The space-time of corporate causation. In: G. Hage, and R. Eckersley, ed. *Responsibility*. Melbourne: Melbourne University Press, 174–186.

Fitzpatrick, L. 2020. Coronavirus and the underserved: we are not all in this together. *Forbes*, 2 April. https://www.forbes.com/sites/lisafitzpatrick/2020/04/02/covid-19-and-the-underserved-we-are-not-all-in-this-together/#4ce654ba5a71 [Accessed 18 July 2020].

Gaztambide-Fernández, R. 2020. What is solidarity? During coronavirus and always, it's more than 'we're all in this together'. *The Conversation*, 14 April. https://theconversation.com/what-is-solidarity-during-coronavirus-and-always-its-more-than-were-all-in-this-together-135002 [Accessed 18 July 2020].

Gibson-Graham, J., 2008. Diverse economies: performative practices for 'other worlds'. *Progress in human geography*, 32 (5), 613–632.

Goodman, M., 2004. Reading fair trade: political ecological imaginary and the moral economy of fair trade foods. *Political geography*, 23 (7), 891–915.

Guarnieri, M. 2020. Stop saying 'we're all in this together'. You have money. It's not the same. *The Washington Post*, 18 April. https://www.washingtonpost.com/outlook/2020/04/18/coronavirus-retail-jobs-inequality/ [Accessed 18 July 2020].

Guterres, A. 2020. We are all in this Together: Human Rights and COVID-19 Response and Recovery. *United Nations*, 23 April. https://www.un.org/en/un-coronavirus-communications-team/we-are-all-together-human-rights-and-covid-19-response-and [Accessed 18 July 2020].

Hacking, I., 1982. Biopower and the avalanche of printed numbers. *Humanities in society*, 5 (3-4), 279–295.

Haq, R. 2020. Corona: BGMEA President deliver Massages to International Buyers to stay with Bangladesh RMG. *YouTube*, 23 March. https://www.youtube.com/watch?v=iwB6vlTvdgg [Accessed 29 March 2020].

Horton, K., 2018. Just use what you have: ethical fashion discourse and the feminisation of responsibility. *Australian feminist studies*, 33 (98), 515–529.

Industriall. 2020. COVID-19 – an existential crisis for the garment industry. *Industriall Global Union*, 23 March. http://www.industriall-union.org/covid-19-an-existential-crisis-for-the-garment-industry 23 March 2020. [Accessed 21 June 2020].

International Labour Organisation. 2020. COVID-19: Action in the global garment industry, 22 April. https://www.ilo.org/wcmsp5/groups/public/—ed_dialogue/—dialogue/documents/statement/wcms_742371.pdf [Accessed 1 June 2020].

Jackson, S.J., Bailey, M., and Foucault Welles, B., 2020. *#Hashtag activism: networks of race and gender justice*. Cambridge, Massachusetts: MIT Press.

Jane, E. 2020. How to support your local designers amid Covid-19. *Russh*, 14 April. https://www.russh.com/supporting-australian-fashion-designers-coronavirus/ [Accessed 30 June 2020].

Kelly, A. 2020. Primark and Matalan among retailers allegedly cancelling £2.4bn orders in 'catastrophic' move for Bangladesh. *The Guardian*, 2 April. https://www.theguardian.com/global-development/2020/apr/02/fashion-brands-cancellations-of-24bn-orders-catastrophic-for-bangladesh [Accessed 12 April 2020].

Khan, R., 2019. 'Be creative' in Bangladesh? Mobility, empowerment and precarity in ethical fashion enterprise. *Cultural studies*, 33 (6), 1029–1049.

Le Baron, G., Lister, J., and Dauvergne, P., 2017. Governing global supply chain sustainability through the ethical audit regime. *Globalizations*, 14 (6), 958–975.

Legesse, K. 2020. Racism is at the heart of fast fashion – it's time for change. *The Guardian*. 11 June. https://www.theguardian.com/global-development/2020/jun/11/racism-is-at-the-heart-of-fast-fashion-its-time-for-change [Accessed 11 December 2020].

Lewis, M. 2020. Opinion: Big brands have mistreated their workers throughout the Covid-19 crisis. *Thomson Reuters Foundation News*, 13 November. https://news.trust.org/item/20201113123916-2hj8y/ [Accessed 7 December 2020].

Mason, P. 2020. Will coronavirus signal the end of capitalism? *Aljazeera*, 3 April. https://www.aljazeera.com/indepth/opinion/coronavirus-signal-capitalism-200330092216678.html [Accessed 30 June 2020].

Miller, L. 2020. Coronavirus outbreak hits Los Angeles Apparel with more than 300 infections, 4 employee deaths. *Los Angeles Times*, 11 July. https://www.latimes.com/california/story/2020-07-12/coronavirus-outbreak-hits-los-apparel-with-more-than-300-infections-4-employee-deaths [Accessed 12 July 2020].

Nesvig, K. 2020. Reformation Founder Yael Aflalo Resigns after Allegations of Racism. *TeenVogue*, 14 June. https://www.teenvogue.com/story/reformation-founder-yael-aflalo-apologizes-for-past-racist-behavior [Accessed 11 December 2020].

O'Connor, S. 2020. Leicester's dark factories show up a diseased system. *Financial Times*, 4 July. https://www.ft.com/content/0b26ee5d-4f4f-4d57-a700-ef49038de18c [Accessed 12 July 2020].

Ong, A., and Collier, S., 2005. *Global assemblages: technology, politics, and ethics as anthropological problems*. Oxford: Blackwell.

Patrona, M., ed. 2018. *Crisis and the media: narratives of crisis across cultural settings and media genres*. London: John Benjamins Publishing Company.

Pham, M.T. 2017. The High Cost of High Fashion. *Jacobin*, 13 June. https://www.jacobinmag.com/2017/06/fast-fashion-labor-prada-gucci-abuse-designer [Accessed 11 July 2020].

Politzer, M. 2020. 'We are on our own': Bangladesh's pregnant garment workers face the sack. *The Guardian*, 9 July. https://www.theguardian.com/global-development/2020/jul/09/we-are-on-our-own-bangladeshs-pregnant-garment-workers-face-the-sack [Accessed 24 July 2020].

Saha, P., 2019. *An empire of touch: women's Political labor and the fabrication of East Bengal*. New York: Columbia University Press.

Samman, A., 2015. Crisis theory and the historical imagination. *Review of international political economy*, 22 (5), 966–995.

Uddin, M. 2020. Why fashion must help Bangladeshi workers survive coronavirus. *Business of Fashion*, 21 March. https://www.businessoffashion.com/articles/opinion/op-ed-why-fashion-must-help-factories-and-their-workers-survive-coronavirus [Accessed 12 April 2020].

Wright, R., and Nillson, P. 2020. How Boohoo came to rule the roost in Leicester's underground textile trade. *Financial Times*, 11 July. https://www.ft.com/content/bbe5dfc5-3b5c-41d2-9637-50e91c58b26b [Accessed 23 July 2020].

Zombie capitalism and coronavirus time

Elmo Gonzaga

ABSTRACT

At the onset of the COVID-19 pandemic, essays and memes likened its social and temporal conditions to the zombie apocalypse visualized in popular media. Circulating through Facebook, Instagram, and YouTube, dystopian photos and videos of abandoned streets, plazas, and malls resonated with harrowing scenes of attacking hordes of zombies in the Netflix series *Kingdeom* (2019-2020), whose second season premiered when most Southeast Asian cities experienced lockdowns. Global news agencies reported on the unsettling anxiety about contagion from foreign migrants and tourists, from which, despite intensifying social tensions, many 'developing' or 'emerging' economies in Southeast Asia derive their vitality. If the scholarship about zombie narratives tends to focus on the docile, subjugated bodies of mass labour, critiques of neoliberal capitalism highlight their insatiable, irrational consumerism. In contrast, this article explores how the steep downturns from travel restrictions and citywide lockdowns to fight the outbreak have exposed the dependency of developmental state capitalism for its rapid pace of material growth not only on the flexibility of migrant labour but also on the contingency of speculative investment from overseas. Whereas state capitalism is typically understood to deploy its resources in protected industries and state-owned enterprises to consolidate its political rule, its use of authority now appears to centre on reducing market risk. The resilient temporality of the novel coronavirus has led to a new cyclical capitalist normalcy of surging, declining, and resurging infections, which governments have struggled to manage through varied forms of lockdown and quarantine such as Circuit Breakers (CB) in Singapore, Movement Control Orders (MCO) in Kuala Lumpur, and Enhanced Community Quarantines (ECQ) in Manila, with the failed aspiration of economic stability.

One of the biggest Netflix-produced hits on the global streaming site among Southeast Asian audiences during the novel coronavirus pandemic was *Kingdeom* (2020), a zombie thriller set during the Joseon period. Exploring the military and ethical actions to quell the spread of the zombie virus, the Netflix series narrates a conspiracy to wrest control from the legitimate

imperial successor, who has a democratic affinity for the marginalized to preserve the stability of the established order. Whereas its debut season focuses
on the self-sacrifice of ordinary heroes to safeguard vulnerable and poor villagers from hordes of attacking zombies, its second season highlights how
government ministers, who are willing to sacrifice the lives of these villagers
in their struggle for greater authority, exhibit the monstrosity of zombies. A
serial thriller that unfolds over multiple episodes, the second season first
aired in mid March when lockdowns were implemented in many Southeast
Asian cities, which forced their residents to turn to online media not only
for information and connection but also for entertainment and solace to alleviate their boredom, loneliness, and anxiety.

Millennial zombie narratives in popular media such as *28 Days Later* and *28
Weeks Later* (2002 and 2007), the *Dawn of the Dead* remake (2004), the *Resident Evil* video game (1996-) and film series (2002-2016), *The Walking Dead*
comic book (2003-2019) and television series (2010-), *World War Z* (2013),
Ojuju (2014), and *Busanhaeng* (2016), *Seoul Station* (2016), and *Bando*
(2020) are typically set in a speculative, post-apocalyptic future, where the
sudden catastrophe of a biomedical laboratory experiment gone awry
brings about the extermination of most of the world's population. Centred
on the desperate fight by the human civilization for survival without recourse
to the protection of the law, these storylines about a zombie apocalypse are
characterized by their harrowing atmosphere of anxiety, hopelessness, and
brutality.

With the onset of the pandemic, many writers likened the COVID-19 lockdowns around the world to the zombie apocalypse visualized in popular
media (Drezner 2020, Moore 2020, Teo 2020). At the beginning of the first
wave in East Asia in the weeks immediately after the 2020 Lunar New Year,
the hysteria over catching the unknown virus was shaped by the horror
among local communities that migrants and tourists might be its carriers.
In one of the more extreme examples of this hysteria, viral rumours circulated
in Malaysia that people who became exposed to these stigmatized carriers
would mutate into zombies (Star 2020). This harrowing dystopian vision resonated in photos and videos on news and social media of abandoned streets,
plazas, and malls under different forms of lockdown emptied of the characteristic congestion and bustle of megalopolises. Evoking scenes of the desperate survivors of a zombie apocalypse ransacking supermarket shelves like
ravenous monsters, Hong Kong artist Tommy Fung shared a digital image
on his Instagram account #surrealhk of hordes of pro-democracy protesters
scrambling upward for scarce surgical masks. As the measures to fight contagion varied across national governments, memes spread on Facebook and
YouTube equating leaders with authoritarian aspirations to the zombie
emperor in *Kingdeom* whose dominion meets its limit against the unpredictable temporality of the virus.

In the early phase of the pandemic, the virus was believed to originate from overseas, leading to irrational physical and verbal violence against individuals with seemingly 'foreign' features. The fear of foreign migrants and tourists translated to demands by local citizens for their governments to tighten border restrictions, which would safeguard the community. After the Philippines' Inter-Agency Task Force for the Management of Emerging Infectious Diseases (IATF) abruptly barred all overseas contract workers and permanent residents from departing in early 2020, angry rumours spread in their StrandedPH Facebook page about the continued arrival of ghost flights from Mainland China bringing illegal workers for Philippine Offshore Gaming Operators (POGO), which had been established by the Duterte government to cater to overseas Chinese-language consumers (Robles 2020). While press conferences of Singapore's People's Action Party 4G (fourth-generation) leaders emphasized the safety of the 'community' in fighting contagion, news reports (Cai and Lai 2020) and opinion essays (Stark 2020) noted that approximately 90% of the total infections in the city–state had been contained by quarantining transient construction workers from India and Bangladesh in cramped, unsanitary dormitories. Amid a surge in pro-democracy protests against the institutional abuse of authority, a new wave of the novel coronavirus in Thailand was murderously blamed by Prime Minister Prayut Chan-o-cha, leader of its military junta, on migrants from Myanmar, who constitute two-thirds of the foreign workforce, for their purported illegal border crossings (Apinya *et al.* 2020).

Situating the proliferation of zombie narratives amid the intensification of neoliberal capitalism at the turn of the millennium, Jean and John Comaroff (2002) write that the increased mobility of transnational flows of finances and bodies has deepened anxieties over the entry of foreign capital and labour into national economies. The demographics of inequality between local citizens and migrant workers had already produced simmering social tensions in many East Asian cities whose national economies rested on global investment, tourism, and migration for their material growth. Faced with the imminent physical degeneration and mortality of rapidly aging populations, so-called 'advanced industrialized' economies such as the PRC, Japan, South Korea, Taiwan, Hong Kong, and Singapore have grown increasingly dependent for their prosperity on the affective corporeality of migrant labour, especially in their healthcare and service sectors. Because of their lack of job opportunities for young graduates, the 'developing' or 'emerging' economies of Indonesia, Vietnam, Thailand, Myanmar, and the Philippines have accordingly become reliant on the remittances of migrants who are systematically trained and deployed by their governments for work overseas. Among urban residents across Southeast Asia, such anxieties are shaped by the racialized resentment that not only wealthy overseas investors are causing property prices to soar but also low-wage migrant workers are causing job opportunities to shrink.

This intensifying unease about migration is tied to the increasing flexibility of labour. While the steep downturns from COVID-19 lockdowns revealed state capitalism's dependence for its pace of growth on the discrepant temporalities of global investment and migration, they highlighted the rise of the gig economy, which supplies digital transportation, shopping, and delivery platforms through flexible, precarious arrangements of work and service. Already struggling to manage the volatility of global markets and flows, national governments must confront the disruption brought by the gig economy to their protected industries and entrenched regulations. Against the backdrop of zombie cubicles and classrooms, the virus unsettled the established order of institutional bureaucracies by speeding up the passage to the incorporeal instantaneity of digitalization. The materiality and vitality of metropolises rest on the routine and bustle of everyday life, in which residents repeatedly perform life-sustaining activities such as commuting to the office, buying groceries, dining in a restaurant, and watching television. As businesses and schools shifted to conferencing platform Zoom for online meetings amid complaints of a loss in the privacy and immediacy of personal interaction, urban residents fearful about physical contact could easily obtain their daily necessities through smartphone apps such as Lazada, Food Panda, Deliveroo, and GrabFood with door-to-door delivery services. Arlie Hochschild (2012) writes about how individuals have compartmentalized and outsourced the routine activities of their everyday life to other, more precarious workers. Because of the growing congestion and traffic in flourishing Southeast Asian cities, these smartphone apps have become vital for restoring the normative operation of capitalist society. Confined to the fragile safety of their homes, residents must rely for their daily life-sustaining tasks on the vulnerable labour and mobility of low-income and ethnic-minority groups without access to citizenship rights, whose corporeal exposure to contagion serves as a proxy for theirs.

Most of the scholarship about zombie narratives dwells on the docile, subjugated bodies of mass labour. Discussions of capitalism tend to equate zombification with an insatiable, irrational consumerism (Lauro 2017). But zombification could likewise act as a framework for comprehending the parasitic relationship of state capitalism with speculative investment. Critiques of neoliberal globalization unveil how developmental states rely heavily for their material growth on overseas money, which can quickly withdraw if their political and financial fortunes suddenly change. Denoting the undead, which subsist by feeding on the corporeality of living organisms, the trope of the zombie has been used to describe human and non-human entities that continue to exist despite having lost their agency or vitality under the precarious conditions of neoliberal capitalism. Analyses of the 2007–2008 global financial crisis apply the term to refer to zombie companies and organizations in post-industrial economies that were kept alive with debt restructuring despite their lack of productivity, efficiency, or innovation because of their entrenchment in the capitalist system (McNally 2011, p. 1). Alternately, the metaphor of zombie capitalism could be taken to index the uncertainties of development in a volatile global market. Ethnographies about the sudden appearance of the uncanny in Southeast Asian economies typically examine the proliferation of rumours about spirit possessions in modern factories in Selangor (Ong 1987) and spectral hauntings in abandoned skyscrapers in Chiang Mai (Johnson 2014), which reveal a consciousness of the monstrous uncontrollability of the imminent arrival of neoliberal capitalism. In Thai cities, for example, ghost stories that proliferated during the 1997 Asian Financial Crisis illustrate how the order and stability that material growth is supposed to deliver can engender unsettling anxiety about its inevitable catastrophe.

To harness volatile global flows for their national development, so-called emerging economies created Free Trade Zones and Special Economic Zones, which would serve as nodes of manufacturing and assembly in transnational supply chains. Singapore's state capitalism has offered a successful, legible model of economic and material growth with its aggressive, interventionist control over its free market and public sphere. Extolled by international news organizations and policy institutes for enabling Asian Tiger Economies to achieve prosperity at a rapid pace, state capitalism is defined by the strong, overarching authority of the national government to invest its resources in protected industries and state-owned enterprises. No longer strictly defined by a centrally planned economy to boost industrial production, millennial state capitalism, contrary to Bremmer (2010), now appears to deploy its authority less to consolidate its political rule than to reduce its market risk. Having fed on the economical, disempowered corporeality of migrant labour to speed up its pace of growth, governments reliant on state capitalism for their development have been confronted by the anxiety and precarity at its core.

Whereas precarity is typically understood to denote the economic, social, and psychological instability of workers without regular income and career mobility (Berlant 2010), it could likewise refer to the financial and political instability at the core of national sovereignty under neoliberal capitalism. Feeding on the precarious mobility of flows of migration and money, state capitalism could be regarded as zombieseque in how it derives its vitality from the tenuous, fugitive presence of transitory labour and speculative investment. Championing the exceptionalism of an elite vanguard of leaders based on a given race, religion, class, or origin, state capitalism is fearful of cultural and political difference, whose unpredictability and recalcitrance must be suppressed for it to achieve the rapid, linear temporality of material development.

In the first year of the pandemic, the novel coronavirus introduced a discrepant temporality to the workings, processes, and rhythms of Southeast Asian cities, especially among those that experienced the longest lockdowns. Vacillating between economic vitality and human mortality, governments have weighed the costs of prolonged social restrictions or temporary citywide lockdowns to maintain the linear pace of growth. On the expected restoration of capitalist normalcy, governments and businesses have been compelled to take on more debt to survive with a borrowed corporeality. Discussion threads on social networks entertained the assumption that the pandemic would be under control by the summer of 2020 just as the desperate survivors in *Kingdeom* mistakenly waited for the zombie virus to be rendered inactive in the heat of the daytime sun. Faced with multiple waves of outbreaks through the hot and wet seasons, urban residents have been forced to adjust to the new normative temporality of recurrent cycles of lockdown, reopening, lockdown, reopening, and lockdown. Akin to Malaysian cities' Enhanced Movement Control Order (EMCO), Semi Enhanced Movement Control Order (SEMCO), Conditional Movement Control Order (CMCO), and Recovery Movement Control Order (RMCO), the Philippines' financial capitals and coronavirus hotspots Manila and Cebu have experienced an amalgam of General Community Quarantines (GCQ), Modified General Community Quarantines (MGCQ), Enhanced Community Quarantines (ECQ), Extreme Enhanced Community Quarantines (EECQ), and Modified Enhanced Community Quarantines (MECQ), which have been interchangeably imposed, lifted, and reimposed without an overarching, rational framework for conquering the virus.

The zombie narratives that circulated through popular and viral media in Southeast Asian cities during the COVID-19 pandemic have been resonant less for visualizing the fear of contagion from migrant labour than for uncovering the precarity of sovereignty under state capitalism. Memes posted and shared in social networks with hashtags such as #nasaanangpangulo (#whereisthepresident) joked about how Duterte's shrunken, ashen visage, kept alive by fentanyl injections, mimicked *Kingdeom*'s zombie emperor (Dimaculangan 2020). Amid accusations of incompetent leadership and unbridled corruption, the Philippine government adopted the tagline #laginghanda (#alwaysprepared) to conjure the tenuous impression that it was in control of the crisis. It is this analogous backdrop of contagion and catastrophe from an uncontrollable outbreak in which the *Kingdeom*'s conspirators keep alive a zombie emperor so that the hollow, decaying visage of his authority would prolong the borrowed stability of an imminent capitalist normalcy.

Disclosure statement

No potential conflict of interest was reported by the author(s).

Further information

This Special Issue article has been comprehensively reviewed by the Special Issue editors, Associate Professor Ted Striphas and Professor John Nguyet Erni.

References

Apinya, W., Wassana, N., and Pencham, C. 2020. We cannot stop them all. *Bangkok Post*, December 22. Available from: https://www.bangkokpost.com/thailand/general/2039171/we-cannot-stop-them-all.

Berlant, L., 2010. *Cruel optimism*. Durham, NC: Duke University Press.

Bremmer, I., 2010. *The end of the free market: who wins the war between states and corporations?* New York: Portfolio.

Cai, W., and Lai, K.K.R. 2020. Packed with migrant workers, dormitories fuel coronavirus in Singapore [online]. *New York Times*, April 28. Available from: https://www.nytimes.com/interactive/2020/04/28/world/asia/coronavirus-singapore-migrants.html.

Comaroff, J., and Comaroff, J., 2002. Zombies, immigrants, and millennial capitalism. *South atlantic quarterly*, 101 (4), 780–805.

Dimaculangan, J. 2020. Netizens draw analogy between Netflix's Kingdom and COVID-19 crisis [online]. *PEP.ph*, March 15. Available from: https://www.pep.ph/guide/tv/150075/netizens-draw-analogy-between-netflix-s-kingdom-and-covid-19-crisis-a2670-20200315.

Drezner, D.W. 2020. What I learned about coronavirus world from watching zombie flicks. *Foreign Policy*, April 11. Available from: https://foreignpolicy.com/2020/04/11/what-i-learned-about-coronavirus-world-from-zombie-movies/.

Hochschild, A.R., 2012. *The outsourced self: intimate life in market times*. New York: Metropolitan Books.

Johnson, A.A., 2014. *Ghosts of the new city: spirits, urbanity, and the ruins of progress in Chiang Mai*. Honolulu: University of Hawaii Press.

Lauro, S.L., 2017. *Zombie theory: a reader*. Minneapolis: University of Minnesota Press.

McNally, D., 2011. *Monsters of the market: zombies, vampires, and global capitalism*. Leiden: Brill.

Moore, L. 2020. Experiencing the coronavirus pandemic as a kind of zombie apocalypse [online]. *New Yorker*, April 6. Available from: https://www.newyorker.com/magazine/2020/04/13/the-nurses-office.

Ong, A., 1987. *Spirits of resistance and capitalist discipline: factory women in Malaysia*. Albany, NY: State University of New York Press.

Robles, A. 2020. Coronavirus: travel ban keeps up to 30,000 Filipinos away from Hong Kong jobs [online]. *South China Morning Post*, February 17. Available from: https://

www.scmp.com/week-asia/economics/article/3051002/coronavirus-travel-ban-keeps-30000-filipino-workers-away-hong.

Star. 2020. Oh, please! – coronavirus won't turn you into a 'zombie', says Malaysia [online]. February 2. Available from: www.thestar.com.my/news/regional/2020/02/02/oh-please—coronavirus-won039t-turn-you-into-a-039zombie039-says-malaysia.

Stark, M.K. 2020. A sudden coronavirus surge brought out Singapore's dark side [online]. *New York Times*, May 20. Available from: https://www.nytimes.com/2020/05/20/magazine/singapore-coronavirus.html.

Teo, Y.Y. 2020. In this zombie apocalypse, your homework is due at 5pm [online]. *Academia.SG*. April 9. Available from: www.academia.sg/academic-views/in-this-zombie-apocalypse-your-homework-is-due-at-5pm/.

No time for fun: the politics of partying during a pandemic

Nicholas Holm ⓘ

ABSTRACT

In 2020, in the face of the unparalleled epidemiological threat posed by Covid-19, multiple governments around the world sought to contain the spread of the virus by imposing strict lockdown measures that dramatically limited the movement and gathering of citizens. Not only did these restrictions severely curtail the regular patterns of economic, political and cultural life, they also made it very hard to *have fun*. While this last point may appear flippant, this article proposes that a proper accounting for fun is absolutely necessary if we are to understand not just the challenges passed by lockdown measures, but also the legal and biomedical risks people were willing to take to engage in activities like hosting parties, surfing and attending raves, during a pandemic. Arguing against the idea of fun as a form of displaced political practice, I instead suggest that fun is best understood as an example of contingent, non-transcendent aesthetic value that is absolutely central to everyday desire and the appeal of popular culture. Often easy to overlook, the experience of lockdown brought the appeal and importance of fun into sharp relief in ways that point towards the powerful role fun plays in shaping our lives both during a pandemic and (hopefully) after.

In response to the growing threat of the global Covid-19 pandemic, on 25 March 2020, Aotearoa New Zealand entered into what was, by many accounts, the most stringent lockdown in the over-developed world (Blavatnik School 2020; Douglas 2020). With only two days' notice, almost all residents were confined to their homes for what would turn out to be just over a month. They were only allowed to venture out for groceries and medical supplies, and to engage in exercise in their local areas. Once it became apparent that this strong and swift action had enabled the island nation to not only 'flatten the curve', but actually to begin a process that would see the first wave of active infections eliminated by early June, the actions of the New Zealand population and its leadership were subject to extensive praise and coverage in a range of global media outlets (Baggaley 2020; BBC 2020; Brockett 2020; Conforti 2020).

In contrast, local defiance of the lockdown orders received relatively little international attention, although it was the subject of acute concern, even conniptions, in local news media. Reports of private parties, social mixing and casual sports stoked furious commentary and public outrage (Alves, 2020; Manch 2020; Ritchie 2020). The general opinion seemed to regard such behaviour as inconsiderate at best, treacherous at worst in the context of wider sacrifices being made. A website, established to allow New Zealanders to report suspected breaches of lockdown to police, crashed due to high demand (RNZ 2020). This anger was only compounded by ambiguities in official guidelines regarding travel limits and sanctioned behaviour. Was swimming allowed? What about surfing? (No, and no, it would turn out) (Leahy 2020). Was it acceptable to drive to a nearby park or beach for exercise? (No, said the Police commissioner. Perhaps, said the Prime Minister) (Geddis, 2020; Sadler 2020). When hunting was initially prohibited, exemptions were sought for those groups who engaged in hunting for subsistence, rather than recreation (Hurihanginui 2020). The overarching theme of these decisions appeared to be that New Zealanders could only leave lockdown for the serious business of maintaining the basics of biological life: woe betide those who appeared to take pleasure in their exercise or provision. Best not to smile while out for your daily constitutional.

Moreover, Aotearoa New Zealand was not alone in witnessing such conflicts around the limits of officially sanctioned behaviour imposed against the backdrop of surging global death counts. In neighbouring Australia, Sydney's famous Bondi Beach became the centre of national concern and anger as surfers and swimmers were reported scaling fences in order to access the ocean after barricades were erected (Doherty 2020). When the beach reopened and the fences were removed, the surf breaks became so crowded that distancing measures became impossible (BBC 2020b). In the UK, as the pandemic continued to rage in June, police cracked down on illegal raves held in contravention of social distancing guidelines (Grant and Okpattah 2020). As the global death count climbed, particular ire seemed reserved for those who prioritized their personal pleasure over epidemiological solidarity.

No doubt many factors are at play in such conflicts over permissible behaviours: not least longstanding tensions over race and class tied up with practices such as surfing and raves (McRobbie 1994; Gilbert and Pearson 1999; Hough-Snee and Sotelo Eastman 2017). However, such debates also point towards an often-overlooked aspect of our social and cultural lives: the idea, the experience, the desire that we call *fun*. Even amidst the spectre of global death and collapsing health systems, evidence of a desire for fun persisted in both discrete and disruptive ways. On the one hand, there has been a constant low-level concern with what it might mean *to have fun* under quarantine conditions: from the novel phenomenon of the Zoom party and online workout classes to the booming fortunes of streaming and video game industries and beyond. More dramatically, on the other hand, the idea of fun also informed many instances of determined opposition to official declarations and state edicts. From the defiant surfers at Sydney's Bondi Beach to police crackdowns on private parties in Aotearoa New Zealand, the pull of fun would seem to be such that it can motivate citizens to defy the will of the state and even risk exposure to a potentially fatal illness. By limiting and distorting the ways and means by which people were accustomed to experiencing fun, stay-at-home and lockdown orders paradoxically made fun, and the ways in which the pull of fun shapes our everyday life, more visible.

The desire for fun during a pandemic will likely strike many as inappropriate or irresponsible, even inhuman. In legal and biomedical terms, the strictures of lockdown orders and the facts of disease transmission effectively forbade almost all those forms of social contact associated with fun. Meanwhile, on a moral level, it would seem indecent to seek out frivolous enjoyment while others are dying or engaging in the grim business of trying to prevent others from dying. Even though this simultaneity is an inescapable fact of the human condition at any time, the ever-present awareness of covid-19 brought into sharp relief the uneven distribution of access to fun. Essential workers of all stripes – from health professionals to low-wage stockers of supermarket shelves – were compelled to labour under conditions widely perceived to put them at risk of infection, while others suffered extreme material hardship as the economy collapsed and businesses closed. At a time when others suffer or are subject to undue risk, fun can certainly seem inappropriate. However, although lockdown was certainly not widely regarded as the time for having fun, *fun* can nonetheless help us make sense of popular responses that defied the predictions of both economic and epidemiological models. In doing so, such an investigation also sheds light on the wider and often taken-for-granted role of fun under the regular conditions of taken-for-granted consumer capitalism. Thus, while the idea of fun might seem a world away from the realities of life during a pandemic, the rapid social transformations implemented in response to Covid-19 instanced a deep, powerful and widely distributed desire for fun.

Even during the best of times, fun can seem like a trivial concern. *Fun* is not only a deeply complex and contested term; it is also fundamentally ineffable. Attempts to nail down or reduce fun to an expression of popular politics or a manipulative concoction of the culture industry risk neglecting the term's apparent lightness. Consequently, it is almost by definition difficult to take fun seriously, and harder still to discuss it in any sustained and rigorous way. This difficulty perhaps goes some way to explaining the term's relative absence in cultural studies, even as related terms such as *pleasure, jouissance,* and *play* have been the subjects of extensive consideration in the field's history (if not as much in recent years) (c.f. Bahktin 1984; Stallybrass and White 1986; de Certeau 1988; Stam 1989; Radway 1991; Harris 1992). As Joanna Zylinska notes, 'fun' is one of those terms that threatens to evoke the 'cultural studies bashing' attitudes of infamous figures like Alan Sokal and Richard Dawkins (2005, p. 26–28). Fun thus functions as something of a limit case: a topic that is potentially too 'embarrassing'. To speak of fun would seem to risk presenting oneself for ridicule and rejection. And yet, the desire that we call fun is an ever-present and often powerful part of our lives: at once the ostensible output of multibillion-dollar media industries, and a powerful object of individual desire that drives everyday sociability and communal experience (Fincham 2016; McKee 2016). Fun sits at the heart of our affective lives in highly mediated contexts as a means by which popular legitimacy, desirability and taste are produced and contested.

Extant studies of fun, predominantly situated in the behavioural sciences, tend to conceive of it in fundamentally apolitical terms: as a desirable but minor form of social experience that can be applied to the instrumental ends of motivation and social integration, or codified as a set of media design principles (Roy 1959; McManus 2010; De Koven, 2013; Blythe and Monk 2018). What such behaviourist models fail to account for, however, is the paradoxical nature of fun. Although almost by definition without conse- quence, the desire, the drive, the appeal of fun is such that, in practice, it can become deeply consequential. This meaningfulness of fun was on full display as large sections of the global population become subject to lockdown orders, or local variants. Under such conditions, fun would appear to be of extremely minimal importance in the face of epidemiological, economic, and even existential threats. And yet, even amidst the spectre of global death and collapsing health systems, commentators yearned publicly for a return to everyday practices and experiences of passing human contact, unburdened movement, and diverse forms of consumption: not only because of the economic benefit associated with the 're-opening' of society, but also because of a deep desire for the pleasures of everyday life. As noted above, some people were even willing to defy public health and police notices in order to experience the fun of communal gathering and physical movement. In this context, fun emerges as an intense desire for what would customarily be regarded as the non-meaningful or the non- serious, the ostensibly trivial and the flippant. Under such circumstances, inherited distinctions between that which is serious and that which is not begin to become shaky, if not untenable.

What such disruptive fun-seeking behaviour demonstrates is how fun can mark particular instances of culture and social life as simultaneously worth- while and potentially trivial, both deeply important and absolutely unimpor- tant at the same time. Accounting for this paradox is the key to understanding how fun functions as a fundamental and deeply consequential source of both social attraction and repulsion: that is, as a force that motivates particular practices, communities, and relationships. In doing so, fun reaches out beyond the limits of recreation and entertainment, such that the promise and possible pleasures of fun become drivers of socially and politically mean-ingful behaviour. This does not mean that fun is inherently progressive or reactionary, but simply that it is implicated in some of the most pressing pol-itical questions of our moment in ways that demand attention.

For example, it is fun, I am arguing here, that informed unexpected instances of resistance to biomedical discipline and regulation during lock-down orders. While much of the formal debate surrounding the desirability of lockdown was couched in terms of economics versus public health, it would be a stretch to attribute the bio-medically defiant actions of surfers, ravers or illicit partiers to purely or even primarily economic concerns. Although there are certainly economic interests tied up with such activities, they are not reducible to them. To argue that ravers rave in spite of stay-at-home orders because they have been conned into doing so by profit-seeking organizers, or that surfers are the pawns of Big Surf, is to reductively characterize the motivations of those subcultures and surrounding econom-ies: it is to deny the agency of the participants so deeply as to slip from a model of false consciousness into misanthropy.

Nor does it make particular sense to attribute the choice to surf or rave or party to a desire to express political opposition to stay-at-home orders through indirect social or cultural means. Such an argument would be fam-iliar to those conversant with those forms of populist cultural studies ascen-dant in the 1980s and 1990s, where 'resistance' to the dominant order could be found in innumerable acts of popular consumption, display, and amateur production (Fiske 2011; Jenkins 2013). However, although forms of prohibited behaviour like partying no doubt acted as indirect challenges to the hegemo-nic consensus under lockdown conditions – particularly in Aotearoa, New Zealand, where the commonsense acceptance of the public health paradigm reigned almost unchallenged – the context of those actions here mitigates an emphatically political reading. In contrast to the USA, where protestors openly declared their opposition to lockdown orders as an impingement of their freedom (DeBrabander 2020), those who took part in clandestine socia-lizing or swimming were almost always attempting to conceal rather than publicize their actions. They relied on neighbours and passers-by to turn a blind eye, rather than escalate the response to their situation. Such reticence challenges any assumption that these are best understood as purposively agonistic communicative actions, instead suggesting that their motivations were private and directed inwards, rather than performative (to the extent that such a distinction makes sense). Thus, while such behaviour certainly has wider ramifications in terms of the negotiation and contestation of

state power in unusual times, I suggest that their motivation is best characterized not as obliquely political or self-deceptively economic, but instead
as a desire for fun as an end in itself.

Fun is usually understood as a self-sufficient justification for engaging in an
activity or behaviour: as in the idea of 'doing something for fun' (McKee 2016,
p. 29–40). To understand fun as something that is desired as an end in itself is
potentially to characterize it as 'autonomous': a term that is historically more
closely associated with the study of art rather than popular entertainment. An
autonomous account of art and artistic practice conceives of them as motivated and directed towards their own internal ends, as opposed to a heter-
onomous conception that regards art as either determined by or directed
towards the conditions of its production (Rancière 2011). However, fun is
not autonomous in this sense: it does not mark a transcendent break with
its social and cultural context. Rather, fun is absolutely bound up with and
shaped by the concrete conditions, the economic and social muck and stink
of the environment in which it is found. In foundational aesthetic terms, fun
aligns more closely with what Immanuel Kant called the 'agreeable': a term
against which he then defined the more promising and powerful notion of
'beauty' (2000, p. 91–98). It is Kant's beauty which has since captured
almost all attention of those who seek to understand the political force of cultural work. Beauty has formed the basis of a critical aesthetic theory that seeks
to understand the political relevance of art and cultural expression through
reference to the negation of everyday interests and investments in favour of
transcendence (Brown 2019). In contrast, fun points towards a different
model of critical aesthetics: one that is non-transcendent, but rather firmly
rooted in the material limits of the everyday. Like beauty, fun is purposeless;
but unlike beauty, fun is not alien to the everyday. Fun lacks the redeeming
sense of social status or betterment that has historically attached itself to
that privileged category of beauty, and as a result, it perhaps carries less
baggage, less sense of Bourdiuesian distinction and pretension (Bourdieu
1984). To paraphrase Raymond Williams, fun is ordinary (2014).

Fun is also terrifying. It not only opens one up to charges of being overly
concerned with that which is *really, actually* trivial, it also refuses to sit neatly
within established models of cultural theory. This is almost certainly the
reason why cultural and critical studies have had no time for fun: a
concept that is deeply rooted in everyday life and popular experience.
However, this is also exactly the reason why the varied experiences of fun
during lockdown conditions are so important: they sharpen attention to
the too often overlooked importance of fun in explaining the motivations,
priorities and decisions of our everyday lives as they relate to questions of cultural consumption, social interaction, and community engagement. Lockdown conditions revealed how important fun is, and how necessary it is
that we take fun into account when trying to explain the consequences

and complications of topics like everyday life and popular culture, or perhaps even when formulating public health policy. Illegal parties and forbidden surfing were undeniably tied up with the forging, negotiating and challenging of hegemonic consensus but cannot be easily understood as politically motivated or directed in any straightforward way. These instances were not primarily indirect statements about the role of the state: they were expressions of the continued pull of fun under dramatically changed circumstances.

To claim that people took part in these activities because they *were fun* is thus to begin to find a way to acknowledge how those actions had political meaning – that they constituted a meaningful intervention in relation to the exercise of authority under largely unprecedented conditions of biomedical regulation – without reducing them to overt political statements. In place of the familiar terms such as *transgression*, *resistance*, and *discipline*, the experience of fun-during-lockdown provides examples of how everyday behaviours and popular culture can constitute forms of meaningful action without being reduced to simply the practice of politics by other means. This is a political aesthetics of texts and practices that are desirable and enjoyable, but that do not mark a profound break with established ideology or epistemology: a cultural politics of the ordinary and the agreeable, in order to complement the well-established cultural politics of the radical and the transcendent. Nor is this simply a lesson for a world in lockdown. Looking beyond a world shaped by the demands and priorities of epidemiological response, making time for fun will enable us to account for new and different ways in which politics is being done: from the utopian impulse of Acid Corbynism to the gleeful disrespect at the heart of the alt-right and the rise of a new class of comedian-politicians (Nagle 2017; Fisher 2018; Milburn 2019). Drawing on an established tradition in cultural studies (Williams 1988), we might therefore even consider *fun* a 'keyword' for pandemic, and hopefully post-pandemic, times: a way to reimagine how we account for political force of popular culture and everyday life. Before and after a world in lockdown, there is a pressing need to attend to the ways in which fun has become entangled in our political lives: not only informing new forms of political action and association, but also potentially altering broader ideas of what politics is, and of how it can and should work.

Disclosure statement

No potential conflict of interest was reported by the author(s).

Further information

This Special Issue article has been comprehensively reviewed by the Special Issue editors, Associate Professor Ted Striphas and Professor John Nguyet Erni.

ORCID

Nicholas Holm ⓘ http://orcid.org/0000-0003-0391-939X

References

Alves, V. 31 Mar 2020. Why we should be mindful of dobbing in our neighbours. *Stuff.co.nz*. Available from: https://www.nzherald.co.nz/nz/news/article.cfm?c_id=1&objectid=12321036.
Baggaley, K. 10 June 2020. What we can learn from New Zealand's successful fight against COVID-19. *Popular Science*. Available from: https://www.popsci.com/story/health/new-zealand-coronavirus-eliminated/.
Bakhtin, M. 1984. *Rabelais and his World*. Trans. Iswolsky, H. Bloomington: Indiana University Press.
BBC. 8 June 2020. New Zealand lifts all Covid restrictions, declaring the nation virus-free. *BBC*. Available from: https://www.bbc.com/news/world-asia-52961539.
BBC. 9 April 2020b. Surfing: Coronavirus lockdown advice leaves room for confusion. *BBC*. Available from: https://www.bbc.com/news/world-australia-52225031.
Blavatnik School of Government. 2020. Coronovirus Government Response Tracker. *University of Oxford*. https://www.bsg.ox.ac.uk/research/research-projects/coronavirus-government-response-tracker.
Blythe, M., and Monk, A., 2018. *Funology: from usability to enjoyment*. Cham: Springer.
Bourdieu, P., 1984. *Distinction: a social critique of the judgement of taste*. Cambridge: Harvard University Press.
Brockett, M. 8 June 2020. New Zealand ends social distancing after eliminating Covid. *Bloomberg*. Available from: https://www.bloomberg.com/news/articles/2020-06-08/new-zealand-eliminates-covid-19-with-zero-active-cases-reported.
Brown, N., 2019. *Autonomy*. Durham: Duke University Press.
Conforti, K. 8 June 2020. Jacinda Ardern Says, 'Thank You, New Zealand,' as Country Crushes Coronavirus. *Forbes*. Available from: https://www.forbes.com/sites/kaeliconforti/2020/06/08/jacinda-ardern-says-thank-you-new-zealand-as-country-achieves-alert-level-1/#68e865195beb.
de Certeau, M. 1988. *The Practice of Everyday Life*. Trans. Rendall, S. Berkeley: University of California Press.
de Koven, B., 2013. *The well-played game*. Cambridge, MA: MIT Press.
DeBrabander, F. 13 May 2020. The Great Irony of America's Armed Anti-Lockdown Protesters. *The Atlantic*. Available from: https://www.theatlantic.com/ideas/archive/2020/05/guns-protesters/611560/.
Doherty, B. 22 Mar 2020. Quiet, with some defiance, as Bondi Beach succumbs to coronavirus closure. *The Guardian*. Available from: https://www.theguardian.com/

world/2020/mar/22/quiet-with-some-defiance-as-bondi-beach-succumbs-to-coron
avirus-closure.

Douglas, J. 23 May 2020. Measuring the strictness of your Lockdown: A University Boils
It Down to One Number; Researchers at Oxford University use 17 variables to
develop a 'stringency index.' *Wall Street Journal*. Available from: https://www.wsj.
com/articles/measuring-the-strictness-of-your-lockdown-a-university-boils-it-down
-to-one-number-11590246001.

Fincham, B., 2016. *The sociology of fun*. London: Palgrave MacMillan.

Fisher, M., 2018. *K-Punk*. London: Repeater Books.

Fiske, J., 2011. *Reading the popular*. New York: Routledge.

Geddis, A. 30 Mar 2020. Lockdown policing can't work well while there's still confusion
over rules. *The Spinoff*. Available from: https://thespinoff.co.nz/politics/30-03-2020/
lockdown-policing-cant-work-well-while-theres-still-confusion-over-rules/.

Gilbert, J., and Pearson, E., 1999. *Discographies: dance, music, culture and the politics of
sound*. London: Routledge.

Grant, P., and Okpattah, K. 5 June 2020. Secret raves in London 'put lives at risk.' *BBC*.
Available from: https://www.bbc.com/news/uk-52923321.

Harris, D., 1992. *From class struggle to the politics of pleasure*. London: Routledge.

Hough-Snee, D.Z., and Sotelo Eastman, A., 2017. *The critical surf studies reader*.
Durham: Duke University Press.

Hurihanginui, T. 22 Apr 2020. Whānau relying on hunting for food should have exemp-
tion – leaders. *RNZ.co.nz*. Available from: https://www.rnz.co.nz/news/te-manu-
korihi/414888/covid-19-whanau-relying-on-hunting-for-food-should-have-exempt
ion-leaders.

Jenkins, H., 2013. *Textual poachers*. New York: Routledge.

Kant, I., 2000. *Critique of the power of judgement*. Huyer, P., ed. New York: Cambridge
University Press.

Leahy, B. 5 Apr 2020. New lockdown law officially bans swimming, hunting, surfing. *NZ
Herald*. Available from: https://www.nzherald.co.nz/nz/news/article.cfm?c_id=
1&objectid=12322512.

Manch, T. 30 Mar 2020. More than 4000 reports of possible lockdown breaches in a
day. *Stuff.co.nz*. Available from: https://www.stuff.co.nz/national/health/coronav
irus/120676405/coronavirus-more-than-4000-reports-of-possible-lockdown-breach
es-in-a-day.

McKee, A., 2016. *Fun! what entertainment tells Us about living a good life*. London:
Palgrave.

McManus, I.C., and Furnham, A., 2010. "Fun, fun, fun": types of fun, attitudes to
fun, and their relation to personality and biographical factors. *Psychology*, 1 (3),
159–168.

McRobbie, A., 1994. Shut up and dance: youth culture and the changing modes of
femininity. In: A. McRobbie, ed. *Postmodernism and popular culture*. London:
Routledge, 135–154.

Milburn, K., 2019. The comedian as populist leader: postironic narratives in an age of
cynical irony. *Leadership*, 15 (2), 226–244.

Nagle, A., 2017. *Kill All normies*. London: Verso.

Radway, J., 1991. *Reading the romance: women, patriarchy and popular literature*.
Chapel Hill, NC: University of North Carolina Press.

Rancière, J., 2011. "The aesthetic revolution and its outcomes." *In*: S. Corcoran, ed.
Dissensus: On politics and aesthetics. New York: Continuum, 115–133.

Ritchie, O., 6 Apr 2020. Crusaders players caught breaking lockdown rules. *Newshub*. Avaialable from: https://www.newshub.co.nz/home/sport/2020/04/coronavirus-crusaders-players-caught-breaking-lockdown-rules.html

RNZ, 31 Mar 2020. Nearly 10,000 reports of suspected lockdown breaches made. *RNZ.co.nz*. Available from: https://www.rnz.co.nz/news/national/413052/nearly-10-000-reports-of-suspected-lockdown-breaches-made

Roy, D.F., 1959. 'Banana time': Job satisfaction and informal interaction. *Human organization*, 18, 158–168.

Sadler, R. 26 Mar 2020. Police 'absolutely discourage' all driving during lockdown that isn't Essential. *Newhub.co.nz*. Available from: https://www.newshub.co.nz/home/new-zealand/2020/03/coronavirus-police-absolutely-discourage-all-driving-during-lockdown-that-isn-t-essential.html.

Stallybrass, P., and White, A., 1986. *The politics and poetics of transgression*. Ithaca: Cornell University Press.

Stam, R., 1989. *Subversive pleasures*. Baltimore: John Hopkins University Press.

Williams, R., 1988. *Keywords*. London: Fontana Press.

Williams, R., 2014. Culture is ordinary. In: J. McGuigan, ed. *Raymond Williams on culture and society*. London: Sage, 1–18.

Zylinska, J., 2005. *The ethics of cultural studies*. London: Continuum.

Un/knowing the Pandemic

Enduring COVID-19, nevertheless

Rebecca A. Adelman

ABSTRACT

This pandemic is a season of *nevertheless*; we are exhausted from all kinds of labour, but keep labouring nevertheless. This labouring, I suggest, takes three forms: doing (the productive and reproductive labour required to sustain life through a pandemic), undoing (the tedious processes of postponing and cancelling plans, or abandoning the process of planning altogether), and not-doing (passing the time left over between doing and undoing). Of course, the particularities of our doing, undoing, and not-doing will vary by our circumstances even as we operate within these general patterns of behaviour. I want to think through these *neverthelesses* as a way of mapping orientations toward the future fractured by the pandemic, and our collective persistence despite those fractures. Under normal circumstances, doing is an expression of optimism about the future, but the pandemic has quickened the tempo and increased the frequency of disappointment and continually forecloses possibility. Undoing is tiresome and painful, the necessary labour that amounts to less than nothing, begetting a collection of losses that often remain private and invisible. Not-doing is an intensified experience of boredom, with no obvious end or relief. Against the calls, which abound in the public culture of the pandemic, to treat COVID-19 as an opportunity to cultivate resilience, I posit endurance as an alternative framework. Resilience implies a better future if only we would learn how to suffer more productively. By contrast, endurance makes no such promises but fully acknowledges all the ways we might hurt, even as it functions as the nameless capacity that carries us through our doing, undoing, and not-doing – nevertheless.

The last thing I didn't have to cancel before I had to cancel everything last spring was a mid-March backpacking trip in Shenandoah National Park. My partner and I arrived at the trail worn out, having spent the previous days frantically doing and undoing. *Doing* entailed both the productive labour demanded by our jobs and the reproductive labour of buying necessaries and otherwise making our homes pandemic-ready.[1] The primary outcome of *undoing* was a long list of cancellations and postponements as I arranged my calendar for a long stretch of *not-doing*. When all of this – a labour that was, in many ways, the opposite of labour insofar as it amounted to less than nothing – was accomplished, it seemed safe for us to spend a few nights in the backcountry. And so we went. Our hiking route took us across the peak of Hawksbill Mountain, the highest one in the park. Weighted by our packs, we were moving relatively slowly; a runner passed us a few times as he ran up to the summit and back down again. Our paths crossed again at the base, where he had stopped to catch his breath. I asked about his running; he answered that he was training for a series of races, his usual springtime routine. Shrugging, he said he was all but certain the races would be cancelled, but was continuing with his scheduled workouts nevertheless.

This pandemic is a season of *nevertheless*. We are aware that everything we might look forward to is newly precarious, but the idea of a future beckons nevertheless. We are exhausted from all kinds of labour, but keep labouring nevertheless. Perhaps our griefs are relatively small – what, after all, wouldn't pale by comparison with the staggering counts of infections, deaths, and lost jobs? – but they are lamentable nevertheless. I want to think through these *neverthelesses* as a way of mapping orientations toward a future that has been fractured by the pandemic, and our collective persistence despite this fracturing.

In a recent auto-ethnographic piece called 'Writing Pandemic Feels,' Mathew Arthur asks, 'How to write out a pandemic?' and summarily answers, 'Lately, everything comes up short' (2019–2020, p. vi). Writing this essay, I'm attempting to attend both to the universal dimensions of this moment – the *pan* in pandemic – and the recognition that it will settle on every individual in a unique way, an experience conditioned by structural patterns of inequality and privilege and the specifics of our biographies. The 'we' and the 'us' I invoke here are meant to reference our common, if disparate, inhabiting of a world remade by COVID-19 as a shared atmosphere. Ben Anderson (2014, p. 152) writes that atmospheres hold things together, if only temporarily, binding bodies, practices, and dispositions.[2] Though they tend to dissipate eventually, in the moment, they are often inescapable, sometimes oppressively so. The notion of an atmosphere makes it possible to speak of a collective, if only loosely. In referencing that collective I do not intend to analyse or erase the specifics of individual experiences, and I do not purport to speak for everyone.

I recognize too that different people will experience the pandemic imperative to stay home in radically different ways. My everyday frame of reference is that of a white, cis-gendered woman who makes a comfortable living as an academic in the United States, and I have so far been insulated from the most damaging consequences of the pandemic. As Arthur (2019–2020, p. vi) notes, 'For some, quarantine is an opening up. For others, a dragging-on of debility.' While this season has not been easy, my experience is much more the former than the latter. I am also aware that, as Nandita Sharma (2020) notes, the 'we' of the widespread insistence that 'we're all in this together' can quickly become weaponized and exclusionary. So I proceed cautiously in an attempt to think about the cultural and affective phenomena that have emerged in response to COVID-19's radical foreclosure of spatial and temporal possibilities. The number of deaths suggests that many of us know someone killed by COVID-19, while the quantity of lost jobs suggests that many of us know someone who is struggling or scared. Then there are those who are, or were, sick and don't know why because they can't get tested for COVID-19, those who have been diagnosed but can't afford proper care, those who have technically recovered from the virus but are still unwell. Given the partisan fracture in American public culture, which COVID-19 has apparently widened, many of us in this country will find ourselves disagreeing, sometimes sharply, with others about both the significance of all this suffering and the appropriate responses to it.[3]

My theorization of the pandemic as a season of *nevertheless* is grounded in two key conceits. First, I assume that most people alive and sentient today are more exhausted than they were before the pandemic; this exhaustion was never evenly distributed, and still isn't, but the pandemic has amplified whatever exhaustion pre-existed. Second, I assume that most people now face more precarious futures than they had before COVID-19. For many – indeed, likely for most of the world – precariousness is nothing new. But COVID-19 has compounded the precariousness of those who were already vulnerable, and distributed precariousness (or at least the feeling of precariousness) widely, and to quarters where a feeling of deep uncertainty about the future was far less common before. The experience of precariousness is relative, and not all forms of precarity constitute emergencies. My invocation of 'we' and 'us' here is simultaneously an effort to name patterns and to acknowledge a shared – if unevenly allocated – bodily vulnerability.[4]

With these caveats in place, I understand the fundamental *nevertheless* of this moment as follows: despite our exhaustion and the new precariousness of our futures, we continue to labour nevertheless. This labouring, I suggest, takes three main forms: *doing* (the productive and reproductive labour required to sustain life through a pandemic), *undoing* (the tedious processes of postponing and cancelling plans, or abandoning the process of planning altogether), and *not-doing* (passing the time left over between doing and undoing). Of course, the particularities of our doing, undoing, and not-doing will vary by our circumstances even as we operate within these general patterns of behaviour.

In and of itself, *nevertheless* is nothing new, and there are long theoretical tradition attempting to explain how humans exist with their *neverthelesses*. Psychoanalysis made one such attempt to explain discrepancies between knowledge, feeling, and behaviour. Freud (1927), for example, wrote about the structure of the fetish, describing it as a condition wherein the fetishist simultaneously inhabits two 'currents' of mental life, believing in a particular fantasy while also recognizing the fantasy as such. Later, Octave Mannoni offered the influential formulation '*Je sais bien, mais quand-même*,' usually translated as 'I know very well, but nevertheless ...' For their part, cultural theorists have employed concepts like tension, contradiction, ideology, and paradox to interpret the various *nevertheless*es that shape our thoughts and practices. The first clause of a *nevertheless* sentence contains the heavy truth that the speaker is trying to accept: death, exploitation, insufficiency, loss, a virus. The second clause reveals their concessions to that truth: grieving, working, making-do, coping, whatever one does to sustain herself through a pandemic. *Nevertheless* is the transit between them, always freighted with sadness that it carries from one side to the other.

Lauren Berlant (2011) has proposed 'cruel optimism' to explain widespread adherence to various 'fantasies of a good life' in neoliberal conditions designed to make that good life inaccessible to the vast majority; 'cruel optimism' is *nevertheless* by another name. She writes (p. 1), 'A relation of cruel optimism exists when something you desire is actually an obstacle to your flourishing.' The object of desire, she contends, is 'really ... a cluster of promises we want someone or something to make us and make possible for us' (p. 23). Optimism is, fundamentally, an orientation toward the future detectable in the 'built and affective infrastructure of the ordinary' (p. 49). It enables, or compels, the optimist to do: to work/persevere/subsist through a present that is exhausting/unsafe/unsatisfying in the pursuit of a future that might be better.[5]

While Berlant published *Cruel Optimism* nearly a decade before COVID-19, the lens of cruel optimism illuminates much about the present juncture, as the desire for a certain experience of freedom creates the very conditions in which the virus spreads. Cruel optimism manifests itself, for example, in the widespread refusal to wear masks in public, as well as the rush to return to normal patterns of work, education, and especially consumption. Coronavirus, and the wild mismanagement of it in the United States, begets unique forms of *nevertheless* as it demands that we do, undo, and not-do. *Doing* is a way of preparing for the future; *undoing* entails mourning that lost future; *not-doing* protracts that mourning further. None of these available pastimes offers much promise, but we occupy ourselves with them nevertheless.

Under normal circumstances, optimism is a motivator for *doing*, whispering that if you do this thing, tomorrow is likely to be better for it, especially if it's a thing you don't feel like doing in the first place. Such optimism is often a tiny private echo of capitalism's promises of constant improvement and limitless progress, always made in bad faith and bound to disappoint. But nevertheless this optimism can be helpful for getting through the day.

The pandemic has quickened the tempo of disappointment, and also increased its frequency. Widespread unemployment, underemployment or overwork for those (essential and otherwise) who are still employed, and the intersection of these pressures with added demands of child and family care, combined with a lack of opportunities for rest or pleasure, nullify even the flimsy good-life aspirations that might otherwise have been helpful for getting out of bed.[6]

With the emphasis on personal responsibility for mask-wearing, hand-washing, and social distancing, public discourse around coronavirus advances a typical neoliberal approach that 'responsibilizes' citizens and insists that their health is simply a 'product of [their] own choices' as opposed to a consequence of circumstance or structural inequality (Godrej, 2017, p. 907). However, coronavirus has also diluted individual agency. Whether or not someone will have access to the vaccine, for example, depends largely on factors beyond their control. In the meantime, partici-pation in public health practices might keep me and those nearest to me safe, but they have no direct or substantial bearing on when I will be able to resume the routines I might wish to resume because the conditions for those activities depend on the population as a whole.[7] Nevertheless, I feel compelled to engage in these practices, wishing for a clear conscience, a modicum of agency, a figment of control. Arthur's (2019–2020, p. x) analysis of doomscrolling is instructive here; he writes, 'Doomscrolling is killing time as an investment in feeling on top of things – a feedback loop of testing for encroachment. *How close, how long, how much, how bad?*' In other words, even the meagre comforts afforded by cruel optimism might be out of reach at this moment.[8] Yet because the job must be preserved, the children must be educated, the house must be cleaned, the dog must be fed, we keep doing nevertheless, prodded through this day, and the next, and the next, by something else.

Simultaneously, pandemic restrictions – if we choose to abide by them – require us to undo: scale back our ambitions, reschedule again or cancel altogether, hope for refunds and settle for credits. As the weight of the pan-demic devolves onto individuals, *undoing* is a way of taking action in response to events far beyond individual control. If we are lucky, we undo on our own terms. If we are less so, we get undone by a misfortune happen-ing to us. Losses of the things that can be quantified and that officials are capable of tallying, like jobs or lives in the aggregate, receive at least some glancing acknowledgement in public culture, inadequate though it might be. Yet these big numbers – millions of cases, hundreds of thousands of deaths, billions of dollars – obscure the personal ramifications of each data point, while other losses remain invisible and uncounted altogether, borne quietly or alone. Even if we are fortunate enough to evade the most costly or catastrophic of losses, presumably we have all lost something.[9] And of course, losses unrelated to COVID-19, both structural and individual, continue to accumulate as well. Every form of discrimination and violence persists. People we love fall ill or die from things that aren't coronavirus, relationships fall apart, we fail at things we care about. Inevitably, someone muses that it could always be worse, but this is supremely unhelpful; these losses hurt nevertheless.[10]

Product shortages, unprecedented delays, higher-than-normal call volume: because doing takes extra effort now and undoing is time-consuming, the off hours between these two kinds of work are rarer than before, and also entail the challenge of *not-doing*.[11] The experience of not-doing something I had planned and hoped to do is the spiky inverse of the pleasure I had expected that experience to provide. Plus there is the tedium of not being able to do the fun, discretionary things that I want to do as a respite from my doing, and not wanting to do the things that I can. Not-doing is surprisingly enervating. The early pandemic genre of motivational advice literature was flush with suggestions on how to optimize not-doing, grounded on the assumption that the pause necessitated by coronavirus in the spring of 2020 would surely be brief, singular, and precious. For those commentators and influencers who dispensed that guidance about how to fill the hours that had newly been emptied out, this little hiatus from the pressures of our usual routines appeared as an ideal opportunity to get organized, take up baking, do some serious home-improvement, learn another language, adopt a shelter pet, reconnect with old friends, establish a yoga practice, or spend more time appreciating nature.

All of this now seems naïve at best, underestimating how much people would still have to work and how tiring pandemic life would be.[12] The initial round of postponements gave way to cancellations, and that rash of cancellations threw into doubt the status of everything that had not yet been cancelled, while also making scheduling anything at all seem less and less thinkable. Whether because circumstances do not permit it or we are too despairing to even try, the horizon beyond which most of us can plan keeps receding, and so it seems that there is more undoing and not-doing to be done. Trends like plotting 'revenge travel' for later in 2021, a year laden with hope for a return to normal, are one way of dealing for those who have the means. Smaller, more modest and immediate pleasures – like inflatable pools, Oreos, *365 Days*, and puppies – are another (Faus and Appel 2020, Giorgis 2020, Heath 2020, Neighmond 2020).

Not-doing is shot through with a current of boredom. Standard, garden-variety, non-pandemic boredom is taxing in its own right, but pandemic boredom has fuzzier boundaries, threatens to creep into any available space or activity, and is much harder to assuage. Annie McClanahan (2019, p. 378) wagers that the condition of being stalled, stilled, or exhausted is seeded with possibility, the 'certainty that what comes next cannot be the future that always came before but must instead be something altogether different'. But it may be difficult to see through or past boredom in this way when days become indistinguishable from one another – #blursday – and the future looks so hazy.[13]

Boredom is a side effect of immobility. Lars Svendsen (2005, p. 19) writes that 'boredom normally arises when we cannot do what we want to do, or have something we do not want to do'. It 'always contains an awareness of being trapped, either in a particular situation or in the world as a whole' (Svendsen 2005, p. 93). Compared to stronger, more urgent feelings of despair, suffocation, or claustrophobia that might also arise when one is or feels stuck, boredom, in Ben Anderson's (2004, p. 749) terms, 'comes to exist as an index of mild dissatisfaction that provides, first and foremost, the impetus to enter into different relations'. He continues, 'it takes place as a form of affectively based imperative to something-else where that movement is possible. There is therefore a weak hope for a not-yet elsewhere or elsewhen internal to boredom'. Boredom is an itchy kind of looking forward, whether to a future in which one's life is more glamorous and exciting than it is at present, or just to the escape from a seemingly endless meeting. But the pandemic, with its restrictions on mobility and lack of a clear endpoint, has made those else-wheres and elsewhens abstract, detached from any specific means for acces-sing them. I know I really ought to do something, but nevertheless.

Part of the affective difficulty of the COVID-19 present – spent toggling between doing, undoing, and not-doing – is that most of the feelings readily available to us are, in a word, shitty. They are also muted. In the absence of, or doldrums between, more intense feelings of screaming rage or howling grief, there are so many less dramatic, and less cathartic, ways to feel. These are akin to what Sianne Ngai (2007) has theorized as 'ugly feelings' and 'minor affects'.[14] Because these feelings are subtle, diffuse, attached to nothing specific, they are also difficult to discharge. I think of my own tiny transgressions, misbehaviours as tempting as they are unsatisfy-ing, and those that friends have confessed to me through this season: quar-antine-quibbling with partners, snapping at children, snarkily side-chatting during online meetings, dodging phone calls from loved ones, missing work-outs, letting the sourdough starter die.

Cue, then, the exhortations to resilience from virtually every quarter. To name just a few: a human-interest compendium of 'tales of pandemic resili-ence' that the New York Times published on Christmas Eve, 2020. A podcast by the American Psychological Association (APA) featuring an interview with a resilience expert (Mills 2020). Tips from the Harvard Center for the Developing Child (2020) on how to make families more resilient during the pandemic. A long list of resilience and mental health resources from The American Hospi-tal Association (AHA) (2020) and accompanying content on 'caring with limited resources'. The rhetorical question posed by transnational consulting firm Deloitte (2020), 'How can businesses thrive post-COVID-19 and beyond?' with answers grouped under the heading 'Connecting for a Resilient World.' And Bloomberg's global 'resilience ranking' to determine which countries are the best and worst 'places to be' during COVID (Chang *et al.* 2020).

The pandemic is only the latest crisis, like climate change before it, to inspire advocacy of resilience. As Sarah Bracke (2016, p. 52) notes, 'resilience has friends in high places,' and is neoliberalism's preferred prescription in response to any kind of catastrophe, whether personal or collective. Resilience assures that the demands of capital will be met, no matter the suffering that threatens to interfere. Resilience, Bracke (p. 52) continues, 'is a powerful idea whose deployment spans the macro level of ecological and economic systems to the micro level of selves, and the complex circuits of power that connect and constitute these different levels of social reality'. Bracke (p. 54) notes that the denotative definition of resilience refers to the capacity of a material to return to its original shape after 'deformation caused by compressive stress'; in other words, resilience is a form of 'shock absorption'. In essence, resilience makes a reward of returning uncritically to the status quo ante. Consequently, resilience can only be demonstrated after the damage has been sustained, while the meantime of resilience is simple misery.

In a recuperative reading of resilience, Nikolas Rose and Filippa Lentzos (2017, p. 34) argue that resilience is valuable because this posture 'responds to a perception that our futures are not predictable and calculable' as discourses of risk management suggest. To be resilient, for Rose and Lentzos, is to preserve the capacity to be surprised, and I surely see the value in this, insofar as it keeps us awake to the possibility of better things. But the pandemic present is surprisingly short on surprises, as more bad news scarcely counts as a surprise anymore and much of it – like the spike in cases after Thanksgiving in the United States – is predictable.[15] The days ooze together in repeating patterns of doing, uninterrupted by the diversions that undone plans would have provided; not-doing is as accessible as Netflix and creeps into any unclaimed hour. The idea of resilience is rooted in an underhanded kind of optimism; it acknowledges adversity, but insists that anyone can overcome adversity if only they try hard enough, and that this overcoming will position them for future success. But pandemic time is less an arrow than a loop, and agency is complicated these days.[16]

So something other than resilience might be in order. I think a lot about the trail runner I met, the *nevertheless* of his routine of training for the possibility, even the likelihood, of nothing. I don't know the details of his story, but his practice illuminates something about how we might find our ways forward, and so I'd like to propose endurance as an alternative to resilience. Cruel optimism sustains itself through the instances where we get close to our objects of desire, just before they swerve out of reach again (Berlant 2011, p. 48). It runs on the resilience required to withstand chronic disappointment and insufficiency. Endurance, however, does not require optimism. While resilience can only be demonstrated after the fact and offers very little in the way of sustenance during a trial, endurance is accessible in the moment. Resilience, the preferred euphemism for neoliberalism's extraction of value from suffering, demands that good subjects actively 'lean in' to scarcity, exploitation, or unsustainability. The posture of endurance is much more a shrug: knowing, defiant, and tired. Whereas resilience insists that the future will be better, at least until the next inevitable crisis, endurance is not predicated on a linear vision of time and makes no promise of improvement. Resilience thrives on crisis, but endurance survives boredom. Resilience suggests that we capitalize on our grief; endurance allows us to carry it rather than attempting to exchange it for something else. Resilience denies damage and minimizes loss. By contrast, endurance acknowledges that things hurt now, makes no guarantee that things will hurt less in a minute or tomorrow or next week, and is totally open to the possibility that things might actually hurt more later. But nevertheless.

Advocates of resilience often exhort us to suffer better, more productively. The goal of resilience is to bear suffering without any trustworthy promise of amelioration. While there is some element of this in training for endurance sports, the goal of training to become more endurant is actually to minimize suffering – perceived or actual – in the long run. As it happens, there have been plenty of stories about what lessons everyday people might draw from endurance athletes to help them get through the pandemic (Braverman 2020, Hutchinson 2020, Minsberg 2020). These stories are interesting, and I read them too, but endurance as I understand it is more than a lifestyle hack.

Endurance is an existential *nevertheless*, but one that doesn't require a resilient second clause to the *nevertheless* construction, in which the speaker attests to everything she is doing despite her pain. Endurance is not the resilient work-no-matter-what imperative of capitalism, which is a *nevertheless* that serves the doer only incidentally (Wołodźko 2019–2020, p. 213). The *nevertheless* of endurance is an end in itself, and requires no product to qualify as such. The notion of endurance enables us to invest all our pandemic labours – the doing, undoing, and not-doing – with meaning as a simple but undeniable record of persistence. In this way, recognition of our own endurance can make all of that amount to something even when it feels like nothing, or worse. And if you're here, at this moment, your endurance is happening; you've already done, and are doing, it.

Notes

1. There was a certain satisfaction in that process, the comfort of having purchased security, or the sense of security that lasted as long as our inventory of consumables remained comfortably high. Marita Sturken's (2006, 2007)

work on the purchase of security, and the imperative that citizens provide security for themselves, is instructive, even though it preceded the current crisis.

2. See Anderson (2014, pp. 119–121) for a reappraisal of Raymond Williams's notion of a 'structure of feeling', which Anderson describes as a common affective orientation that organizes 'otherwise disparate practices, events, or processes' (p. 119).

3. As Rushing (2020, p. S-54) notes, 'perceptions of risk and threat' have become 'factionalized.'

4. On the importance of recognizing shared vulnerability in COVID times, see Rushing (2020).

5. Anderson's (2014, p. 41) definition of 'morale' as mobilized by states bears some similarities to this. He describes morale as the property that 'enables bodies to keep going *despite the present* – a present in which morale is either targeted directly or threatens to break.' See also Sara Ahmed (2010). For a critique of hope, see McManus (2011).

6. On the collision of care with the demands of capital, see Micki McGee (2020).

7. As Armstrong (2015, p. 181) notes in his work on the etymology of 'precarity', the Latin *precārius* 'refers to something requested or obtained by entreaty or favor', which means that a 'precarious situation depends on the will of another to concede to a request, an uncertainty in the sense of a person or another situation on which one cannot fully depend.' In the case of coronavirus, we are dependent not just on a sovereign authority, but also on one another, which leaves us all in a doubly precarious position.

8. I've always appreciated critiques of futurity, like Edelman's *No Future: Queer Theory and the Death Drive* (2004). But then I ran out of things to look forward to, and I suddenly found myself hungry for something that would anchor me to a time beyond this one.

9. In an attempt to give these losses a place to live, I created a public archival project called *Coronavirus Lost and Found* (pandemicarchive.com), a site where anyone can log anything they've lost – or, more happily, found – during the pandemic.

10. On the political potential of 'resting in sadness', see Thelandersson (2018). She writes (p. 17), 'But the mere act of resting in sadness … might function as an impasse, where the refusal to move forward becomes a protest of the neoliberal demands of becoming a labouring and 'happy' subject.'

11. For an analysis of the politics of waiting, see Sharma (2014).

12. On the trends that arose in the first weeks of the pandemic, see Marcus (2020) and Jung (2020).

13. 'Time', Arthur (2019–2020, p. vi) writes, 'feels caught between aftermath and looming recurrence: impasse, interruption, repeat'.

14. According to Ngai (2007), these ugly feelings arise at the site of blocked or suspended agency.

15. As Bracke (2016, p. 59) notes, when threats themselves become resilient, the difference between a threat and resilience collapses.

16. Connecting resilience to cruel optimism, Bracke (2016, p. 65) argues, 'resilience becomes a symptom of the loss of the capacity to imagine and do otherwise, and cruelty is one of the more politically cautious names for such a condition'.

Disclosure statement

No potential conflict of interest was reported by the author(s).

Further information

This Special Issue article has been comprehensively reviewed by the Special Issue editors, Associate Professor Ted Striphas and Professor John Nguyet Erni.

References

Ahmed, S., 2010. *The promise of happiness*. Durham, NC: Duke University Press.

American Hospital Association. 2020. Well-being resources addressing resilience during COVID-19. Available from: https://www.aha.org/well-being-covid-19 [Accessed 2 January 2021].

Anderson, B., 2004. Time-stilled space-slowed: how boredom matters. *Geoforum*, 34, 739–754.

Anderson, B., 2014. *Encountering affect: capacities, apparatuses, conditions*. London: Routledge.

Armstrong, P., 2015. Precarity's prayers. *The Minnesota review: a journal of creative and critical writing*, 85, 180–188.

Arthur, M., 2019–2020. Writing pandemic feels. *Capacious: journal for emerging affect inquiry*, 2 (1-2), vi–vii.

Berlant, L., 2011. *Cruel optimism*. Durham, NC: Duke University Press.

Bracke, S., 2016. Bouncing back: vulnerability and resistance in times of resilience. *In*: J. Butler, Z. Gambetti, and L. Sabsay, eds. *Vulnerability and resistance*. Durham, NC: Duke University Press, 52–75.

Braverman, B. 2020. What my sled dogs taught me about planning for the unknown. *The New York Times*, 23 Sep. Available from: https://www.nytimes.com/2020/09/23/sports/sled-dogs-mushing-unknowns-planning.html [Accessed 2 January 2021].

Chang, R., Hong, J., and Varley, K. 2020. The best and worst places to be in Covid: U.S. sinks in ranking. *Bloomberg*, 24 Nov. Available from: https://www.bloomberg.com/graphics/covid-resilience-ranking/ [Accessed 2 January 2021].

Deloitte. 2020. Connecting for a resilient world. Available from: https://www2.deloitte.com/global/en/pages/about-deloitte/articles/connecting-for-a-resilient-world.html [Accessed 2 January 2021].

Edelman, L., 2004. *No future: queer theory and the death drive*. Durham, NC: Duke University Press.

Faus, J. and Appel, T. 2020. Pool sales skyrocket as consumers splash out on coronavirus cocoons. *Reuters*, 6 Aug. Available from: https://www.reuters.com/article/us-health-coronavirus-pools/pool-sales-skyrocket-as-consumers-splash-out-on-coronavirus-cocoons-idUSKCN2520HW [Accessed 2 January 2021].

Freud, S., 1927. Fetishism. *In*: J. Strachey, ed./trans. *The standard edition of the complete psychological works of Sigmund Freud, volume XXI*. London: The Hogarth Press and the Institute of Psychoanalysis, 147–157.

Giorgis, H. 2020. Why people are obsessed with a terrible polish erotic thriller. *The Atlantic*. 26 Jun. Available from: https://www.theatlantic.com/culture/archive/2020/06/why-365-days-is-netflixs-surprise-summer-hit/613576/ [Accessed 2 January 2021].

Godrej, F., Oct 2017. Gandhi, Foucault, and the politics of self-care. *Theory & event*, 20 (4), 894–922.

Heath, T., 2020. Big food brands, some out-of-favor for years, see sales and stock prices jump on stay-at-home grazing. *Washington Post*, 11 May. Available from: https://www.washingtonpost.com/business/2020/05/11/big-food-brands-out-of-favor-years-see-sales-stock-prices-jump-stay-at-home-grazing/ [Accessed 2 January 2021].

Hutchinson, A. 2020. COVID-19 is like running a marathon with no finish line. What does sports science say about how we can win it? *The Globe and Mail*, 21 Nov. Available from: https://www.theglobeandmail.com/opinion/article-covid-19-is-like-running-a-marathon-with-no-finish-line-what-does/ [Accessed 2 January 2021].

Jung, E.A. 2020. Nothing made sense this year – unless you were on the Internet. *Vulture*, 7 Dec. Available from: https://www.vulture.com/article/quarantine-brain-quarries-2020.html [Accessed 2 January 2021].

Marcus, E. 2020. Leave it in 'early quar'? *New York Times*, 14 Dec. Available from: https://www.nytimes.com/2020/12/14/style/early-quar-covid.html [Accessed 2 January 2021].

McClanahan, A., 2019. Life expectancies: mortality, exhaustion, and economic stagnation. *Theory & event*, 22 (2), 360–381.

McGee, M., 2020. Capitalism's care problem: some traces, fixes, and patches. *Social text*, 142 (38.1), 39–66.

McManus, S., 2011. Hope, fear, and the politics of affective agency. *Theory & event*, 14 (4), n.p. [online journal].

Mills, K. (host), Apr 2020. Speaking of psychology: The role of resilience in the face of COVID-19 with Ann Masten, PhD. Episode 105 [Podcast]. Available from: https://www.apa.org/research/action/speaking-of-psychology/human-resilience-covid-19 [Accessed 2 January 2021].

Minsberg, T. 2020. Build mental endurance like a pro. *new York Times*. 7 Nov. Available from: https://www.nytimes.com/2020/11/07/well/mind/athletes-pandemic-advice.html [Accessed 2 January 2021].

Neighmond, P. 2020. Pet adoptions bring some joy during coronavirus pandemic. *NPR*. 11 Nov. Available from: https://www.npr.org/2020/11/11/933754536/pet-adoptions-bring-some-joy-during-coronavirus-pandemic [Accessed 2 January 2021].

New York Times. 2020. A flying elephant, a teacher's hugs: 12 tales of pandemic resilience. 24 Dec. Available from: https://www.nytimes.com/2020/12/24/world/coronavirus-resilience.html [Accessed 2 January 2021].

Ngai, S., 2007. *Ugly feelings*. Cambridge: Harvard University Press, 27–48.

Rose, N. and Lentzos, F., 2017. Making us resilient: responsible citizens for uncertain times. *In*: S. Trnka and C. Trundle, ed. *Competing responsibilities: the ethics and politics of contemporary life*. Durham, NC: Duke University Press.

Rushing, S., Oct 2020. On bodies, anti-bodies, and the body politic in viral times. *Theory & event*, 23 (4 supplement), S53–S60.

Sharma, N., Oct 2020. The global COVID-19 pandemic and the need to change who we think 'we' are. *Theory & event*, 23 (4 supplement), S-19–S-29.

Sharma, S., 2014. *In the meantime: temporality and cultural politics.* Durham: Duke University Press.

Sturken, M. 2006. Weather media and homeland security: selling preparedness in a volatile world. *Understanding Katrina: Perspectives from the Social Sciences.* 11 Jun. Available from: http://understandingkatrina.ssrc.org/Sturken/ [Accessed 2 January 2021].

Sturken, M., 2007. *Tourists of history: memory, kitsch, and consumerism from ground zero to Oklahoma city.* Durham, NC: Duke University Press.

Svendsen, L., 2005. *A philosophy of boredom,* trans. John Irons. London: Reaktion Books.

The Harvard Center for the Developing Child. 2020. How to help families and staff build resilience during the COVID-19 outbreak. Available from: https://developingchild.harvard.edu/resources/how-to-help-families-and-staff-build-resilience-during-the-covid-19-outbreak/ [Accessed 2 January 2021].

Thelandersson, F., 2018. Social media sad girls and the normalization of sad states of being. *Capacious: journal for emerging affect inquiry,* 2 (1), 1–21.

Wołodźko, A.A., 2019–2020. Living within affect as contagion: breathing in between numbers. *Capacious: journal for emerging affect inquiry,* 2 (1–2). Available from: http://capaciousjournal.com/cms/wp-content/uploads/2020/04/capacious-wolodzko-contamination.pdf [Accessed 2 January 2021].

The dead-end of ad-hocracy

Charles R. Acland

ABSTRACT

Since the 1960s 'ad-hocracy', an approach to organizations that values provisionality and is especially advantaged by new technological systems, has been understood as a 'radical' challenge to the rigidity of bureaucratic institutions. This essay argues that commonsense championing of the temporary, the anti-institutional, and the flexible in corporate, political, educational, and daily life established the conditions that preordained the disastrous handling of the COVID-19 crisis in the United States. Most hazardously, a powerful strain of Left critique also advances on a comparable tack, one that too easily embraces temporary and flexible organizational structures over lasting institutional ones, resulting in unintended ideological support for 'ad-hocracy'.

I heard a man tell in a monotone how he couldn't get a doctor while his oldest boy died of pneumonia but that a doctor came right away after it was dead. It is easy to get a doctor to look at a corpse, not so easy to get one for a live person. It is easy to get a body buried. A truck comes right out and takes it away. The state is much more interested in how you die than in how you live.

John Steinbeck (1996a [1938]) 'Starvation under the orange trees', p. 1026

The COVID-19 pandemic is our health and economic crisis; it is of our making and of our time. For all the science fiction analogies that our recent experience conjures up – the space suit encumbrances of personal protective equipment (PPE), the virus as a planetary enemy, the confrontation with the unimaginable – our pandemic did not come from outer space or the future. It is entirely a product of this moment in history, our global movement, our relationship with animals, our technological and analytical fragility, and our systemic priorities and neglects.

Still, past encounters with health crises, economic devastation, and societal collapse have left us with portraits that speak of the human experience of such hardship and help us grasp the specificity of our current situation. As a deep economic winter settles in the United States, ruining the livelihood of African-American and Hispanic communities disproportionately while a stratum of the professional-managerial class enjoys the sourdough-breaded misfortunes of uninterrupted paychecks, we can prepare intellectually and affectively by returning to those portraits. John Steinbeck's *The Grapes of wrath* (1996b [1939]), a monumental tale of the injustices that reigned over mass migrant labour during the American Great Depression, remains surprisingly shocking, frank, and resonant with our comparable economic catastrophe. His documentary-realist novel casts the reader with the prideful, hard-working, poor set down Route 66 by a cruel financial calculus. The immediacy of the novel's dirt and hopelessness grew out of the years Steinbeck spent understanding and chronicling the struggles of Californian agricultural labour, which included newspaper articles about migrant farm workers. The source of the opening quotation above is one such article, 'Starvation under the orange trees,' which appeared in *The Monterey Trader* in 1938. It took as its focus the horrifying contrast between the bounty of Californian farming and the literal starvation of those hired to work the land.

Hunger was but one threat. Exposure to disease was part of migrant life, made only that much more dangerous due to the inaccessibility of doctors and health care facilities. As Steinbeck put it, the official governmental agencies, those agencies that might be arranged to supply the needed medicine and medical attention, and that might build support services for labour as much as they did for corporate owners, instead left the suffering alone. The dead, though, were another matter; attention was paid, promptly so. 'The state is much more interested in how you die than in how you live'.

As it was during the Great Depression, and as it was for its legions of migrant workers, so it is today worldwide. In Canada, migrant agricultural labour has similarly been recognized as a population, beyond their conventional economic exploitation, that is especially at risk of COVID-19 spread, without secure medical programmes, safety procedures, and enforcement of precautionary measures found elsewhere in Canadian society. Lockdown measures have made some domestic and health care professionals on Canada's Temporary Foreign Worker programme vulnerable to abuse and without access to emergency assistance. These workers consist of racialized populations, with large numbers coming from Mexico, Jamaica, and the Philippines. Ethiopian migrant labour in Yemen has been blamed for viral spread and then had to endure threats of violence and summary deportation. But few situations are as dire as that of the United States. The shambles of U.S. health care, with its low regard for public health and high regard for health profit, has performed as expected during this pandemic, leaving economically and physically vulnerable people casualties while celebrities and elites swapped silver spoons for swabs, design-forward masks, and personal services, all needed to ride out the crisis in maximum comfort and style. With the absence of adequate health coverage for many temporary workers, digital proletarians, newly unemployed, and millions of others with simply no medical insurance at all, the crushing weight of a global pandemic is not borne equally.

While supply chains for medical masks, virus testing, and PPE were ill-formed with ruinous consequences in the United States, despite weeks of notice about SARS-CoV-2 and years of assessments warning about the need for pandemic preparedness, refrigeration trucks were parked outside hospitals to serve as mobile morgues. Yet again, attention to the living lagged behind the urgency of the corpse.

Moments of crisis are terrific mechanisms for revealing infrastructural weaknesses and damage. Comparing the different national responses provides us with ample evidence of differential institutional priorities. The lack of preparedness for a health emergency of this kind in the United States has been scandalous and has resulted in an inability to adapt on the fly, to launch rapid mobilization plans, and to make decisions about who is supposed to make decisions based on what information. This virus similarly slammed other countries. The U.S. was among the least effective, proving itself dismally incapable of navigating the crisis humanely.

There are many reasons for this criminally poor performance. One infrastructural weakness deserves special attention as a determining force, namely, the widespread embrace of gig work, devalued labour, and just-in-time supply that left the country devastatingly unprepared. The temporary and the flexible have been, paradoxically, permanent features of how we have imagined the coming technological age from at least the 1960s onward, when Alvin Toffler (1970) popularized 'ad-hocracy' in *Future shock* as an alternative to the rigidity of bureaucracy. Of the many forces that constitute our historical conjuncture, especially powerful is the link between the deglobalizing economic depression of the COVID-19 pandemic and the short-term contract work that has helped make human energy insecure, whether migrant agricultural labour or digital migrants who rabbit from one task to another while enriching software overlords and financial speculators. Economic exploitation, and the programmes to make labour inexpensive and insecure in order to further advantage the financially stable, makes our situation a repeat experience, echoing the hardship of earlier eras of struggle. Put bluntly, the commonsense championing of the temporary, the anti-institutional, and the flexible in corporate, political, educational, and daily life established the conditions that preordained the disastrous handling of the COVID-19 crisis in the United States. Ironically – or fatally – a powerful strain of Left critique, as this essay explores, also advances on a comparable tack, one that too easily embraces temporary and flexible organizational structures over lasting institutional ones, resulting in unintended ideological support for ad-hocracy.

Educational systems are one major arena in which this contradictory pressure can be observed. Schools have been preparing for years for adaptation to flexible economies, with neo-liberal and progressive voices often overlapping in their appeals to 'universally' individualized training. The various remote teaching programmes that valiantly tried to recover terms, courses, and credits for students following the shut-down of face-to-face instruction in the Winter of 2020 had a welcoming landing pad. That jerry-rigged educational transformation was made possible by a consensus about the utility of technological platforms as well as an infrastructure of materials and priorities, which itself sat on the back of decades of discursive preparation about the inevitability of the technological society.[1] We witnessed great institutions dissolving into privately-owned platforms because they are available, not because they are good or sufficient. When the pandemic lifts, remaining with be the dust of apps and websites, recordings and access codes, that will continue to radiate influence for an untold half-life.

Economic divisions are immediately consequential during a crisis, and they are more visible than ever. So many, by all counts an historically high number, who live one pay-cheque away from homelessness and the food bank have had that thin line cut. Economic injustice, as much a founding principle of ad-hocracy as flexibility and convenience, overlaps with racial injustice. The transient tune of the heroic front-line worker – the cashier, the nurse, and the delivery driver – sung in earnest and with sincere marvel, just can't rise above the noise of racial divide that produced the disparities and whose sub-living wages we will continue to pay when our collective melancholic appreciation has been expended. The intersection of pandemic and protest that transpired at the end of May 2020 was no random occurrence. Both speak of overlapping forces and conditions. Again, there was no novelty there, and Keeanga-Yamahtta Taylor (2016) has comprehensively historicized Black Lives Matter as part of a multi-generational American struggle against racism, poverty, and capitalism. The popular pressure released following the circulation of the images of George Floyd being killed – revelatory for some, but maddeningly predictable for others – tells us that we too arrive on the scene where police brutality, anti-Blackness, and structural economic impossibility all collide. The state doesn't just show up for a corpse, as Steinbeck put it; it has a hand in producing one.

Authoritarian libertarianism

In the early days of the American COVID-19 experience, with some marginal efforts to respond, *New York Times* columnist Farhad Manjoo (2020) wrote that 'everyone's a socialist in a pandemic'. Far from bestowing praise on the Trump administration, Manjoo was noting the qualified acceptance of the idea that public health was a shared fate and that responsibility shone best in the context of an emergency. He saw the scramble of corporate players to shore up their patchwork policies for sick employees, wondering hopefully if this momentary socialistic impulse could reverberate into more lasting health care agendas.

But by focussing on such possibilities, Manjoo did not notice a parallel impulse that can be detected in crisis moments. In a pandemic, many, frighteningly, seem to adore an authoritarian, too. Even as suspicions have grown about ulterior motives of the Chinese state and their use of crisis surveillance to supress the democratic movement, authoritarian envy blushed through Western states. China's rapid mass response – mandating highly policed quarantines, secrecy and misinformation about the disease, rolling out high-tech surveillance programmes, eliminating travel and criticism – made some wonder what might be if only we had some of that totalitarian nerve ... !

Witness the awkward authoritarian dance of Donald Trump, a freestyle, shotgun approach to power that left even friendlies bewildered and American political scientists burning received convention on the operations of advanced democracies. Whatever his fascistic twitches, he only ever represents an authoritarian style trapped in a democracy. He is a version of what would have been recognized as *bossism* from the late nineteenth century through the 1940s. This doesn't make him any less dangerous, and his administration's concerted efforts to weaken democratic institutions – regulatory regimes, immigration rights, voting registration procedures, even basic election outcomes – have not been without consequence. But we have been watching a marginally equipped leader perform as a strongman, enabled by a cynical party. In the moments in which we expect, and crave, seriousness, thoughtfulness, inspiration, and gravitas, Trump delivers schtick. The routine, the Trump-classic lines, and the clownish faces are all recognized and, more importantly, appreciated by his supporters. He is doing more than breaking with elitist decorum, itself a source of great pleasure, but he is fulfilling the promise of amusement that speaks his supporters' language. This element is so frequently missed by the critics who are content to isolate clips, expressions, and gestures to point out his wrongness, his dimness, his mendacity, and his bodily excesses. He has been a success because he is funny and strange, and not in spite of it.[2]

History was bound to catch up with him, as was the virus itself. And every crisis-point since the 2016 U.S. election seemed to suggest that, yes, it finally has. Except it hadn't. Well, at long last, in 2020, even with a rising softness on and excuse-making for totalitarianism, the thinness of his authoritarian style meant that he simply could not deflect or joke his way through the deaths of hundreds of thousands of people. Nor could he grasp the rage of millions who took to the streets to say that it is no longer acceptable that the police, an institution of safety, security, and lawfulness, is in actuality for many an institution of threat, harm, and criminality.

Trump's authoritarian style is distinct from that of the familiar totalitarian version, where complete oppressive measures can be exercised with the added benefit of suppression of all criticism and opposition. Instead, Trump has to be content with the chaos he can catalyze, withstanding the endlessly searing but largely harmless jabs of media pundits and shrugging off the limits handed to him by the legal establishment. His desperation following his loss to the Joe Biden-Kamala Harris presidential ticket in 2020, stymied by legal and state powers that his fantastical claims of fraud could not upend, was a continuous expression of his aimless authoritarianism, one that successfully rattled the democratic core of the United States. There is a powerful and underappreciated authoritarian tactic, one that Trump and company have deployed with relish when confronted with the pandemic: the power to do nothing, the power to not be responsible, the power to be irresponsible. The small government strain of American politics embraces this as part of the path to individual responsibility and freedom from the state and from institutional constraint. His incoherence moulded into a new presidential creature that dramatically declared 'it's not my job' and 'grow up, snowflake, do it yourself'. For this reason, Trump might be an odd oxymoronic creature: an authoritarian libertarian, terms which, for traditional political theory, are supposed to be found on opposite poles.

Libertarianism is not particular to Trump. He is but a fine expression of the anti-statist instinct that appeals to the rebellious heart of the American spirit, both on the Left and the Right. Larry Grossberg (2018) has importantly elaborated this in relation to key features of our historical conjuncture, including legitimated racism, changed labour divides, and novel economic forces. Grossberg charted the strategic 'chaos' that has been mobilized to the advantage of Trumpians. The New Chaotic Right has done its best to advance the decentralized, unregulated, and weakened state, and appears supremely comfortable with a decidedly un-conservative form of political engagement. The complicating feature is that some of the self-described Left participates on an adjacent stage, where institutions are seen first and foremost as sites of suspicion, control, and constraint. Where Black Lives Matter has helped mount, organize, and expand an extensive response to structural racism and a coalition of progressives has successfully begun to have traction inside the Democratic Party, there is a powerful techno-utopian lifestyle Left that validates and contributes to a retreat from public institutional engagement, understanding self-organization and micro-communities as the path to influence. This position is, in many ways, a dominant one, requiring the energies of organized political movements to have to engage with and struggle against forces that devalue and treat with suspicion mass socialistic initiatives. These champions of ad-hocracy make the crucial error that we can each on our own, in our self-designated bubbles of convenience and affinity, make it up as we go along, just on a more naturally progressive path. The lifestyle Left cannot deflect ad-hocracy's culture of self-interest; it moves too easily toward a libertarianism that is relatively undifferentiated from that of the Right, surrendering too much that could prove advantageous to popular democratic movements.

Pedagogical masking

Kids these days: human capital and the making of Millennials (2017) is an insightful trade press study of wide-spread generational economic insecurity in the United States, written by cultural and political commentator Malcolm Harris. His date-of-birth is on the cover to boast of his *bona fides* as a Millennial. Another paratextual facet is even more telling. The author's biographical statement gives us a most curious illustration of ideological slippage related to ad-hocracy: 'Malcolm Harris is a communist.' Writing, as he has, for such venues as *The New York Times Magazine*, *Bookforum*, and *The New Republic* hardly assures this claim. Other facets of his biography are better indicators: Harris was one of the key activists in Occupy Wall Street – add three points – notoriously fabricating and circulating the rumour that Radiohead were going to play a free concert in Zuccotti Park in Lower Manhattan to get more people down to the protest site – minus one point. The biographical tidbit of Left-wing political commitment is noteworthy on its own terms. It is a rare sighting. But wait, on the dust jacket is a revised bio: 'Malcolm Harris is a freelance writer.' The substitution of 'freelance writer' for 'communist' is arresting, and this version of Harris's biography is the one chosen for Amazon's website.

As inadvertent as it may be, the substitution of communist for freelancer is noteworthy because it connects with a dominant sensibility that celebrates as progressive the self-organized, the autonomous, the independent, the libertarian, and other forms of supposedly spontaneous social relations associated with ad-hocracy. The linguistic possibility of this substitution is, today, a probability, so powerfully accepted are the ideas about singular technologically-enhanced virtue, rejecting institutions in favour of the ad-hoc and self-organized as de facto 'radical'. The revolt against bureaucracy has made sense, given general experience of institutional tone-deafness and specific unresponsiveness to marginalized voices and concerns. But the expansiveness of this revolt is such that it represents all political stripes and serves as a mobile critique ready to be unpacked at a moment's notice by anyone.

The celebration of ad-hocracy effectively sublimates the actual institutional and public resources deployed. With every app we download, whether at work or at home, we are participating in the triumph of ad-hocracy and its infrastructure. Most urgently – and this is the strain that needs amplifying in our crisis moment – one end of the flexible, self-driven, gig economy translates into a cheapening labour pool (e.g. ride, delivery, micro-contract rental and work services), one that in no way reduces corporate size and institutional complexity, though it does disperse financial risk. Moreover, the self-organized invariably favours those already structurally advantaged with educational, social, and cultural capital, not to mention family wealth. What Angela McRobbie (2014) describes as self-entrepreneurship is part of a highly individualized, competitive environment, where workers are in a perpetual game of promoting themselves as mini-corporate entities. This advantages some who have the resources and skills *not* to make an income while they build their brand. For every story you hear of a gig-hero who made it big in their chosen freelance domain, ask what lasting structure cushioned them economically or prepared them intellectually as they enjoyed the contemporaneity of self-organized autonomy.

The critique just outlined is actually part of the challenge Harris offers in *Kids these days*, however variously his biography is narrativized. The book is an account of how contemporary capitalism built on precarity and technological change has failed the next generation. Harris (2017, p. 12) makes a compelling case for the profoundly structural and systemic dead-end of the current capitalist regime, so much so that he declares that a breaking point will soon be reached and Millennials will be either the first generation of American revolutionaries or fascists. (Not the first; there have in fact been several such of each).

Many have pointed to the cost of post-industrial economies, and the rise of affective and insecure labour markets, supporting Harris's critique. Gig work has taken us into a world of not just cheapened but free labour, doing so by either circumventing or disintegrating the hard-won labour rights of decades past (Terranova 2000, Irani 2015, Duffy 2016, Srnicek 2016). The sharing economy is a smokescreen for labour devaluation. Harris adds to this critique with commentary on the role educational institutions play in preparing the work force for this situation, tilling the mental and emotional soil for personalized flexibility. We agree to individualize the responsibility of building the human capital needed for the economy to run; we agree to compete against one another for a piece of that economy; we agree to career impermanence; we agree to accept the associated economic and health risks; and we agree to pay for our preparation and training for the labour market with our own time, effort, and money.

Harris discusses 'pedagogical masking' – not to be confused with the medical face-masking that has become necessary if not as conventionalized as it ought to be – where the actual resources associated with labour are disguised as learning or knowledge acquisition. In effect, at school a student works for free, preparing themselves to be valuable on a labour market, and to be valuable to someone else's gain. Through all levels of schooling, students absorb the skills deemed essential to their own future economic (in)security. The more anxious you can make these proto-workers, the more you can count on them not getting organized and expect them to settle for small-scale alternative affinity communities and situational self-declared ahistorical micro-identities. The mantra of life-long learning makes your expertise always on the cusp of obsolete. The nervous proto-worker – that is, student – faces scarcity of places in the 'schools that count' and dwindling stable occupational positions, which drive up credentialing and result in 'excellence' inflation. A student body in competition with itself produces an early drive to self-branding – who you are, who are your people, what skills do you offer, which Harris smartly understands as a kind of professionalization of childhood.

These are some of the conditions that drew the contours of the pandemic and how it would slam into people differently.

For that reason, we ought to be alarmed when versions of the gig economy and ad-hocracy are embraced as subversive responses to threatening situations. Everywhere, even as some forms of tentative egalitarian impulses are acceptable in ways that are unusual in the United States – as seen with the inspiring emergence of a progressive wing inside the Democratic Party – anti-communitarian pressures dominate, where making decisions for a collective violates the primacy of self-interest and individual success potential. This anti-communitarian pressure does not just refer to the armed militias that stormed state capitols to demand economic openings, contra all prudent medical advice, nor the Right-wing extremist groups who brutishly demanded the overturning of the 2020 Presidential election results. It describes the individualistic ideals of micro-community affiliation; it describes the technophilic culture of convenience; it describes the 'radical' sneering at regulation, whether pertaining to intellectual property, education, medical care, or finance. The ad-hoc is that which rests upon and deepens inequality; as such, it cannot be sustained as a movement or strategy, operating as it does without the accountability necessary to assure ongoing expanding egalitarian operations.

The slippage between 'communist' – or for that matter 'revolutionary', 'radical', 'alternative', 'progressive' – and 'freelancer' might be read as an insignificant and minor illustration, given the world-historical waves of pandemic and protest we are experiencing. But it is emblematic, and the thinking that produced such a slippage works against a real popular communitarian effort, one that would marshal a broad collective of people you don't know, who don't live nearby, and who are not like you in most ways. Chantal Mouffe (2018) has powerfully advanced the importance of *agonism*, or relations among adversaries, as essential to the building of a progressive democratic movement, or a Left populism. We need to build alliances and assemblies, not divisions that comfort a tightly defined community. Your agonistic relationship with others – which must involve both immediate experience *and* abstract unities – is part of a struggle to find commonalities among differences that will allow us to work and live together.

The future will be critical institutional practice

Pierre Bourdieu (1984) demonstrated after years of study – this was not an insight that arrived instantaneously, and nor should we expect that we can eye-roll and harumph our way forward either – the markers of a class faction and its reproduction include all that is *not* taught in school. There are knowledge formations that are valued but not officially conveyed in the curriculum. This often resides in the realm of taste, social graces, networks, and exposure to worldly experience. This could be travel and museum-visits. This could be the accumulated social capital of networks of people to contact when you have questions that pertain to their domains of influence. It manifests in cultural forms, where previously marginalized practices build their own legitimation processes, in say film, television, music, games, dance, sports, or food and drink connoisseurship. And now it seems that so much is not taught in school, and that school itself tilts to advantage the self-starter who is individually equipped with technology, expanded social and cultural capital, outside interests and priorities, and the means to support them.

What can be done given the hidden power vectors of bespoked life? The self-organized and autonomous actor is a vehicle for class factions to be re-entitled, regardless of whatever branded 'alternative' identities are asserted. How might we push back against our technologically fortified culture of self-interest? Of the many fronts that must be engaged, there is a special need *to find pockets of progressive possibility inside institutions, inside dominant culture, and inside popular forms*; this is what Raymond Williams (1977) discussed as distinctive and specific 'cultural formations' and this is where resources are found to make a popular collective alliance last beyond the heat of a single issue's spark. Let me be clear: I know that many are doing this work, operating to organize and appropriately direct institutional resources to expand critical and egalitarian potential. But there is such a totalizing romanticization of the self-organized, of the individually convenient, of the anti-institutional troubler, that we risk pushing a generation away from lasting and meaningful engagement with actual agents and materials of change.

As a teacher, I see a comfortable encouragement of the anti-institutional anti-intellectual in tremendous abundance at the university. The pursuit of self-authorized and self-legitimized knowledges, against a shared curriculum representing historical intellectual formations and diverse forms of new expertise, slides neatly into the pockets of those who wish to increase the informalization of education, which has a direct effect on the labour needed to run educational programmes. What tries to pass as 'alternative' and 'radical' is often in fact a valorization of the self-taught, the flexible course, and the self-directed student, for which the pandemic's mass remote teaching effort has been a gigantic beta-test.

The language of Paolo Freire's *Pedagogy of the oppressed* (1970) can be found deployed shamelessly in new visions of the university as though the orientation toward convenience and individualism in education is a radical intervention in the hierarchies of standard curricula. Instead, we must confront a serious problem: there is an overlap between 'radical' 'horizontal' education and the techno-educationalist agenda. Make no mistake, for Freire, dialogic teaching between educator and student was never about absence nor standardized technological architecture! And yet, here we are, living through the continuing hegemony of the 'banking' model of education, which Freire critiqued so resoundingly, in which students are containers to be filled with prime deposits of self-reliance, ontological certitude, technophilia, and anxiousness.

The scholarly critiques of media and cultural studies are a case in point. We have an urgent question to answer about our critiques: *when are we delivering the essential critical vehicles for our times and when are we smoothing out the hegemony of the digital age?* The discourse of the gig is entwined with presumptions about media and technological environment, such that when media is taught it is now about informality, decentralization, individuation, micro-niches, micro-branding, self-organization, innovation, creation, radicality, and alternativeness. These themes have no stable essential political or ideological status, and I don't discount the possibility of rearticulating them strategically to serve egalitarianism. Yet today they are all comfortably and prominently part of our dominant economic regime. Singing their song does not guarantee social, cultural, political, or institutional progress. The academy has become the cutting edge of the entrepreneurial self and an unbounded celebration of techno-autodidactism. Media studies has been front and centre of this swing, and it's a site at which students are taught to see and exploit informality, decentralization, individuation, micro-niches, micro-branding, self-organization, innovation, creation, radicality, and alternativeness. Some versions of media and cultural studies are distorting into a form of skills teaching that tacitly accept and affirm the wave of historical and technological change about informality, decentralization, individuation, etc., when they ought to be thorns that prick and trouble those conceits.

We are still where we were before the pandemic, before the mass take-up of #BLM, before the mass confrontation with new experiences of risk and isolation, before the mass removal of whatever epistemological certainty we may have enjoyed about the way we live, that is, in the midst of the long revolution and the multi-generational work of transforming consciousness alongside our governing institutions. This work can be bumped ahead with tactics that lend themselves to the rewards and hazards of public demonstration.

That's one part of the puzzle. Dream of a messianic moment, if you wish; who doesn't need that dream every now and then? But also scale your energy to the ongoing unphotogenic labour of community building and institution changing, one policy, one hiring, one day at a time.

The timeline for meaningful, lasting, progressive change is not that of the software update to fix a few bugs.

This argument is not a plea to wait or to be patient. And I want us to recognize the work of so many people who show up every day to wrestle with these issues. They have been there before this historic moment and they will be there after the crowds go home, after the epic food bank lines have thinned, and after the refrigeration trucks have moved. I invite us all to plan for sustained action wherever you reside, in whatever institutional context you make your contributions, action that will not be visually or sonically impressive, action that will require day after day, year after year, perseverance and action that will move us forward.

The basic humanity of a living wage, the fundamental dignity of certain and continuous employment, is captured nowhere more completely than by Steinbeck in 1938 in 'Starvation under the orange trees.' He wrote,

> If you buy a farm horse and only feed him when you work him, the horse will die. No one complains of the necessity of feeding the horse when he is not working. But we complain about feeding the men and women who work our lands. (1996a [1938], p. 1027)

From this appeal to decency, Steinbeck swung to describe the wide reverberations one can expect from a hungry work force and organized labour. He continued,

> Is it possible that this state is so stupid, so vicious and so greedy that it cannot feed and clothe the men and women who help to make it the richest area in the world? Must the hunger become anger and the anger fury before anything will be done?

We are, many decades later, awake to the fact that we have preferred to find innovative ways to cheapen and individualize labour, to embrace the gig and the convenient, rather than directly and satisfactorily address such injustices. One slice of the economic pyramid scheme benefits enough people who can then gather up resources to protect their advantage, including policing, tax holidays, and celebrations of individualism and racial division. But anger has collectively grown, and we are seeing the alchemic transformation of that energy into fury.

Building alliances across experiences of injustice is work that needs large-scale institutions, asking, after Antonio Gramsci, about the conditions in which a national-popular formation might emerge. Never settle for pat answers and the imagined comfort of virtuous consensus. Use our critical compass to point to features that might provide what we need to build a progressive historic bloc. And know that to do so, at some point, we have to leave the zones of ad-hocracy and return to the tough, incomplete, messy work of building a lasting popular democratic front. This is an analytical and critical quest that involves perpetually taking stock of the cultural and ideological landscape, describing it, understanding it, and acting on it in our differential capacities with empathy, care, and love.

Notes

1. Elsewhere, I have charted the discursive emergence of our contemporary technological situation, with special focus on the role of education. See, Acland (2012, 2017).
2. It's not surprising that it took a television critic, Emily Nussbaum (2017), to nail this dimension early on in the Trump presidency.

Disclosure statement

No potential conflict of interest was reported by the author.

Further information

This Special Issue article has been comprehensively reviewed by the Special Issue editors, Associate Professor Ted Striphas and Professor John Nguyet Erni.

References

Acland, C.R., 2012. *Swift viewing: the popular life of subliminal influence*. Durham: Duke University Press.
Acland, C.R., 2017. American A.V.: Edgar Dale and the information age classroom. *Technology and culture*, 58 (2), 392–421.
Bourdieu, P., 1984 (1979). *Distinction: a social critique of the judgement of taste*. Cambridge, MA: Harvard University Press.
Duffy, B.E., 2016. The romance of work: gender and aspirational labour in the digital culture industries. *International journal of cultural studies*, 19 (4), 441–457.
Freire, P., 1970 (1968). *Pedagogy of the oppressed*. New York: Herder and Herder.
Grossberg, L., 2018. *Under the cover of chaos: Trump and the battle of the American Right*. London: Pluto Press.

Harris, M., 2017. *Kids these days: human capital and the making of Millennials*. New York: Little, Brown and Company.

Irani, L., 2015. The cultural work of microwork. *New media and society*, 15 (5), 720–739.

Manjoo, F., 2020. Republicans want medicare for all, but just for this one disease: everyone's a socialist in a pandemic. *New York Times*, 11 March. Available from: https://www.nytimes.com/2020/03/11/opinion/coronavirus-socialism.html.

McRobbie, A., 2014. *Be creative!: making a living in the new cultural industries*. Cambridge: Polity Press.

Mouffe, C., 2018. *For a Left populism*. New York: Verso.

Nussbaum, E. 2017. Tragedy plus time: how jokes won the election. *The New Yorker*, 23 January, 66-71.

Srnicek, N., 2016. *Platform capitalism*. Cambridge, MA: Polity Press.

Steinbeck, J., 1996a (1938). Starvation under the orange trees. In: R. DeMott, and E.A. Steinbeck, ed. *John Steinbeck: the Grapes of wrath and other writings, 1936-41*. New York: The Library of America, 1023–1027.

Steinbeck, J., 1996b (1939). The Grapes of wrath. In: R. DeMott, and E.A. Steinbeck, ed. *John Steinbeck: The Grapes of wrath and other writings, 1936-41*. New York: The Library of America, 207–692.

Taylor, K., 2016. *Black Lives Matter to Black liberation*. Chicago: Haymarket Books.

Terranova, T., 2000. Free labor: producing culture for the digital economy. *Social text*, 63 (18.2), 33–58.

Toffler, A., 1970. *Future shock*. New York: Random House.

Williams, R., 1977. *Marxism and literature*. New York: Oxford University Press.

The spectacle of competence: global pandemic and the redesign of leadership in a post neo-liberal world

Leon Gurevitch ⓘ

ABSTRACT
This discussion piece examines the role that New Zealand played in the global media narrative about Covid-19 responses. The New Zealand Government's response in general, and Prime Minister Jacinda Ardern's leadership in particular, came to stand as an example of functional governance to a world experiencing the accelerating fragmentation of Western neo-liberal geo-political economy. The 'spectacle of competence' that has characterized Ardern's leadership is bound up in a pre-existing set of political fault lines that the pandemic has served to amplify. New Zealand's geo-political cultural position, and the competence (both spectacular and actual) that its leadership has come to represent reveal something of the fracture of political economy of the global North and West, not least because the construction of New Zealand as representing a successful 'Western' response is geographically, economically and culturally inaccurate. Contrasting the New Zealand government's pandemic response to the failed responses of Western models of governance, this piece argues that Jacinda Ardern's leadership is important, not because it represents an example of Western success but rather because it represents a departure from the deadly consequences of neo-liberal norms.

As the Covid-19-induced global lockdown began to spread in spring 2020, Western media began to analyse the comparative success and failures of national leaders' responses to the growing pandemic. The broad strokes of the narrative that emerged are now familiar: with the American President initially claiming the virus would 'go away' before seeming to effect a partial about-turn when epidemiological data emerged predicting mass deaths, the UK Prime Minister, Brazilian President and other neo-liberal leaders across the Global North and West initially failed to take the disease seriously, with disastrous consequences. In what became a macabre global spectacle of the deadly consequences of incompetence, British Prime Minister Boris Johnson proudly and publicly confessed to ignoring professional hygiene advice on a hospital ward and Britain was left temporarily leaderless. Like a reality TV character with a poorly constructed story arc, Johnson went from visiting hospitalized Covid-19 patients to being one himself (a story arc that was to be repeated by Trump just six months later). Both Britain and America, historically regarded sources of leadership during a crisis within the post-war Western order, offered little except a spectacle of failure and ongoing chaotic confusion. Unsurprisingly, Western media outlets and social media commentators turned to the question of where leadership could now be found, given its conspicuous absence from the traditional heartland (Mishra 2020).

In the tsunami of commentary that followed, a common theme began to emerge: a number of female leaders in countries previously on the margins of traditional geo-political centres of power were outperforming their male counterparts. New Zealand, Iceland, Scotland, Finland and Denmark were all held up as examples of countries where female leaders had taken rapid action on the basis of citizen well-being above all else. Some commentators (Hirsch 2020, Samarajiva 2020) rightly noted that these analyses suffered a significant flaw in their narrative. Indi Samarajiva, in particular, scathingly noted that such media narratives failed by reinforcing structural racism. In upholding those white leaders who had succeeded relative to the abject failures of most European and American administrations, Samarajiva accused Western media discourse of wilful Orientalist socio-political ignorance. For Samarajiva, the bar for 'success' was so low that to focus on Western sphere 'achievements' in comparison to Western sphere 'failures' repeated the mistake of failing to acknowledge, analyse and learn from the actions Asian countries had taken in managing the disease with far greater degrees of success.

With this in mind, this discussion piece examines the role that New Zealand played in the global media narrative about Covid-19 responses. I will argue that the New Zealand Government's response in general, and Prime Minister Jacinda Ardern's leadership in particular, came to stand as an example of functional governance to a world experiencing the accelerating disintegration of Western geo-political economy. This 'Spectacle of Competence' is important, I will argue, because it is bound up in a pre-existing set of political fault lines that the pandemic served to amplify. The slow breakdown of neoliberal political economy, underlying the 2008 global financial crisis and apparent in Brexit and Donald Trump's subsequent election on a nationalist platform had already revealed a rapid shift in the post-war Western order toward populist nationalist sentiment and away from the transnational signature of neoliberalism. New Zealand's geo-political cultural position, and the competence (both spectacular and actual) that this position engendered in its leadership, reveals something of the fracture of the economic order of the Global North and West. Importantly, the construction of

New Zealand as a successful 'Western' nation is questionable. Presented as an English speaking, predominantly white, culturally anglo-European country in the Western sphere of influence, in reality, New Zealand's position is much more complex. Its geographical location, its growing Asia-pacific demographic and its economic integration with the wider Asia-pacific region have led to a situation in which to label the country 'Western' (always a geographical fallacy) is now tenuously reductive and best understood by a brief examination of the country's recent economic history.[1]

From its location in the south pacific, New Zealand suffered economic crises in the 1970s and 80s after its agricultural economy lost preferential trading status with the United Kingdom. In 1973 the UK entered the European Economic Community and consequently entered into the common agricultural policy. The shock saw New Zealand's purchasing power decline from 115% of the Organisation for Economic Co-operation and Development (OECD) average to 80% (Drew 2007), forcing the country to look to its closer Asian neighbours (not least China) for economic growth and integration. These events were defined by three important political and economic variables that set the country apart from its North/Western counterparts. Firstly, it was a Labour party in the 1980s that introduced neo-liberal market reforms, rather than the right-wing parties and politicians of Europe and America who undertook a similar path. Second, New Zealand's economic trauma was caused by a North/Western counterpart, in this case, a former colonial Britain that, in an ironic historical precursor to Brexit, affected a sudden shift in its trading relations resulting in significant disruption. And thirdly, New Zealand's economy during this crisis, like many of the Asian neighbours it subsequently turned to, was predominantly agricultural and in need of diversification. The solution that eventuated was a diversification from agriculture into tourism, creative digital industries (or 'From Wool to Weta' as former Chief Science Advisor Paul Callaghan (2009) characterized it) and a marketized tertiary education sector. In other words, this crisis marked a historical precedent in which the country and its predominantly Labour government experienced an existential national shock that rapidly realigned its political, ideological, economic and industrial orientation. Perhaps more importantly, many of the solutions (neo-liberal or otherwise) to this crisis were found in, and supplied by, a southeast Asian subcontinent itself diversifying beyond agriculture. The consequence of this was not only that solutions to New Zealand's economic crisis were found in rising Asian neighbours, but that such neighbours shared at least some geographic, industrial and economic commonalities that are often ignored in the problematic characterization of the former colony is a purely 'Western' country in the South East Pacific. These historical differences and experiences may explain some of the stark contrasts in response to the pandemic between New Zealand and its North/Western former colonial counterparts, not least of which was the country's immediate willingness to look to Asia for examples of best practice in dealing with the deadly outbreak. To what extent these differences were a matter of geographic fortune (relative isolation), historical divergence from the Global North and West,[2] or differences of leadership is a question that requires a closer examination of contemporary models of neo-liberal governance.

The spectacle of 'leadership' and the failure of neo-liberal governance

The term 'neoliberalism' is often criticized for the breadth and multiplicity of potential meanings that have come to be attached to it. Consequently, the task of defining the term has been undertaken at length by a range of scholars (Harvey 2007, Brown 2019, Cupers et al. 2020, Wilson 2017, Kotsko 2018), discussion of which could consume the rest of this piece. Instead, for purposes of brevity, I will simply use the term to broadly describe the political-economic ideology that saw reduced government, expanded privatization, liberalization of capital movement and the reduction of progressive tax regimes paired with a diminishment of labour rights and an acceptance of the reduced capacity of democratic governments to shield its citizens from rapidly changing employment conditions under the deindustrialization that followed. Crucially, in recent years criticisms of neoliberalism's failures have emerged from within the very institutions that had championed it over the preceding four decades. With the International Monetary Fund publishing criticism that neoliberalism and its austerity-based solutions to the Global Financial Crisis (GFC) have failed (Ostry et al. 2016) and Financial Times editorials (April 4th, 2020) stating that the economic orthodoxy of the past four decades has run its course (with radical reforms, the reversal of policy and redistribution of wealth necessarily back on the table), it is clear a shift in thinking is already well underway. However, it has not so far been the progressive critics of the carnage that neoliberalism has wrought who have benefitted from the rising public backlash. A disarming feature of this shift has been the way in which the right-wing political architects of globalized free movement of capital and production have been the quickest to capitalize on and hasten its collapse: promising angry, impoverished and politically alienated working- and middle-class electorates across the North/West a reversion to nationalist blueprints underpinned by a supposed return to democratic and economic sovereignty. So far, as both Donald Trump and Boris Johnson have demonstrated, this reversion has not materialized beyond rhetoric. It seems likely that both leaders (and others like them) have calculated that in an attention economy (Simon 1971) the spectacle of leadership, imbued with a publicly nationalist economic rhetoric,[3] would be enough to consolidate and wield the power it has provided them.

Against this background, as the Covid-19 pandemic swept the world, neither Britain nor America's leaders initially took the virus seriously, perhaps in part because it did not feature as a functional variable within their calculus of leadership as a fundamentally spectacular process. As Boris Johnson missed multiple emergency UK Government Cobra meetings and Trump shut down international travel from China but failed to take any steps to address the fact that the virus had already arrived in the US, both leaders' behaviour betrayed a central conviction of their leadership: that action was secondary to the spectacle of 'action'. A clue to the seemingly incomprehensible motivation for this behaviour can be found in Aeron Davis' excellent 2018 sociological study of political and corporate leadership and governance in the United Kingdom. In *Reckless opportunists: Elites at the end of the Establishment,* Davis interviewed leaders from across the British elite for three decades regarding the practices and processes that constituted their professional careers. His conclusions are damning: deregulated neoliberal free market economics has created socio-professional conditions that have corroded the capacity for governance. The high degree of precarity (not simply amongst the working class but also amongst political and corporate elites), the rapid turnover of staff (even at the very top of both public and private institutions), and the need to produce short-term economic results (usually achieved through labour restructuring) has led to a culture in which leaders are unable to gain deep expertise in the institutions they govern, but are instead forced to enact sweeping change and move on to new positions before the results are apparent. Davis' conclusion is stark:

> In the modern system of British elite rule, leaders have come to succeed almost by undermining the very institutions they manage. The ethos of venal self-interest has produced a series of individual risk-reward structures that conflict with organisational objectives. Thus modern British-based elites do well by transforming institutions into something they were never meant to be: short-termist organisations for dealing with other elites rather than catering to publics and society. This shift not only erodes social cohesion, it destabilises the same institutional hierarchies and power structures that underpin elite rule itself. (Davis 2018)

Perhaps where Davis' study is most revealing is in his description of the way in which public and private institutional leaders have seen their roles transformed into that of media message managers, whose role it is to constantly construct specific economic signals intended primarily for the consumption of other elites. In an analysis reminiscent of studies revealing that advertising firms direct most effort on industry clients rather than potential consumers, Davis describes a professional sphere in which governing elites continually refine media messaging for other governing elites, with devastating institutional consequences.

It is, then, unsurprising that neither Donald Trump nor Boris Johnson would imagine that Covid-19 required specific action beyond media messaging and the carefully (and more often, not-so-carefully) constructed spectacle of leadership. Donald Trump's nonsensical public claims that the virus would take care of itself and 'just go away' make more sense in the context of a professional life characterized by short-termist messaging to other members of the financial elite, and by spectacular constructions of corporate leadership designed to function for the duration of an *Apprentice* episode. As does the behaviour of Boris Johnson, a man who rose within a Thatcherite geography that claimed there was 'no such thing as society' and initiated sweeping neoliberal reforms to Britain's political and industrial economy. For Johnson, who inherited a financialised economic and political structure scaffolded around spectacle, it seems his mantra shifted beyond Thatcher's famous claim to a philosophy ironically more reflective of Marxist Theorist Guy Debord's assertion that:

> The spectacle appears simultaneously as society itself, as a part of society, and as a means of unification. As a part of society, it is ostensibly the focal point of all vision and consciousness. But due to the very fact that this sector is separate, it is in reality the domain of delusion and false consciousness. The unification it achieves is nothing but an official language of universal separation. (Debord 1994)

In such a context, a global pandemic was not a catalyst for a failure of Western leadership but a crisis that exposed the dysfunctionality of an economic and political structure premised upon the short-term value of the spectacle of leadership devoid of meaningful actions (which require long-term thinking and collective responsibility).[4] By contrast, as the full implications of the pandemic's spread became apparent, the New Zealand Government acted remarkably quickly.

Jacinda Ardern's response to the pandemic was rapid, clearly communicated[5] and far-reaching – a stark contrast to the ambiguous, often contradictory and sometimes entirely absent responses of other governments in the North/Western hemisphere. Ardern's actions were swift and telling: she closed the borders many months before other leaders, a decision uncomfortably reminiscent of Trump's own shock move to block Chinese travel to the United States. This apparent nationalist and isolationist response to a globalized crisis ran contrary to the thinking of many progressive centre left-leaning instincts, as it did for many centre right neo-liberals, but its implementation had precedent in another of Ardern's actions three years earlier. Upon being sworn into office, the New Zealand Labour Party immediately enacted a policy promised on the campaign trail to place a ban on non-New Zealand nationals purchasing houses in the country. New Zealand had been suffering from a long-running and seemingly intractable housing crisis, with some of the highest house price-to-income ratios in the world. The ban on foreign purchase was an (ultimately futile) attempt to buffer

New Zealand citizens from the tsunami of global liquidity, released upon the world by post GFC central banks, increasingly in search of high yield commodities (which New Zealand housing stock had become).

At the time, negative commentary on this move ranged from criticism of its protectionism and potentially risky rejection of global free market capital, to valid concerns that it represented a xenophobic rejection of rising wealthy Chinese investment in the country.[6] The policy did not have the desired effect of curtailing the country's runaway housing bubble,[7] but is worth mention because it marked a clear, early example of a nationally focused protectionist and market interventionist measure that rejected accepted neoliberal norms in favour of responding to citizenship suffering caused by asset price inflation.[8] In common with the rhetoric of rising right-wing parties across America and Europe, in 2017 New Zealand's Labour leadership ran an election on a nationalist rejection of neoliberal market norms.[9] On the eve of taking office, Ardern was asked in a press conference if, as the Deputy Prime Minister in waiting had indicated, she agreed that capitalism was failing New Zealanders. Her response was immediate and unequivocal: yes, it had. How else were we to understand the highest numbers of homelessness per capita in the OECD?[10]

From the spectacle of 'leadership' to the spectacle of competence

In their 2018 book *Network Propaganda*, Benkler et al. depart from frequent popular declarations that the internet in general and social media in particular have upended traditional channels of news curation and consumption by widening access to, and the availability of, disinformation that would traditionally have remained marginal. Instead, they argue that media ecosystems of both left and right are still dominated by major mainstream media sites. However, they are careful to make clear that networked actors have taken advantage of, and partly constructed, what they label a 'propaganda pipeline' (Benkler et al. 2018, p. 226) through which fringe conspiracy theory material and disinformation are able to move to the major outlets. Importantly, Benkler et al argue that the transit of this material is still dependent upon established elite actors with the political, economic, professional and, most importantly, network capital to be able to make it happen/facilitate it. This is significant because the arrival of such material on major media sites, hand-in-hand with the astonishing and (for the liberal establishment) unexpected spectacle of a US president willing to act publicly as a key networked partisan actor of the propaganda pipeline, led to a powerful and concerted pushback from liberal media platforms. Consequently, long before the Covid-19 crisis emerged, Jacinda Ardern began to be elevated across Western media outlets as an important beacon and counterpoint to what

William Connolly describes as 'the aggressive white territorial nationalism of Trump' (Connolly 2017, p. 6). In March 2019, for instance, shortly after the mass shooting of Muslim mosque-goers in Christchurch, New Zealand, the *New York Times* ran an opinion piece by Sushil Aaron titled 'Why Jacinda Ardern Matters', describing her as 'the antithesis to right-wing strongmen like Trump' (Aaron 2019). Aaron was not alone in making this assertion, and a torrent of articles, news media videos and social media posts followed that presented similar conclusions (Fifield 2019, Lester 2019, Malik 2019, Moore 2019, Salam 2019, Tharoor 2019, Wickstead 2019).

By the time the Covid-19 crisis emerged in early 2020, liberally inclined Western news media outlets were already primed to observe Ardern's reaction. It did not disappoint. Appearing on national television to announce that New Zealand would 'go hard and go early', Ardern directly and concisely acknowledged the potential scale of the crisis and prepared New Zealanders to join the effort. Ardern's extraordinary measures were far reaching. Closing the country's borders to all but returning New Zealand citizens and preparing the nation to implement a pre-emptive full-scale lockdown were to have devastating short-term consequences for an economy structured around open global transit of both people and capital. The New Zealand public responded with widespread support for the policy, and the torrent of positive international headlines praising Ardern's leadership resumed. Importantly, the Ardern Government's actions were presented as a very different spectacle of leadership to that of Trump and Johnson (but also Bolsonaro and others). Less frequently noted was the fact that the spectacle of the Ardern Government's functional decisiveness and capacity to take such action revealed a preparedness to think beyond the standard operating procedure of accepted neoliberal market norms.

In a North/Western sphere that looks set to be characterized by a second crisis of its neoliberal financial system in little more than a decade, emergency neo-Keynesian fiscal responses have been quickly proposed. The emergency infrastructural spending regimes enacted across the West to attempt to mitigate what is euphemistically referred to as an 'emerging depression' put into hard reverse the policy norms that have dominated since the 1980s, and seem likely to accelerate the accompanying political paradigm shift. Until now, prevailing discourse across Western economies has articulated a political landscape with a pro-globalisation neoliberal centre that was understood to represent viable political electability on the one hand, and nationalist tendencies on both the far left (with economic sovereignty located in the democratic nation state and philosophical sovereignty to be found in an internationalist mindset) and the far right (economically protectionist and philosophically isolationist) out on the margins. In the wake of the elections of Donald Trump and Boris Johnson, the rhetoric of national economic sovereignty combined with promised (but subsequently reneged upon) infrastructure spending seemed to be emerging as a new tool in the spectacle of leadership that continued to serve the interests of financial capital to the detriment of electorates. Ardern's leadership and its high profile position as a stark contrast to the abject failures of the United States and United Kingdom's shared dysfunction is significant in the sense that it presents a vision of political and economic leadership that can be both nationally orientated in favour of the protection of its citizens, and at the same time progressive and internationally focused.

Recognizing the once-in-a-generation opportunity to shape the economic narrative that must follow this crisis, the Ardern government has moved with striking rapidity to acknowledge that a new economic settlement must be struck. Repeating their mantra of 'go hard and go early' in their economic response as much as they did in their epidemiological one, the New Zealand Government appears to have acted with an awareness that the world beyond their borders has turned an intense spotlight on the country's governance. Announcing a huge expansion of the national budget, the New Zealand Government has sought to direct infrastructural investment into sustainable long-term job creation that looks beyond a carbon-intensive global tourist industry that has all but collapsed for the short to medium term. Unashamed discussion of a return to the 1930s 'Ministry of Works' has been floated, and the country's finance minister has described this moment as an opportunity to reverse the corrosive effects of economic inequality that late-stage neoliberal economics and the global commodity bubble have created.

The extent to which these discourses translate into long-term results remains to be seen. Reminiscent of recent political actors from Tony Blair to Barak Obama, Ardern has also professed an aversion to change she deems 'too radical to stick' (Giovannetti 2020). Similarly, New Zealand's status as the first 'Western' country to react, and therefore the first to emerge from the epidemiological effects of the global pandemic, has left it in a position to present itself as an attractive production hub for American tech and creative industries in need of a Covid-19-free production location. It is still far too early to know what the economic landscape of national and global economies will look like in a year, let alone a decade, but one thing is already clear: In the absence of functional leadership, and in the presence of a Western media sphere that is still largely ignoring the example of Asia and Africa (see also Hirsch 2020) in focusing on Western responses to the pandemic, New Zealand has found itself at the centre of an ideological and economic tug of war over the nature of national leadership in a world riven by geo-political tension. New Zealand's economy, like most others, will suffer significantly. New Zealand's neoliberal economic immigration strategy, until now premised upon 'global body shopping' (Biao 2007, Castles *et al.*

2009, Castles 2011) of privileged and highly educated migrants, is now facing the potentially immovable object of a medium-term bio-political quarantine.

The question of how far New Zealand's economic fortunes will be shaped by its capacity to leverage its unexpected geographical and biological advantage, and to what extent doing so requires the free movement of skilled labour, remains to be answered. The emerging conflict between resurgent nationalist demands of electorates, governments attempting to negotiate an ever more complex global economic environment and the necessity of governance to offer more than lip service to the nationalist tendencies of some voters continues to play out. What is clear, however, is that New Zealand's initial 'gold standard' (Melinek cited in Thomas 2020) response to the pandemic crisis was shaped by a centre-left government that professed nationally-oriented motivations and scepticism regarding neoliberal norms. Such a position placed the government sharply at odds with a conservative opposition that insistently claimed that the country's isolation was too high a price to pay. Among voters, the electoral consequences have been devastating for the opposition.[11] New Zealand and its Covid-19 response point to the possibility of a fluctuating political future characterized by the return of contrasting forms of nationalism: one utilized for rhetorical ends by formerly neoliberal conservative economic elites continually moving right, and the other deployed by progressives to underpin a commitment to their electorate while attempting to negotiate a complex and shifting international economic order. So far the Ardern government's deployment of the latter has been accompanied by international press characterizing her leadership as an astonishing example of competence. But characterizations that have held New Zealand up as an example of 'Western' success elide the reality of New Zealand's geographical, economic and increasingly cultural position in the Asia Pacific. Importantly, Ardern's government has rejected standard neo-liberal operating procedure that places notions of the economy above public health and liberalized faith in market mechanisms above active governance.

Ironically, and largely unnoticed by more recent international media accounts of New Zealand, what started out as a pandemic crisis has turned into an accelerating housing crisis. In the face of a predicted labour market meltdown triggered by the nation's closed borders, and fearful that a correlated house market drop would precipitate a domino effect that triggered severe economic depression, the Reserve Bank followed the global trend and unleashed a new wave of liquidity whilst slashing interest rates. The result of this intervention, alongside the successful eradication of the virus, not only avoided a widely predicted 10% drop in house prices but supercharged an already two-decade old housing bubble resulting in a tulip-mania-like 20% rise in prices. With a narrative circularity that would seem too neatly fabricated if it were fiction, the Ardern government vanquished one crisis only to fuel another in the process: and not just any 'other' but one that Ardern built her rise to power promising to finally resolve. In the closing months of 2020, house prices rose so quickly (up to 3% per month) that the bubble's threat to both social and economic stability replaced the pandemic as the top story nationally. With price inflation so rampant the Labour government found itself presiding over the fastest inequality growth in the country's history, calls for meaningful action have grown across the political spectrum.

Where Ardern was radical in the face of a pandemic, however, she has been equally conservative on house price contagion. Responding to accusations of historic miscalculation Ardern pointed to asset inflation as a global phenomenon, doubled down on a refusal to introduce capital gains tax and asserted her preference for destructively high prices 'not to drop'. Here then, appear to be the limits of New Zealand Labour's challenge to the neo-liberal status quo. With a disproportionate quantity of the country's wealth locked in real-estate, challenging constituents of New Zealand's growing millionaire asset owning elite appears to be a step too far. Where the threat was perceived as external, be it a virus or foreign capital flows, radical, decisive and spectacularly competent leadership was abundant. Where the growing chasm between haves and have nots is an internal affair, such radical and decisiveness is absent.

Both the US Republicans and the New Zealand Conservatives suffered historic defeats in the final months of 2020, and with a Brexit deal now concluded it remains to be seen how long the British Conservative 'Chumocracy' (Mishra 2019) can escape the consequences the ongoing spectacle of incompetent leadership. But with progressive alternatives that seek to 'invent the future' (Srnicek and Williams 2015) still struggling to gain meaningful political-economic policy traction, the waning of the pandemic is at present still a story of rapidly growing, and more importantly *accelerating*, inequality in New Zealand. Convincing analyses of New Zealand's successful eradication of Covid-19 has centred around the fact that the country has been preparing its population for an unprecedented natural disaster for decades. Earthquake preparedness for 'the big one' is an ongoing narrative in the background of daily life and, it has been argued, saw the country ready and willing to make collective sacrifices for the greater good when the pandemic arrived. Another narrative long held dear amongst New Zealand citizens has been that of relative egalitarianism: the country was not rich but neither was it characterized by inequality. To some extent this narrative ignored clear deprivations suffered by its Maori and Pacific Island communities, but with extreme asset inflation now driving inequality far beyond historical averages, it is clear that management of the Covid-19 virus is only the first stage in an environment of proliferating impacts. If New Zealand does stand as a beacon of competent leadership amongst liberal democracies, it is its next act not its previous one, that will be its most crucial.

It is now clear that rising popular discontent fuelled the geopolitical earthquakes of Brexit and the Trump administration long before the initiation of the global pandemic. In their excellent analysis of the limitations of progressive 'folk politics' that have refused to 'invent the future' for fear of discredit risked by failed grand narratives, Srnicek and Williams (2015) argue that we need a new left-wing embrace of the utopian possibilities of the 'future'. Since Covid-19 emerged, claims that the global pandemic presents an opportunity for a 'great reset' (Schwab 2020) have abounded. So far however, though the country avoided a much feared crippling depression, New Zealand's domestic economic landscape has reflected a 'great retrenchment'. With economic policy elites from the Central Bank to Government hosing billions of dollars of liquidity into already inflated assets, claims that Universal Basic Incomes, Universal Basic Services and policy initiatives that share social solidarity after the 'great lockdown' cannot be afforded will face increasingly intense scrutiny.

On Jacinda Ardern's desk sits a photograph of Michael Joseph Savage, Prime Minister of New Zealand's first Labour government from 1935 to 1940. Taking office during the great depression and enacting radical social reforms, Savage is regarded as the architect of modern New Zealand and its post-war welfare state. Like Ardern, Savage's popularity was considered a consequence of his charismatic personality, skilled oration and communication. Savage used his capacities and political capital to enact radical reforms and lay down the foundations of a country that was to be characterized by relative equality during the twentieth century. If Ardern is to follow a similar trajectory she will need to enact policy change currently regarded as 'too radical to stick'. Huge infrastructure spending has already been enacted, but housing for all, income security in the potential face of a second jobless recovery in as many decades and the reaffirmation of the principle of relative economic equality backed up by redistributive taxes all require rigorous political support. New Zealand is much more than a nation state scale bunker for libertarian tech billionaires seeking to escape the social collapse of their North/Western homelands. If the North/West really is looking to New Zealand, the country should effect a disproportionate influence on the shape of the post-pandemic recovery as ambitious as its approach to the pandemic itself, but it will require an economic approach as radical as the failed neo-liberal orthodoxy that has left a vacuum in its wake.

Thanks to:

I have a number of people to thank for support and feedback on this article. Thanks to Kristy Grant, Katie Brennan, Steve McCormick, Nicci Stilwell, Simon Nicholson, Jenny Vickers, Dan Scudder Maja Gutman, Regis Le Moguc dec, Rose Jago, Mo Zareei and Reuven Gonzales who all read and commented on various stage drafts of this article.

Notes

1. New Zealand's refusal to join the five eyes alliance in a joint communique regarding Hong Kong is an example of the increasingly complex geopolitical tightrope act the country is attempting to walk.
2. The phrases 'Global North' and 'West' are used somewhat interchangeably in this article and reveal something of the limitations of both concepts. I have felt it necessary to reference both the 'Global North' and its preceding 'Western' conception though both are limited by their ontological shortcomings as the Post War order wanes.
3. It should be noted that both leaders profess to support the notion of free trade whilst wielding nationalist populism to assert that the current problem lies in the distortion of its original tenets (for the UK in the form of the EU and for the US in the form of a World Trade Organisation that supposedly now favours China).
4. Something of this is encapsulated in Pankaj Mishra's excellent London Review of Books essay 'Flailing States'.
5. Through both traditional national media and social media.
6. However, the enactment of these rules contained a telling signal as to its primary aims. Foreign citizens could in fact own houses in New Zealand but were required to build them first: a move intended to prevent global capital flows inflating housing stock that Labour felt should be a public necessity rather than a global commodity. By forcing foreign capital to build rather than purchase, the government signalled an openness to global capital investment but a rejection of global free market mechanisms for an essential public good.
7. In part because of a failure to implement a subsequently recommended capital gains tax.
8. Comparing the New Zealand government's pandemic response with that of its earlier actions against foreign capital in its housing market is potentially fraught. Not least for its xenophobic potential to associate foreign house buyers with a pathogen. For this reason it is important to stress that this was about capital flows and protection of the country's residents rather than human migration. The New Zealand Ardern government has been active in consistently raising its quota of refugees including during the pandemic itself though admittedly from a low base.
9. So far, amongst the Western nationalist projects that have gained ground since the collapse of the global financial system in 2008, with the exception of Scottish and Catalonian separatist projects, the direction of political travel has seemed to favour a combined strategy of appeals to working- and middle-class voters to reject 'globalist' economic technocracy, mixed with a reactionary protectionism that ultimately serves the interests of elite capital. The result of these incompatible but electorally successful contradictions (Strongly reminiscent of Hannah Arendt's analysis of the European masses' alignment with both capital and elites in the nineteenth century pre-war periods) has been the manifestation of governments in both the United Kingdom and United States that deploy spectacular constructions of national leadership while failing to perform meaningful actions within the social, political and economic frameworks which they rose to power attacking, and which have disenfranchized their voters.

10. The point here is not that the current New Zealand government is a radical one, (that Leilani Farha, UN special rapporteur on housing rights accused the New Zealand government in February 2020 of presiding over a human rights crisis testifies to its continued timidity in intervening in excessive market mechanisms) rather, it is that it is characterized by one significant though so far muted departure from all previous governments since the neo-liberal market reforms of the mid 1980s in being willing to acknowledge a failure of global capital where its citizenry are concerned.

11. As of writing the first draft, polls heading into a September election had placed the Labour government on and unprecedented 54% and the Conservatives on 29%. It had seemed likely that these numbers would shift significantly but, in the end, Ardern's Labour Party won a historic outright majority landslide of 49.1% against the Conservative National party's equally historic 26.8% meltdown.

Disclosure statement

No potential conflict of interest was reported by the author(s).

Further information

This Special Issue article has been comprehensively reviewed by the Special Issue editors, Associate Professor Ted Striphas and Professor John Nguyet Erni.

ORCID

Leon Gurevitch ⬤ http://orcid.org/0000-0002-8124-5856

References

Aaron, S. 2019. Why Jacinda Ardern matters. *New York Times*, 19 March. Available from: https://www.nytimes.com/2019/03/19/opinion/jacinda-ardern-new-zealand.html.
Benkler, Y., Faris, R., and Roberts, H., 2018. *Network propaganda: manipulation, disinformation, and radicalisation in American politics*. Oxford: Oxford University Press.
Biao, X., 2007. *Global body shopping: An Indian labor system in the information technology industry*. Princeton: Princeton University Press.

Brown, W., 2019. *The ruins of neoliberalism: The rise of antidemocratic politics in the west*. New York: Columbia University Press.

Callaghan, P., 2009. *From wool to weta: transforming New Zealand's culture and economy*. Auckland: Auckland University Press.

Castles, S., 2011. 'Migrations, crisis, and the global labour Market'. In *Globalisations, June 2011, Vol. 8, No. 3*, London: Routledge, pp. 311–324.

Castles, S., De Hass, H., and Miller, M., 2009. *The Age of migration: international population movements in the modern world*. 4th ed. Basingstoke: Palgrave MacMillan Press.

Connolly, W., 2017. *Aspirational fascism: The struggle for multifaceted democracy under trumpism*. Minnesota: University of Minnesota Press.

Cupers, K., Gabrielsson, C., and Mattsson, H., eds. 2020. *Neoliberalism on the ground: Architecture and transformation from the 1960s to the present*. Pittsburgh: University of Pittsburgh Press.

Davis, A., 2018. *Reckless opportunists: elites at the end of the establishment*. Manchester: Manchester University Press.

Debord, G., 1994. *The society of the spectacle*. New York: Zone Books.

Drew, A. 2007. New Zealand's productivity performance and prospects. *Reserve bank of New Zealand bulletin*, 70 (1) March 2007. Available from: https://www.rbnz.govt.nz/research-and-publications/reserve-bank-bulletin/2007/rbb2007-70-01-02.

Fifield, A. 2019. New Zealand's prime minister receives worldwide praise for her response to the Mosque shootings. *The Washington Post*, 19 March 2019. Available from: https://www.washingtonpost.com/world/2019/03/18/new-zealands-prime-minister-wins-worldwide-praise-her-response-mosque-shootings/.

Giovannetti, J. 2020. Covid-19, crisis and transformation: an interview with Jacinda Ardern. *The Spinoff*, Available from: https://thespinoff.co.nz/politics/22-05-2020/covid-19-crisis-and-transformation-an-interview-with-jacinda-ardern.

Harvey, D., 2007. *A brief history of neoliberalism*. Oxford: Oxford University Press.

Hirsch, A. 2020. Why are Africa's coronavirus successes being overlooked? *The Guardian*, 21 May. Available from: https://www.theguardian.com/commentisfree/2020/may/21/africa-coronavirus-successes-innovation-europe-us.

Kotsko, A., 2018. *Neoliberalism's demons: on the political theology of late capital*. Stanford: Stanford University Press.

Lester, A. 2019. The roots of Jacinda Ardern's extraordinary leadership after Christchurch. *The New Yorker*, 23 March 2019. Available from: https://www.newyorker.com/culture/culture-desk/what-jacinda-arderns-leadership-means-to-new-zealand-and-to-the-world.

Malik, N. 2019. With Respect: how Jacinda Ardern showed the world what a leader should be. *The Guardian*, 28 March 2019. Available from: https://www.theguardian.com/world/2019/mar/28/with-respect-how-jacinda-ardern-showed-the-world-what-a-leader-should-be.

Mishra, P. 2020. Flailing states. *London Review of Books*, 42 (14), July. Available from: https://www.lrb.co.uk/the-paper/v42/n14/pankaj-mishra/flailing-states.

Mishra, P. 2019. The Malign Incompetence of the British Ruling Class. *New York Times*, 17 Jan 2019. Available from: https://www.nytimes.com/2019/01/17/opinion/sunday/brexit-ireland-empire.html.

Moore, S. 2019. Jacinda Ardern is showing the world what real leadership is: sympathy, love and integrity. *The Guardian*, 18 March 2019. Available from: https://www.theguardian.com/commentisfree/2019/mar/18/jacinda-ardern-is-showing-the-world-what-real-leadership-is-sympathy-love-and-integrity.

Ostry, J., Loungani, P., and Furceri, D. 2016. Neoliberalism: Oversold? In *Finance and Development*, International Monetary Fund. Available from: https://www.imf.org/external/pubs/ft/fandd/2016/06/pdf/ostry.pdf.

Salam, M. 2019. Jacinda Ardern Is Leading by Following No One. *The New York Times*, 22 March 2019. Available from: https://www.nytimes.com/2019/03/22/world/australia/jacinda-ardern-new-zealand-leader.html.

Samarajiva, I. 2020. How Germany is A COVID Failure: the incredibly low bar for white people. *Medium*, 24 April. Available from: https://medium.com/@indica/germany-is-a-coronavirus-failure-7e2a58f5b4fe.

Schwab, K., and Malleret, T., 2020. *Covid-19: the great reset*. Geneva: ISBN Agentur Schweiz.

Simon, H., 1971. Designing organisations for an information-rich world. In: M. Greenberger, ed. *Computers, communications, and the public interest*. Baltimore: The Johns Hopkins Press. Available from: https://digitalcollections.library.cmu.edu/awweb/awarchive?type=file&item=33748.

Srnicek, N., and Williams, A., 2015. *Inventing the future: post capitalism and a world without work*. London: Verso.

Tharoor, I. 2019. New Zealand shooting: The world is Praising Jacinda Ardern's response to terrorist attack. *The Independent*, 20 March 2019. Available from: https://www.independent.co.uk/news/world/australasia/new-zealand-shooting-jacinda-ardern-video-reaction-world-praise-a8832186.html.

The Financial Times. 2020. Virus lays bare the frailty of the social contract: Radical reforms are required to forge a society that will work for all. 4 April 2020. Available from: https://www.ft.com/content/7eff769a-74dd-11ea-95fe-fcd274e920ca.

Thomas, J., 2020. Coronavirus: US pathologist credits NZ leadership for 'gold standard' response. *Stuff*, 10 July. Available from: https://www.stuff.co.nz/national/300053080/coronavirus-us-pathologist-credits-nz-leadership-for-gold-standard-response

Wickstead, E. 2019. Why Jacinda Ardern Is A Leader For Our Times. *Vogue*, 22 March 2019. Available from: https://www.vogue.co.uk/article/why-jacinda-ardern-is-a-leader-for-our-times.

Wilson, J., 2017. *Neoliberalism*. London: Routledge.

The epiphanic moments of COVID-19: the revelation of painful national truths

Mette Hjort

ABSTRACT

Focusing on the small nation state of Denmark, this article considers the implications of responses to COVID-19 for the dynamics of multiple belonging involving Western and Asian nations. The claim is that COVID-19's cultural dimensions include the phenomenon of weakened attachments to an originary homeland on the part, for example, of non-resident Danes and a concomitant strengthening of commitments to adopted homelands in Asia, such as Hong Kong. To understand these shifting allegiances, it is necessary to be attuned to the cultural virulence of COVID-19. In coining the term 'cultural virulence' I seek to draw attention to the ways in which the virus has been not only a source of contagion and illness, but a veritable engine of telling cultural revelations. In COVID-19's *cultural virulence* we discover striking manifestations of painful national truths that we ignore at our peril. Careful scrutiny of COVID-19's epiphanic moments brings to light Western arrogance and exceptionalism, a costly refusal to acknowledge the tried and tested efficacy of Asian practices. Faced with a future marked by pandemics, we must recognize the need for humility in the West regarding the cultural and geographic provenance of best practices as these relate to the containment of serious epidemiological threats.

On December 30, 2019 Li Wenliang, an ophthalmologist working in a hospital in Wuhan, China, alerted fellow doctors to the existence of a new Sars-like disease in a WeChat posting (OT&P). Li, we now know, had identified a novel coronavirus to which he himself would eventually succumb. Dubbed COVID-19 by the WHO, which sought to avoid the blame implicit in geographical namings (examples include US President's Donald Trump's references to 'Kung flu' or the 'Chinese virus'), this infectious disease went on to contribute to a worldwide public health emergency within months and, through this, to a whole host of crises (economic, social, financial, geo-political, and generational, among others) that remain acute almost a year later, with no clear end in sight. I speak of the virus as *contributing* to a global health emergency, rather than simply *causing* it, for many of the causes of the pandemic relate to longstanding cultural factors (e.g. the destruction of natural habitats, the failure to respond to the climate crisis with a shift to non-meat diets on a global scale, and escalating geopolitical conflicts). It is not hard to imagine a counterfactual story in which the novel coronavirus encounters quite different cultural conditions during the various phases of its global transmission, conditions that effectively contain rather than amplify its potent capacity for harm. This brief intervention suggests that parochialism, arrogance, and even racism created a fertile environment for the virus in the West, causing its transformation from a merely serious threat into a fully realized global crisis. Responses to COVID-19, whether official or unofficial, are deeply embedded in cultural frameworks. Indeed, they are even revelatory of such frameworks, for they lay bare, at times with shocking clarity, attitudes and beliefs that pervade a given national space.

What we might call COVID-19's epiphanic cultural virulence has impacted identity formation in countless significant ways. It has, for example, had far-reaching consequences for persons with identities forged through processes of multiple belonging. It is fair to say that for many Western nationals residing in Asia, the cultural dynamics of COVID-19 have had the effect of significantly weakening attachments to an originary homeland and substantially strengthening connections to an adopted home. While general in nature, this proposition is supported by anecdotal evidence derived from pronouncements by a substantial number of Hong Kong-based citizens of the USA, UK, and Denmark.

A Dane by birth who was denied the right to family unification by an anti-immigrant government in Denmark in 2017, I have lived the crises of COVID-19 in Hong Kong, which I have had the privilege of calling home almost without interruption since 2001. Conditioned, like many fellow Hong Kongers, by the earlier SARS crisis of 2003 and immersed in a culture, among other things, of informed, disciplined, and compliant general mask-wearing in response to the virus, I watched with horror as the West, Denmark included, questioned the efficacy of masks. Even as COVID-19 was contained in China (by the end of January 2020, Hong Kong had implemented a suite of effective measures, and, on March 19, 2020, China reported zero new local transmissions), the nations of the West, having failed to prepare for the inevitable arrival of the virus, found themselves facing a full-blown public health crisis (from around February 20, 2020 in Italy, March 6, 2020 in the US, and with the UK locking down for the first time on March 24, 2020) (OT&P 2020).

'Crisis,' as the etymologists tell us, refers to those productive, significant moments that make a critical difference, to a kairotic temporality (Castoriadis 1997) that witnesses the emergence of forking paths, with some prevailing and others fading from view. Viewed through a Hong Kong lens, the multiple national failures in the West to engage appropriately with Asia and Asian practices have effectively become a series of epiphanic moments, each of them a revelatory source of national truths that must be stated and recognized, however painful, if we hope to avoid future pandemics, some of them possibly more virulent and deadly than COVID-19. In what follows I focus on the specific case of Denmark, regularly (self-)described as the happiest country in the world, although many immigrants, asylum seekers, returning non-resident Danes, Danes married to non-Danes, and any number of other persons falling outside a bureaucratized template culture of deep, ancestral belonging would be hard pressed to agree. The point about happiness ascriptions is worth making, as it highlights a wider cultural context for COVID-19's reproduction in this specific instance, one that is inward-looking, self-congratulatory, exceptionalist, and ethnic nationalist.

The absence of transnational sympathy: COVID-19 as an engine for national humour

COVID-19 entered the national space of Denmark through the portal of a much favoured tradition of affluence, more specifically, the northern Italian ski vacations enjoyed by well-heeled Danes during their so-called *vinterferie* (Winter holidays). The first Danish COVID-19 case was registered on February 27, 2020. But let us look at the period just prior to the first Danish case. After all, an important part of the cultural picture of COVID-19's spread relates to responses to news of the virus' existence prior to its penetration of a given national space.

A small nation that instills beliefs about the superiority of its state, systems, and nationals in its citizens from cradle to grave, Denmark initially regarded itself as protected from COVID-19 by some unspecified amalgam of hyper-positive traits. In the parochial mindset of Danish exceptionalism, COVID-19 could only be a problem of, and for, 'the Other.' The role of Danish humour during the early outbreak of COVID-19 in China is highly symptomatic of the cultural dysfunctions of Danish exceptionalism. Instead of preparing seriously for the inevitable arrival of COVID-19, by making reference, for example, to developments in other jurisdictions, such as Hong Kong, Taiwan, or Korea, Danes indulged their nationalist predilection for a particular species of disrespectful humour.

An object of tremendous pride in Denmark, Danish humour, far from being the expression of enlightened freedom as Danes would have it, in fact merits description, now through a Hong Kong lens, as a profoundly oafish and often cruel lack of civility, sympathy, and respect. On January 27, 2020, *Jyllands-Posten*, the daily that provoked the life-costing 'Cartoon Crisis' in 2005 with a series of depictions of the prophet Muhammad, one of them a drawing of the religious figure with a bomb protruding from his head, took the initiative to publish a 'cartoon of the Chinese flag with virus-like figures in place of the symbolic yellow stars.'[1] In response to objections from China, Editor-in-chief Jacob Nybroe defended the newspaper's provocation by evoking diverging cultural traditions: 'As far as I can see, we are dealing with two different cultural views …. We have a strong tradition of freedom of expression and caricature in Denmark, and we will continue to have it in the future' (Oelze 2020).

That the deployment of Danish humour in response to the initially Chinese tragedy of COVID-19 was ultimately an unacceptable manifestation of a profound lack of transnational sympathy was not lost on one UK-based academic who was teaching a Scandinavian Studies course to a number of students from China at the time. Acutely well informed about the ravages of the virus, these students were worrying about their own health and that of loved ones in their home country. Dr Claire Thomson, Senior Lecturer in Scandinavian Studies at University College London, intervened admirably on Facebook as follows:

> the same Danish newspaper responsible for the so-called 'Cartoon Crisis' has published this vile cartoon. While I accept and respect that the right to offend is central to Danish culture, and promoting and mediating Danish culture is part of my job, the people being cruelly reduced to cartoon viruses here are my students and my friends. I am not going to be defending or 'contextualising' this. I am going to write to my students tomorrow—all the 24 students from all over the world, a majority of them from China, who have freely and enthusiastically chosen to spend a term studying Nordic Cinema—and apologise. (Thomson 2020)

Jyllands-Posten was not the only newspaper to encourage the cruel superficiality of Danish humour at a time when serious-minded citizens of Asian countries were battling the virus on all fronts, for example through a host of imaginative citizen-driven initiatives aimed at mitigating the risks to which the poor and elderly were exposed (at Hong Kong Baptist University, staff and students donated increasingly precious surgical masks to those in need, while the School of Chinese Medicine distributed herbal concoctions, designed to strengthen immunity, to the elderly). On February 21, 2020, *Politiken*, much favoured by readers who self-identify as part of the Danish intelligentsia, published a costume guide ahead of *Fastelavn*, a carnival tradition that is greatly enjoyed by children. The title of the piece in *Politiken* was 'Er du klar til krænkelsesfastelavn?' (Are you ready for an offensive carnival?). The idea of dressing up as COVID-19 – as a yellow ball with protruding crowns – figured in the list of suggestions that could be adopted with an eye to being maximally offensive and provocative during the carnival period. COVID-19 called for deeply serious responses, ones informed by authentic attempts at understanding, including through processes of empathy and sympathy. Instead, Danes saw fit to exploit the crisis through self-congratulatory attempts at bravado humour that could only become self-defeating, given the nature of COVID-19.

Discounting Asian practices and knowledge: questioning the utility of masks

At the time of writing, the Danish authorities are inching their way towards acknowledging what has long been known in Hong Kong and Asia more generally, namely that a generalized adoption of masks across the population offers a decisive tool for combatting COVID-19. Yet, there is still a long way to go, for as of early August 2020 the Minister of Health only requires masks when using the public transport system, and only in the town of Århus. The government's early rejection of masks described the humble object in question as insufficiently researched, ineffective, and as creating a false sense of security. Months later a concession to best practices elsewhere was made: masks should be worn when travelling to be tested for COVID-19 and could even be worn by persons of an especially 'worried' disposition. The small minority of mask adopters in Denmark, most of them of bi-cultural or foreign background or with a personal history of 'non-resident Dane' status, rightly described the reference to a state of worry as an act of false categorization with ramifications for how they would be perceived when in public space.

The authorities' refusal of masking practices over a period of many critical months was admittedly not entirely home-grown, in as much as it made reference to the WHO's changing and often highly questionable positions on the matter. Slow to recognize the value of masks, the WHO implicitly acknowledged the highly divergent attitudes towards the humble objects in question in its 'Interim Guidance' dated 6 April 2020 (WHO 2020): 'In some countries masks are worn in accordance with local customs.' Apparently sceptical of the validity of such customs, or, perhaps more accurately, fearing the consequences of a shortage of masks in the medical sector, the WHO went on to advise 'decision makers on the use of masks for healthy people in community settings' as follows: 'the wide use of masks by healthy people in the community setting is not supported by current evidence and carries uncertainties and critical risks' (Ibid). Proffering this advice, the WHO effectively continued to deny the true and justified beliefs of citizens in countries throughout Asia, knowledge of the efficacy of general masking having been mobilized with good results in such places as Taiwan (through government actions) and Hong Kong (as a result, initially, of citizen activism). Instead of validating the evidence afforded by remarkably low rates of infection and death in places such as Taiwan and Hong Kong, where generalized maskwearing was adopted, the WHO gave a country like Denmark a convenient license to reject masks as, variously, unnecessary, a risk in themselves, culturally alien, and unproven.

The WHO-endorsed possibility of rejection found fertile ground in Denmark, where facial coverings have long been a matter of significant controversy (in connection with non-Western immigrants and asylum seekers of Islamic faith and culture), and where citizens are taught from the earliest age to celebrate their country as the 'best in the world.' Danish citizens who had experienced a wider world, for example as exchange students at Asian universities or as long-term residents of China, repeatedly reported that their attempts to discuss the utility of masks with peers, colleagues, room mates, and even family members were generally met with hostility and, in some cases, even accusations of having 'gone native' or having been 'brainwashed' (for example by Hong Kong) after a period abroad.[2] Allegedly shielded from the ills of less developed countries, Denmark, the pervasive attitude would have it, had no compelling need to look beyond national borders for knowledge, best practices, or solutions, and certainly no need to look beyond the West. It is safe to say that COVID-19's continued (and, as of early August 2020, accelerating) diffusion in a deeply mask-resistant culture brings Denmark's parochialism to light, just as it lays bare the (in this case, deadly) serious limitations of the inward-looking mindsets.

Issues of belonging: blood and soil during during the COVID-19 pandemic

COVID-19's epiphanic cultural virulence has also made itself felt in the area of national belonging, with actions, decisions, and interventions bringing to light some of the ways in which the imagined community of the Danish nation is constituted and even officially 'managed.' Like many other countries in the West, Denmark has witnessed a surge in racist abuse, with victims singled out purely on the basis of putatively Asian features. This chapter in the story of COVID-19's cultural virulence certainly deserves to be explored more fully.[3] In the present context, however, I wish to focus on the curious cultural twists and turns of state power as the government sought to defend its populist commitment to what it had previously constituted as an especially potent expression of deep belonging, the handshake. Here too, the novel coronavirus had the effect of exposing parochialism and a profound lack of empathy, this time in the very dynamics of citizenship. I am referring to the curious handshake crisis, one relating specifically to immigrants and asylum seekers who were on the cusp of becoming Danish citizens when COVID-19 prompted the Danish government to introduce social distancing measures. These individuals, it should be noted, had met the most stringent of criteria over a significant period of time, including the criterion of passing a citizenship test that most Danes with Danish ancestry are unable to pass without a substantial amount of preparation.

Under a Danish law introduced on January 1, 2019 (nr. 1767 regarding the requirements of constitutional ceremonies at the level of local government), a flesh against flesh (no gloves are allowed) handshake is part of the formal ceremony of bestowing Danish citizenship on new Danes. Introduced by an anti-immigrant government as a means of testing the depth of the cultural commitments of the soon-to-be Dane, the handshake must occur, irrespective of gender and originary cultural/religious background. That is, according to the law of 2019, any Muslim woman who aspires to become Danish must accept in advance that she will be required to shake the hand of the officiating mayor, whether or not the individual in question is male. Faced with the challenges of COVID-19, the government initially ruled that all citizenship ceremonies would be cancelled until further notice, it being the case that handshakes were no longer possible. Confounded by the lack of empathy and the profound lack of imagination on the part of the government, a number of rebel mayors announced the intention to forge ahead with the planned ceremonies. Eventually, on May 5, 2020 'L 180,' a proposal relating to the citizenship ceremony, was debated in Parliament, the outcome being that the handshake requirement would be temporarily suspended. At issue during the debate was, precisely, the question of culture. Thus, for example, Peder Hvelplund (belonging to Enhedslisten, the Red-Green Alliance) indicated support for the initiative but also proposed to make it lasting rather than temporary, on the grounds that culture is 'dynamic.' His argument was that COVID-19 had had a profound impact on culture and that some cultural practices pre-dating the virus would now arguably be ill advised on a permanent basis. Tellingly, the response from Rasmus Stoklund, a social democrat, was as follows:

> For centuries it has been customary in Denmark to shake hands, as a gesture, when we greet one another. I believe this is a completely natural way of greeting each other and of conducting a ceremony, when it is a matter of something as momentous as becoming a Danish citizen. (Folketinget/Parliament 2020)

Advocates of the handshake repeatedly linked the practice to Denmark's putative commitments to social norms of openness, transparency, and trust. At the time of writing, the ruling is that the handshake will be reinstated once the challenges of COVID-19 have been met.

The epiphanic moments of COVID-19's cultural trajectories offer opportunities for reflection and change, and even lessons for the future. There has been much talk of China's failings, especially during the early period of the outbreak in Wuhan. Yet, the West has much to answer for too. While the mortality rate in Denmark has been less grim than in other parts of Europe, there can be no doubt that, moving forward, the country, but also the global community to which it belongs, would be well served by Danish efforts to foster a far greater capacity for transnational sympathy and empathy, to curtail a powerful sense of exceptionalism, and to counter small-nation tendencies in the direction of parochial inwardness and small-mindedness. If future pandemics are to be avoided, the perspectives that multiple belonging afford must be instilled and taken seriously. Respect for other cultures, a willingness to learn from and about other cultures, these are capacities that must be cultivated. Art and Humanities subjects, including Cultural Studies, have much to offer in this regard. For this reason alone, it is imperative that they survive the crises of COVID-19.

Notes

1. See Jorgensen (2006) for a timeline of how the cartoon crisis unfolded.
2. Radhika Vang Jensen, a student of Film and Media Studies at the University of Copenhagen and an exchange student at Hong Kong Baptist University in the Fall of 2019, has provided extensive testimony along these lines over a period of months.
3. See Sven Holms Skov (2020) for a relevant discussion of racism experienced by Asian Danes during COVID-19.

Disclosure statement

No potential conflict of interest was reported by the author(s).

Further information

This Special Issue article has been comprehensively reviewed by the Special Issue editors, Associate Professor Ted Striphas and Professor John Nguyet Erni.

References

Castoriadis, C., 1997. *The imaginary institution of society*. Cambridge: Polity.

Folketinget/Parliament, 2020. L 180 Forslag til lov om indfødsrets meddelelse (L 180 Proposal with reference to communiqué regarding citizenship). Available from: https://www.ft.dk/samling/20191/lovforslag/l180/index.htm.

Holms Skov, S., 2020. Coronavirus får racisme mod dansk-asiatere ud i lys lue (Coronavirus brings racism against Danish-Asians into the open). *Politiken*, 2 April. Available from: https://politiken.dk/indland/samfund/art7737522/Coronavirus-får-racisme-mod-dansk-asiatere-ud-i-lys-lue.

Jorgensen, I., 2006. Timeline: How the cartoon crisis unfolded. *Financial Times*, 21 March. Available from: https://www.ft.com/content/d30b0c22-96ee-11da-82b7-0000779e2340.

Oelze, S., 2020. China angry over coronavirus cartoon in Danish newspaper. *DW*, 30 January. Available from: https://www.dw.com/en/china-angry-over-coronavirus-cartoon-in-danish-newspaper/a-52196383.

OT&P, 2020. COVID-19 Timeline. Available from: https://www.otandp.com/covid-19-timeline.

Thomson, C.C., 2020. Facebook posting, January 29.

WHO, 2020. Advice on the use of masks in the context of COVID-19. Available from: https://apps.who.int/iris/bitstream/handle/10665/331693/WHO-2019-nCov-IPC_Masks-2020.3-eng.pdf?sequence=1&isAllowed=y.

Collective disorientation in the pandemic conjuncture

Alexander J. Means and Graham B. Slater

ABSTRACT

In its far-reaching impacts on global life, encroaching upon seemingly every aspect of social totality, the COVID-19 pandemic is an urgent topic for cultural studies. This article situates the pandemic within a historical conjuncture in which various post-neoliberal formations are being struggled over. These emergent formations will in turn be indelibly impacted by the pandemic's social, cultural, and political economic dimensions. Key to this uncertain future is a phenomenon we call collective disorientation, a concept that is implicated in the emergence, experience, and effects of the pandemic, as well as the political prospects for surviving the cascading crises of the pandemic conjuncture. Though the pandemic is a historically disorienting force, the cultural studies tradition is remarkably well-equipped to contribute to collective struggles seeking loci for new articulations beyond the COVID-19 conjuncture.

> The domain of culture and ideology is where those new positions are opened and where the new articulations have to be made. And in that domain, people can change and struggle. (Hall 2016, p. 190)

Despite the SARS-CoV-2 pathogen's viral novelty, the COVID-19 pandemic that has erupted following its cross-species transmission to humans did not emerge from nowhere. Experts have warned of the likelihood of such an event for years. Indeed, what is perhaps most surprising about the global pandemic is its delayed arrival relative to scientific anticipation. The necessary preconditions for the emergence of a global pandemic afflicting humanity have been in place for quite some time, and despite the increasing likelihood of a pandemic outbreak – registered almost to exhaustion within mass culture – preparatory or suppressive measures have proven startlingly insufficient. The restless expansionary drive of global capitalism, unabated resource extraction and environmental degradation, and heedless urban sprawl have all placed humanity into closer contact with non-human animal habitats and various species, increasing the risk of zoonotic leaps like the one that occurred with COVID-19 in Wuhan, China late in 2019 (Davis 2020). As climate change transforms ecologies, social landscapes, and the interactions between humans and non-humans in new and often unpredictable ways, the emergence of new viruses like COVID-19 is almost certain to increase in frequency and impact. In this regard, the current coronavirus does not alone constitute the totality of the pandemic conjuncture.

Nevertheless, the coronavirus pandemic has provoked a disorienting rupture, revealing stark pathologies in social, economic, cultural, and environmental relations, while at the same time catalyzing novel patterns of daily life marked by profound historical uncertainty. This is reflected in how the pandemic is represented and responded to. For instance, in the United States, right-wing politicians and pundits have actively stoked conspiracy theories, ignorance, and denial regarding the pandemic, meanwhile in other Western societies, even those taking the pandemic far more seriously, the response has often adhered to a well-established technocratic framework which seeks to contain and mitigate crises without critically linking them to the socio-historical processes out of which they emerge (see White 2020). These viral irrationalities and insufficiently historicized responses are morbid symptoms (Gramsci 1971) of collective disorientation, in which the ideological, political, and biomedical collide.

The morbid symptoms of pandemic disorientation

The general inability to locate the emergence of the pandemic within the hypermodern systems immanent to global capitalism is symptomatic of a profound sense of disorientation that haunts contemporary cultural formations and social life. The coronavirus pandemic has unleashed a cascade of crises, exacerbating underlying tensions and inequalities already present within and across societies. GDP has cratered worldwide with some economists predicting a ten-year pandemic depression for global capitalism (e.g. Roubini 2020). Oxfam International predicts that half of the world's 7.8 billion people may be living in poverty by the time the pandemic subsides (Oxfam 2020). While some societies such as South Korea and Italy nearly contained the coronavirus, at least during its first 'wave', others, most glaringly the United States, the richest nation in world history, as well as India and Brazil, have failed on almost every conceivable level to ensure public health and social welfare. Millions of people have lost their jobs and millions more face the threat of eviction and immiseration in the coming months. Lines for food banks sometimes stretch for miles in major cities and small towns alike. Ambient anxieties have become more deeply embedded in daily life. Conspiracy theories abound. The temporality of economic production and social reproduction have been dramatically altered. The acceleration of news cycles collides with the monotonous requirements of simply 'getting by' in the pandemic – educating and caring for children, securing food and other basic necessities, attempting to plan for the future, all in a moment of extreme unpredictability that increasingly takes on the character of the durative. Indeed, it is difficult to predict how the social, political, and economic impact of the pandemic will develop between the time of our writing and publication. When we first drafted this essay, the highest total of new cases in a day globally had not yet topped 250,000. Only a few months later, and after so many societies abandoned their lockdown protocols, mainly for 'economic' reasons, new cases worldwide regularly reached twice that number.

Ironically perhaps, the sense of disorientation that has accompanied the pandemic is not due to a sense of historical closure, an end of history, or the stubborn persistence of what Mark Fisher (2009) referred to as capitalist realism: the conviction that there is no temporal horizon other than an endless neoliberal present. On the contrary, the pandemic arrived at a particular moment in Western societies where the dominant myths, narratives, sensibilities, and affects that bound the neoliberal project together had largely collapsed at the level of popular legitimacy. The 2008 economic crisis and the ensuing explosion of austerity, debt, and inequality has led to a fracturing of neoliberal hegemony, a destabilizing process which has fostered the resurgence of neo-fascist identifications and growing support for ethnonationalist right-wing authoritarian leaders. Yet among many elites there is a nostalgic longing for neoliberalism, manifested in attempts to revive the mainstream consensus that married deregulated finance capitalism to meritocratic multicultural inclusion (Fraser 2017). Simultaneously, we also see a growing desire and identification with egalitarian alternatives that directly challenge the irrationality, violence, and unsustainability of the current global system. Resistance to neoliberal austerity and right-wing nationalism across Europe, protests against monarchic rule in southeast Asia, the explosion of social protest over police brutality in the US, Nigeria, and many other nations is emblematic of these egalitarian energies and desires, as is the growing force of resistance against the looming eviction crisis.

The pandemic has heightened anxieties concerning the uncertainty of the future, yielding an emergent structure of feeling (Williams 1977) that the pandemic, both as manifestation of ecological crisis and catalyst of economic crisis, constitutes a historical moment of acceleration toward catastrophe. But how do we make sense of this disorientation within the pandemic? And how might we articulate collective disorientation to a common horizon in order to survive the pandemic? These two questions are intimately related. The absence of a common horizon signifies the fundamental source of collective disorientation. On one hand, disorientation reflects the startling depth of reification within the contemporary condition. Here the existential patterns of vulnerability and the concrete crises we face, those associated immediately with the pandemic and more generally with climate change, are either apprehended as floating signifiers abstracted from their historical sources and material consequences or denied altogether (Latour 2018). On the other hand, disorientation takes the form of what William Connolly (2017) refers to as 'passive nihilism': the recognition that things are out of control, perhaps irrevocably, however, we suspect, or at least have been educated to believe falsely, that we are powerless to intervene. The social, economic, and cultural conditions catalyzed by the pandemic amplify conflict, denial, and anxiety, but they also foster imagination and resistance. Thus, the task of cultural studies in the pandemic conjuncture remains one of articulation, of forging social and political pathways through which we might (re)-orient ourselves toward common horizons, collective agency, and livable futures.

The political economy of post-Neoliberalism and the cultural politics of disorientation

Despite its particularities, the pandemic has intensified an already established sense of collective disorientation within an emerging post-neoliberal order (see Means & Slater 2019). In the political economic register, the pandemic has accelerated patterns of oligarchic plunder and systemic crisis within capitalism. With fewer avenues for productive investment, capitalism has come to increasingly rely on the upward redistribution of wealth through political means, eroding its underlying basis of expansion by immiserating workers and draining collective wealth from societies. Robert Brenner (2020) illustrates these dynamics within the pandemic by detailing how the economic crisis that has followed the outbreak of COVID has been handled at the highest levels of federal policy within the United States. He estimates that the Coronavirus Aid and Relief and Economic Security Act (or CARES Act), the massive stimulus package issued by the US congress in March 2020 with bipartisan cooperation, transferred $4.5 trillion (out of $6.2 trillion total) in public money to the nation's largest corporations through no-strings-attached payouts, bond purchases, and other investments. Thus while mercilessly slashing employment and reinvestment, top corporate managers and stockholders were given the green light to line their own pockets through stock buybacks, dividends, and executive salaries, fuelling an unsustainable bubble in corporate debt and stock valuation.

The oligarchic plunder of collective wealth during the pandemic has been largely obscured from public view, left largely unremarked upon within the mainstream media. However, the impacts are felt in the disorienting abandonment of civil society and the crumbling of public infrastructure including public health capacities necessary to address the coronavirus. Along with the plunder of collective wealth, the pandemic has amplified disorienting conditions of precarity. Thirty million workers lost their jobs in the United States in the first phase of lockdowns. According to one estimate by economists at the University of Chicago, 42 percent of jobs lost during the pandemic may vanish forever in a cascade of business failures and corporate bankruptcies.[1] This will likely accelerate the trend toward precarious gig work and heightened monopolistic concentration, for instance, as social distancing practices and a wave of brick-and-mortar retailer bankruptcies allow platform corporations like Amazon to grow precipitously. The pandemic has also aided industrial deregulation and the shredding of labour protections. As Jane Mayer (2020) details in the *New Yorker*, Ronald Cameron, a billionaire poultry tycoon, leveraged his connections to the Trump administration to ignore federal guidelines, speed up meat packing production, and declare his largely immigrant labour force to be 'essential' in the pandemic, effectively forcing them to work through the explosion of the coronavirus pandemic in what was already one of the most dangerous and low-paid jobs, leading to the infection of up to thirty thousand meat packers in three months and killing several hundred.

The pandemic is accelerating a disorienting realignment of power within the sphere of work that includes not only the precaritization of livelihoods, processes of flexibilization and automation, and the rise of platform capitalism and gig labour, but also the global production of vast labour surpluses and disposable populations (Bauman 2004, Srnicek 2018). Simultaneously, the pandemic has intensified a disorienting crisis of care and social reproduction. In the United States, the underlying necessities for survival have been increasingly privatized, defunded, and financialized including health care, social support, affordable housing, public schools and universities (Weeks 2011, Fraser 2017). The pandemic has been particularly acute and mismanaged in the United States precisely because it is a rapidly deteriorating social order, designed to secure profit over and above human need. As the lockdowns proceeded there was an accelerated privatization of risk and care, the impact of which fell most heavily on working class families, women, people of colour, and immigrant communities. For those who have lost jobs and income, support from the state, such as unemployment benefits, will not last forever. With job and income loss, millions will soon be unable to maintain their health insurance during a virulent and deadly pandemic with no clear terminus. At the same time they cannot continue to make mortgage and rent payments to maintain shelter. For professionals who are able to work remotely from home, distinctions between work and the domestic sphere collapse as schooling children and other non-waged duties compete with the demands of employers.

The pandemic intensifies disorienting systems of power, complexity, precarity, and social fragmentation. We see this perhaps most starkly within digital space, under what Shoshana Zuboff (2018) refers to as 'surveillance capitalism', in which illiteracies and resentment are manufactured via corporate algorithms, designed to capture value from attention, data mining, and the addictive tweaking of fear and other libidinal drives. Forms of disoriented consciousness are produced through manipulative ecosystems of digital hyper-reality. The sense of unreality is so thick that conspiracy films such as *Plandemic* inspired a large number of people to refuse mask wearing and to act out violently against scientists and other health experts, politicians (most notably the failed plot to kidnap Michigan Governor Gretchen Whitmer), not to mention low-wage employees in stores, shops, and restaurants, who encourage the practice. These forms of pathogenic disorientation obscure real material power, including how Silicon Valley platforms such as Youtube, Facebook and Google, manipulate fear as a means of furthering market domination. Such conditions are ripe for the growth of neo-fascism. As both the Frankfurt School and Hannah Arendt noted from different vantage points, fascism thrives on the disorientation of autonomous thought, as critical reflection melts into a vortex of detached systems, images, sounds, and lies. Indeed new neo-fascist groups have emerged more fully onto the public scene during the pandemic. We also see how these movements are synergizing with state power in disturbing ways as unmarked federal paramilitary forces intermingled with right-wing militias and local police in response to the persistent Black Lives Matter protests against police brutality and white supremacy, and supporters of Donald Trump baselessly decried a stolen election, clamoring for a coup.

The fundamental condition undergirding all of these phenomena is a disorienting sense of ecological fragility. The pandemic has only heightened this sense of vulnerability demonstrating how a tiny microbe leaping from species to species, at a particular time and place, can instantly alter the historical trajectory of social life on the planet. The pandemic itself has also triggered new environmental threats, stealing precious time from the mobilization of urgent efforts to address climate change. One particularly vivid example of the disorienting ecological reality can be found in the decimation of the United States fracking industry as energy prices have plummeted. Ostensibly this would be cause for celebration, however, the initial effect has been the proliferation of over two million abandoned and unplugged fracking wells leaking 'the methane equivalent of the annual emissions from more than 1.5 million cars' into the atmosphere, meanwhile failed fracking companies cash in on their unregulated freedom, filing bankruptcy while rewarding the executives who oversaw their failure (Tabuchi 2020).

Articulating a common horizon against disorientation

Conjunctures are often fraught with ambivalence, and the historical trajectories that emerge from struggles within conjunctures are dependent upon the characteristics and power of the various formations operating within them. This is why the fundamental distinction between residual, dominant, and emergent formations within the cultural studies tradition is so crucial to understanding the political necessity of articulation (Williams 1977). As Stuart Hall (2016, p. 206) put it, '[t]he conditions within which people are able to construct subjective possibilities and new political subjectivities for themselves are not simply given in the dominant system. They are won in the practices of articulation which produce them'. Yet as we have argued, the collective disorientation that has become increasingly prevalent within the pandemic conjuncture is a significant obstacle to emancipatory articulations.

If cultural studies remains committed to 'the contemporary struggle over thought, imagination, and the possibilities for action' (Grossberg 2010, p. 3), then it is indeed crucial to the struggle to overcome collective disorientation in the pandemic conjuncture, and to articulate collective capacities and forms of agency – obscured and obstructed, but nonetheless present – through cultural politics and ideological struggle. Our argument is essentially that it is unsurprising that the pandemic is collectively disorienting: the material conditions produced through state and corporate power, and the cultural and ideological conditions of reification it magnifies and mobilizes, are powerful forces of obfuscation. Thus, the struggle for political articulation simultaneously necessitates an educational project, one that is multifaceted and goes beyond traditional forms of institutionalized schooling alone (the call to 'reopen' schools and universities being itself a manifestation of contemporary disorientation), aiming instead at the reorientation of consciousness and collectivity. Social movements and cultural struggles are also part of a collective learning process reflective of underlying disorientation and a political desire for reorientation toward that which is and should be held in common. In a brutal capitalist society such as the United States, it is clear that any solution to the social suffering produced in concert with the pandemic, or indeed measures to stem the spread of the pandemic itself, will not come from the state or capital. It will emerge from struggles within the sphere of culture and ideology, the realm in which social subjects are formed, reformed, and brought together in the material pursuit of egalitarian alternatives and livable futures.

Note

1. https://www.cnbc.com/2020/05/20/most-americans-see-layoffs-as-temporary-but-research-shows-otherwise.html

Disclosure statement

No potential conflict of interest was reported by the author(s).

Further information

This Special Issue article has been comprehensively reviewed by the Special Issue editors, Associate Professor Ted Striphas and Professor John Nguyet Erni.

References

Bauman, Z., 2004. *Wasted lives: modernity and its outcasts*. Malden, MA: Polity Press.

Brenner, R., 2020. Escalating plunder. *New left review*, 123 (May–June), 5–22.

Connolly, W.E., 2017. *Facing the planetary: entangled humanism and the politics of swarming*. Durham, NC: Duke University Press.

Davis, M., 2020. *The monster enters: COVID-19, avian flu and the plagues of capitalism*. New York: OR Books.

Fisher, M., 2009. *Capitalist realism: Is there no alternative?* London: Zero Books.

Fraser, N., 2017. From progressive neoliberalism to Trump – and beyond. *American affairs*, 1 (4), 46–64. https://americanaffairsjournal.org/2017/11/progressive-neoli beralism-trump-beyond/ [Accessed 13 May 2020].

Gramsci, A., 1971. *Selections from the prison notebooks* (trans. Q. Hoare and G. N. Smith). New York: International Publishers.

Grossberg, L., 2010. *Cultural studies in the future tense*. Durham, NC: Duke University Press.

Hall, S., 2016. *Cultural studies 1983: A theoretical history*, eds. Jennifer Daryl Slack and Lawrence Grossberg. Durham, NC: Duke University Press.

Latour, B., 2018. *Down to earth: politics in the new climatic regime*. Medford, MA: Polity Press.

Mayer, J., 2020. How Trump is helping tycoons exploit the pandemic. *The New Yorker*, 20 July. https://www.newyorker.com/magazine/2020/07/20/how-trump-is-helping-tycoons-exploit-the-pandemic [Accessed 8 August 2020].

Means, A.J. and Slater, G.B., 2019. The dark mirror of capital: On post-neoliberal formations and the future of education. *Discourse: studies in the cultural politics of education*, 40 (2), 162-175. doi:10.1080/01596306.2019.1569876

Oxfam, 2020. Half a billion people could be pushed into poverty By COVID-19. *Oxfam America*, 8 April 8. https://www.oxfamamerica.org/press/half-billion-people-could-be-pushed-poverty-covid-19/ [Accessed 26 May 2020].

Roubini, N., 2020. Ten reasons Why a 'Greater Depression' for the 2020s is inevitable. *The Guardian*, 29 April. https://www.theguardian.com/business/2020/apr/29/ten-reasons-why-greater-depression-for-the-2020s-is-inevitable-covid [Accessed 26 May 2020].

Srnicek, N., 2018. *Platform capitalism*. Medford, MA: Polity Press.

Tabuchi, H., 2020. Fracking firms fail, rewarding executives and raising climate fears. *New York Times*, 12 July. https://www.nytimes.com/2020/07/12/climate/oil-fracking-bankruptcy-methane-executive-pay.html [Accessed 14 August 2020].

Weeks, K., 2011. *The problem with work: feminism, marxism, antiwork politics, and post-work imaginaries*. Durham, NC: Duke University Press.

White, J. 2020. Technocracy after Covid-19. *Boston Review*, 27 April. Available from: http://bostonreview.net/politics/jonathan-white-technocracy-after-covid-19 [Accessed 10 November 2020].

Williams, R., 1977. *Marxism and literature*. Oxford, UK: Oxford University Press.

Zuboff, S., 2018. *The age of surveillance capitalism: the fight for a human future at the new frontier of power*. New York: PublicAffairs.

Mistranslation as disinformation: COVID-19, global imaginaries, and self-serving cosmopolitanism

Sheng Zou

ABSTRACT
This article delves into the politics of the U.S.-China blame-game regarding COVID-19's origin, particularly Chinese disinformation narratives attributing the virus's root to the United States. The blame-game is symptomatic of contradictory global imaginaries circulated within distinct geopolitical spaces. This article approaches Chinese disinformation narratives as transnational and intertextual constructs, which involve the practices of (mis)translating and referencing foreign source texts to paradoxically delegitimate the foreign, especially Western, Other; they reinforce what I call self-serving cosmopolitanism, a narcissistic and locally conditioned sense of global consciousness that is oriented towards the consolidation of self-identity and pride. It is my contention that, to combat global disinformation about COVID-19, we should foreground the politics of translation, enhance cross-cultural sensibility, and most importantly, mobilize a kind of counter-politics against the xenophobic nationalism that disinformation narratives often parasitize. Cultural scholars with comparative perspectives are well positioned to take the initiative in revealing the structural issues at play within a global context and in promoting genuine cosmopolitan openness.

Introduction

Concomitant with the outbreak of COVID-19, swirls of misinformation and disinformation[1] regarding the pandemic – infodemic, as it were – swept across the world, embroiling major global powers and straining international relations, not least the tension between the United States and China. From Trump's labeling the pandemic a 'Chinese virus' to a Chinese foreign ministry spokesperson associating the virus with the U.S. military, governments on both sides sought to discredit each other, to deflect blame for their own coping of the pandemic, and to discursively contain the pandemic's social impact. Much more than a biomedical occurrence, the pandemic confronts us as a complex conjuncture where various political, economic, and ideological forces wrestle with one another at national and global levels. The (re)naming of the coronavirus and the (re)framing of its origin are symptomatic of contradictory global imaginaries circulated within distinct geopolitical spaces, challenging the rosy vision of a singular cosmopolitan world order.

This short article looks into Chinese disinformation narratives around the origin of COVID-19, which both feed on and reproduce an ethnocentric imagination of self and other. As a number of viral fake news stories involve manipulative appropriation of or attribution to Western media coverage and information sources, this article approaches disinformation narratives as transnational and intertextual constructs that need to be examined in a global context, with emphasis on the politics of translation. In particular, I construe the intertextual practice of (mis)translating and referencing foreign source texts as a strategic legitimating device deployed to paradoxically delegitimate the foreign, especially Western, Other, while reinforcing what I call *self-serving cosmopolitanism*. In so doing, I seek to relate the infodemic to the perennial discussion on the unresolved tension between nationalism and cosmopolitanism.

COVID-19, Chinese disinformation, and the 'epidemic of signification'

Soon after its outbreak, the novel coronavirus was casually named after the Chinese metropolis, Wuhan, where the virus had been first identified. Despite the official renaming of the virus, labels such as 'Wuhan virus' and 'Chinese virus' continued to be used, sometimes intentionally, as shorthand for the pandemic. The term 'Wuhan virus' was used by a number of conservative politicians including Secretary of State Mike Pompeo, Senator Tom Cotton of Arkansas, and Representative Paul Gosar (Levenson 2020), while the label 'Chinese virus' was popularized by Trump (Moynihan and Porumbescu 2020). The deliberate use of such names reflects an attempt to spatialize and racialize the disease not only to deflect blame but also to symbolically confine it to an externalized Other. The U.S. administration's use of the term 'Chinese virus' is an outcome of a protracted blame game with the Chinese government that started in February 2020, which included U.S. Senator Tom Cotton's speculation that linked the virus to a Wuhan-based lab and Chinese foreign ministry spokesperson Zhao Lijian's tweets in March, suggesting that the virus was likely introduced to Wuhan by American military personnel who attended the Military World Games in October.

In Zhao's tweets, he backed up his theory with references to not only a controversial piece by a dubious Canadian-based organization named Global Research, but also a subtitled video from a U.S. congressional hearing on the country's response to the pandemic, where Robert Redfield, director of the U.S. Centers for Disease Control disclosed that some patients previously diagnosed to have died from the seasonal flu were later found to have died from the coronavirus (Molter and Webster 2020). The conclusions of Global Research's article were translated and summarized by Chinese social media accounts, and the video of Robert Redfield's speech, with Chinese subtitles, also circulated on China's Internet. The anti-U.S. conspiracy theories did not start with Zhao, but had been spreading on China's social media since as early as January 2020 (Molter and Webster 2020). Fake news stories attributed their 'evidence' to foreign sources such as a Japanese TV station; screenshots of the Japanese news program spread across Chinese social media. The Chinese official outlet, *Global Times*, also drew on this Japanese source in a report that discussed the U.S. origin theory (*People's Daily Online 2020a*).[2] It was later debunked that content from the Japanese source had been misrepresented to fit into the conspiracy theory (Poynter 2020).

American media sources were also frequently referenced and misrepresented in disinformation narratives, including a *New York Times* article on the suspension of certain germ research at the U.S. military lab in Fort Detrick, an *ABC* report indicating that intelligence officials warned of the coronavirus as far back as late November, and a *CNN* story confirming the first U.S. coronavirus case of unknown origin. A screenshot of the CNN coverage was circulated widely on Chinese social media, which retained the original English headline: 'CDC confirms first coronavirus case of 'unknown' origin in U.S.' The headline, however, was accompanied by a Chinese mistranslation that said, 'CDC in the U.S. confirms that the first coronavirus case originated from the U.S.' (Author's translation of the Chinese text that goes, '美国cdc疾控确认，首例冠状病毒源于美国'). Although the original source of this Chinese mistranslation and its underlying intentionality remain unknown, the possibility that it was a piece of maliciously crafted disinformation could not be readily ruled out.

Such blatant incongruity between the English source text and the Chinese mistranslation deeply upset me as a U.S.-based Chinese diasporic scholar uneasily caught between two ideological-discursive fields, receiving conflicting 'news' updates on the pandemic from both Chinese and American sources. The conflicting and schizophrenic narratives around the origin of COVID-19 lay bare the struggle between competing claims to the power of framing the pandemic. For a more in-depth understanding of this struggle, it is instructive to revisit the social constructionist approach to science and technology and, in particular, Treichler's (1987) conception of AIDS as an 'epidemic of signification'.

According to Pinch and Bijker's (1984) elaboration of the social construction of scientific facts, the emergence of new scientific findings is often surrounded by interpretive flexibility, where different interpretations of scientific facts are available. Dominant social groups participate in negotiating the interpretive flexibility so as to achieve rhetorical closure, where consensus over the given scientific facts is reached. As Latour and Woolgar (1985, p. 285) put it astutely, 'interpretations do not so much inform as perform'. Interpretations of scientific facts shape people's belief about and response to the outside world. Informed by this perspective, Treichler (1987, p. 264) examines AIDS as a social and linguistic construction, arguing that it is at once 'an epidemic of a transmissible lethal disease and an epidemic of meanings or signification'. The profound ambiguity and uncertainty around AIDS are managed socially and linguistically through semantic work. Popular and biomedical discourses around AIDS reflect people's attempts to make the epidemic intelligible, and they are saturated with power dynamics. Treichler shows how discourses around AIDS constructed by dominant social groups – including scientists – attached the epidemic to primarily gay male bodies and reproduced homophobia. Of course, in Treichler's discussion, the fragmentary and conflicting discourses around AIDS are less a result of deliberate attempts of disinformation but more an outcome of entrenched social stereotypes. Nonetheless, like AIDS, COVID-19 triggers public emotions such as fear, anxiety, and hostility towards minoritized and exoticized subjects, and consequently messy interpretations around its etiology. It is, like AIDS, a nexus of conflicting meanings, discourses, and interests, albeit one at a new historical conjuncture marked by changing geopolitical landscapes and technological conditions.

From day one, COVID-19 has been bound up with anti-Chinese and anti-Asian sentiment; as the pandemic reached a global scale, the social construction of its etiology has been a project laden with political and economic interests, and a contest between major global powers invoking their respective geopolitical and global imaginaries. To dissect the cultural politics of COVID-19, we need what Treichler (1987, p. 287) calls 'an epidemiology of signification', namely a mapping of the multiple meanings associated with it. This epidemiology of signification entails a closer scrutiny of the disinformation mechanism at play as well as the economy of emotions on which it thrives. It is evident that the current epidemic of signification that confronts us is deeply entwined with nationalist politics and global consciousness. In the following, I briefly explore the social and linguistic construction of COVID-19 in relation to the perennial paradox between nationalism and cosmopolitanism, with particular emphasis on Chinese fake stories about the pandemic's origin.

Fake news, translation, and self-serving cosmopolitanism

Chinese disinformation campaigns around COVID-19 are often condemned by Western media as government-led operations. What is in fact at work is a complicated assemblage of both top-down campaigns and bottom-up practices, which involve not just government organs and official media, but unidentified grassroots sources and average users. While the misleading screenshot of CNN's coverage circulated on social media, which came from an unidentifiable source, is arguably a grassroots fabrication, the foreign ministry spokesperson's tweets serve the top-down maneuver to regain control of the narrative. State-run media *CGTN* (Wang 2020) and *People's Daily Online (2020b)* also ran op-eds to hint at the possibility that the virus may have originated from the United States. Both pieces cited much-trumpeted conspiracy theories, such as the appropriation of Robert Redfield's remarks on misdiagnoses and the shutdown of a military lab in Fort Detrick, among others.

These disinformation narratives share some common features. First, they feed on and reproduce nationalist emotions at a very personal level, trumping one's interest for veracity. Second, they often appropriate texts and images from foreign sources to fake an aura of legitimacy and authority. A fake news story about COVID-19 is, in this light, a bricolage comprised of exotic texts and visuals, (mis)translation of these foreign sources, and (mis)representations of their meanings. Paradoxical as they may seem, references to apparently legitimate Western/American sources are utilized to delegitimate and overturn the ideological hegemony asserted by the West, particularly the United States. Fake news about COVID-19, as transnational and intertextual bricolage, fulfills and reinforces what I call *self-serving cosmopolitanism*, a narcissistic and locally conditioned sense of global consciousness that is oriented towards the consolidation of self-identity and pride.

My conception of the self-serving cosmopolitanism is informed by Ong's (2009) cosmopolitan continuum that encompasses different degrees of openness to the outside world. Cosmopolitanism, a capacious yet nebulous term, is 'both description and normative program' (Calhoun 2008, p. 429), hence the fuzziness of its definition and usage. Silverstone's (2006) conceptualization of cosmopolitanism, for instance, has strong normative valence in that it foregrounds 'a duty of care, obligation, and responsibility' towards others (p. 47). In this sense, cosmopolitanism is a desirable ethical orientation in an increasingly globalized world, which entails 'a positive recognition of difference and signals a conception of belonging as open' (Delanty 2006, p. 359). Media are considered instrumental in building this sense of openness towards distant others. Hannerz (1990, p. 249) notably argues that 'the implosive power of the media may now make just everybody a little more cosmopolitan'.

Although cosmopolitanism as an orienting ethical norm could inform international news coverage (Chouliaraki 2006), the rise of mediated cosmopolitanism is never guaranteed. For one thing, the heightening of global consciousness does not necessarily translate into positive recognition of otherness, but may, just as likely, become 'a source of fear and defensiveness' (Calhoun 2008, p. 429). For another, in lieu of a singular 'mediapolis'

(Sliverstone 2006) where contemporary political life is lived out at both national and global levels, most of the people are still deeply embedded in local and national contexts, with their perceived realities of the world shaped by local and national media and sources. Significant linguistic and cultural barriers remain despite the ease of mobility of people and resources across borders.

Ong's cosmopolitanism continuum differs from the view of cosmopolitanism as a stable orientation, and proffers a vocabulary with which we are able to discuss different degrees and expressions of cosmopolitan openness. Cosmopolitanism as a stable orientation entails not only willingness to engage with others, but also a certain level of social and cultural competence (Hannerz 1990, Beck 2006), which reveals the latent association between cosmopolitanism and capital or class positions. However, Ong's continuum lowers the threshold of cosmopolitan expressions, and enables us to empirically examine the actually-existing cosmopolitanism(s). This bottom-up view of cosmopolitanism recognizes the complex identity politics in concrete local struggles, and jettisons the dichotomy between nationalism and cosmopolitanism. Under this framework, nationalism and cosmopolitanism can be perceived as flexible identity frames of which subjects move in and out. In particular, Ong uses the oxymoronic term 'closed cosmopolitanism' to denote the rejection of the ideal of openness and the recourse to the self-other distinction; he uses 'instrumental cosmopolitanism' to capture a 'selfish' expression of cosmopolitan openness, which 'makes use of one's knowledge of the world to promote oneself' so as to 'further delineate self from other' (pp. 454–456). Instrumental cosmopolitanism is in line with what Hannerz (1990, p. 240) regards as the 'narcissistic streak' of cosmopolitanism, where individuals pick from other cultures only those pieces that suit themselves. Building upon Ong's typology, I intend to highlight, with the notion of self-serving cosmopolitanism, the paradox between the recognition and the simultaneous delegitimation of the Western-dominated world order, the consciousness of the global arena not as a level playing field but a hierarchical one, and the consolidation of national identity and pride.

Self-serving cosmopolitanism is but one side of the multifaceted globalization process, and differs from anti-cosmopolitanism due to its ambivalence and seeming contradiction. This kind of consciousness becomes salient with the deepening of globalization, and is performed through everyday experiences such as material consumption. One's fervor of transnational travels and shopping, for instance, may co-exist well with their inclination to deprecate the foreign other and, in turn, to reinforce their identification with their home country. When it comes to news production and consumption, one's reliance on high-status global outlets and sources for first-hand information on current affairs may go hand in hand with their propensity to confirm parochial and xenophobic beliefs.

COVID-19-related fake news stories circulated on Chinese social media satiate this paradoxical demand. By associating the origin of the virus with Western countries such as the United States, they tap into pre-existing popular hostility towards the Western hegemony as well as the vehement popular demand to defend China from external biases and criticisms. Zhang (2020) observes, in her research on right-wing populist discourse on Chinese Internet, that the rhetoric of Western-style right-wing populism is appropriated by some Chinese netizens to paradoxically challenge the Euro-American-centric world order, and to buttress their own vision of a declining West in rivalry with a rising China. She documents that racial nationalists in China internalize Eurocentric notions of race, nation, and progress while embracing Western right-wing ideas and vocabulary, such as the aversion towards progressive values (e.g. feminism, multiculturalism, diversity) and liberal elites. They use the same ideological language to express their criticism of the Western powers' promotion of universal values and of these 'superior' forces' vulnerability and decline, which they attribute to the rise of Western liberal elites and the threat of ethnic minorities.

Likewise, Chinese disinformation narratives about the possible origin of COVID-19 mobilize people's discontent towards the U.S. administration's criticism of Chinese government's handling of the pandemic. These sensational narratives around COVID-19, either top-down or bottom-up, are also narratives of an imagined global order and geopolitical rivalry. They either intentionally shore up or inadvertently coincide with the Party-state's attempt to reframe the outbreak of the pandemic. Most importantly, they thrive on a surging economy of emotions characterized by retaliatory motives and exclusionary nationalism. Although much hope has been reposed in the cosmopolitanizing potential of media, the bleak reality that confronts us is one in which people are enmeshed in discrete media spaces demarcated largely by national boundaries. From Anderson's (1983) 'imagined community' to Billig's (1995) 'banal nationalism', much has been said about the nexus between media and nationalism. COVID-19-related disinformation exemplifies a pernicious facet of this nexus in the extreme, exploiting the existing linguistic and cultural barriers across nations as well as the opacity of translation. To better understand the workings of disinformation in a global context, we need to foreground the politics of translation.

Translation has long been obscured in the dominant discourses of globalization that emphasize the instantaneity of global communication and transmissibility of information flows; under this framework, translation is seen as a transparent and technical process, which 'merely facilitates linguistic and cultural transfer without leaving any traces of its intervention' (Bielsa 2014, p. 393). However, far from being automatically transparent or simply technical, translation often involves varying levels of intelligence and labor, and can be profoundly political. The (mis)translated CNN coverage is a compelling case in point. Ironically, the English source text is retained in this piece to conjure up a fake aura of authenticity and legitimacy; it is juxtaposed with a subtly inaccurate – and deeply unethical – translation, where a minor omission of words leads to a fundamental alteration of meanings. The politics, ethics, and the generative power of translation should be foregrounded in order to deconstruct the disingenuous design of the disinformation narrative.

Translation is not only linguistic transfer, but also what Bielsa (2014, pp. 395–396) calls the 'experience of the foreign', a key process mediating our encounters with alterity. As much as it can bridge cultural differences, translation can also operate as an ethnocentric act (Venuti 2008, Bielsa 2014), which involves violent replacement of linguistic and cultural differences. Translation is a craft of selection and re-creation, which structures, assembles, and even creates information to render a text intelligible to the target audience (Bielsa and Bassnett 2009). Despite its potential to cosmopolitanize a local culture, translation can also distort the image of the foreign. Translation and trans-editing are commonplace in news practices, which entail various kinds of 'textual manipulation, including synthesis, omission, explication and a host of other textual strategies' (Bielsa and Bassnett 2009, p. 8). These strategies could also be maliciously deployed to construct fake news stories. A diagnosis of (mis)translation in fake news stories should not restrict its attention to the technical, but should probe into the social and political conditions in which the labor of translation takes place, the role of translation in cross-cultural interactions, as well as the connections between (mis)translation, nationalism, and cosmopolitanism.

Concluding remarks

Disinformation about COVID-19 is symptomatic of conflicting global imaginaries and geopolitical rivalry, and is intricately intertwined with a larger project of national and political identity formation. Although this article focuses on Chinese disinformation in this regard, the same can be said about the U.S. side as well. Not only did Trump claim that he had high confidence that the virus had originated from a virology lab in Wuhan (Mason 2020), but the U.S. Secretary of State Mike Pompeo also claimed that there was 'enormous evidence' supporting this idea (U.S. Department of State 2020). In September 2020, The Fox News show 'Tucker Carlson Tonight' aired an interview with Chinese virologist Li-Meng Yan, who made the misleading claim that the COVID-19 virus was man-made in a lab (Hsu 2020). The interview exploited and reproduced the Western stereotype of China as the authoritarian Other.

Countering the assumption that cosmopolitan openness is a naturally occurring trend, I argue that openness to alterity is not automatically activated. Nor are media and communication technologies some sort of *deus ex machina* (Lindell 2015), eliminating cross-cultural barriers or misunderstandings on their own. Rather than treating cosmopolitanism as a coherent and unifying concept, I underline the messiness and paradoxes of its expressions in everyday practices. Chinese disinformation narratives about COVID-19, as transnational and intertextual constructs, fulfill and reproduce a kind of self-serving cosmopolitanism that at once recognizes and delegitimates the Western-dominated world order.

To combat disinformation about COVID-19 and about anything of global relevance, journalists, educators, public figures, policy makers, scientists, and cultural scholars all have vital roles to play at national and global levels. To begin with, we need to promote a heightened sensitivity towards the politics of translation in the production of transnational disinformation. That will enable us to dissect the intertextual design of disinformation narratives circulating across cultural-linguistic and geopolitical boundaries, and to lay bare the political interests, agendas, and power dynamics lurking behind those narratives.

To identify disinformation in the era of social media, we need not only improved media literacy and digital savviness, but also enhanced cross-cultural understanding and sensibility. What needs to be cultivated is a genuine kind of cosmopolitan openness, characterized by unbiased recognition of cultural differences, a sincere quest to understand the realities of other cultures and societies, and a genuine appreciation of the global interconnectedness. More importantly, we should mobilize a kind of counter-politics against the xenophobic nationalism that disinformation narratives often parasitize. This is, of course, a formidable undertaking. And comparative media/cultural scholars are well positioned to act as public intellectuals to intervene into the parochial nationalist politics by revealing the pitfalls of self-centered global imaginaries and signaling the promises of a genuine sense of cosmopolitan openness. In an era of global risks, the only way out of our predicament is opening up cross-cultural dialogues and transnational cooperation on all fronts, rather than retreating into cocoons of self-delusion.

Notes

1. Although 'misinformation' and 'disinformation' are variously defined, I follow the definition of misinformation as inadvertent sharing of false information, and disinformation as deliberate creation and sharing of false information (Bakir and McStay 2018).
2. The *Global Times* story was reprinted by *The People's Daily Online*.

Disclosure statement

No potential conflict of interest was reported by the author(s).

Further information

This Special Issue article has been comprehensively reviewed by the Special Issue editors, Associate Professor Ted Striphas and Professor John Nguyet Erni.

References

Anderson, B., 1983. *Imagined communities: reflections on the origin and spread of nationalism*. London: Verso.
Bakir, V. and McStay, A., 2018. Fake news and the economy of emotions: problems, causes, solutions. *Digital journalism*, 6 (2), 154–175.
Beck, U., 2006. *The cosmopolitan vision*. Cambridge: Polity Press.
Bielsa, E., 2014. Cosmopolitanism as translation. *Cultural sociology*, 8 (4), 392–406.
Bielsa, E. and Bassnett, S., 2009. *Translation in global news*. London: Routledge.
Billig, M., 1995. *Banal nationalism*. London: Sage.
Calhoun, C., 2008. Cosmopolitanism and nationalism. *Nations and nationalism*, 14 (3), 427–448.
Chouliaraki, L., 2006. *The spectatorship of suffering*. London: Sage.
Delanty, G., 2006. Nationalism and cosmopolitanism: the paradox of modernity. *In*: G. Delanty and K. Kumar, eds. *The SAGE handbook of nations and nationalism*. London: Sage, 357–368.
Hannerz, U., 1990. Cosmopolitans and locals in world culture. *Theory, culture & society*, 7 (2), 237–251.
Hsu, T., 2020. Facebook and Instagram flag tucker carlson virus posts. *The New York Times*. 16 September. Available from: https://www.nytimes.com/2020/09/16/business/media/facebook-instagram-tucker-carlson-virus-posts.html.
Latour, B. and Woolgar, S., 1985. *Laboratory life: the construction of scientific fact*. Cambridge: Cambridge University Press.
Levenson, T., 2020. Conservatives try to rebrand the coronavirus: the term Wuhan virus treats COVID-19 as a Chinese scourge – and ignores an ugly history. *The Atlantic*, 11 March. Available from: https://www.theatlantic.com/ideas/archive/2020/03/stop-trying-make-wuhan-virus-happen/607786/.
Lindell, J., 2015. Mediapolis, where art thou? Mediated cosmopolitanism in three media systems between 2002 and 2010. *International communication gazette*, 77 (2), 189–207.
Mason, J., 2020. Trump confident that coronavirus may have originated in Chinese lab. *Reuters*, 30 April. Available from: https://www.reuters.com/article/us-health-coronavirus-trump-china/trump-confident-that-coronavirus-may-have-originated-in-chinese-lab-idUSKBN22C3TB.

Molter, V. and Webster, G., 2020. *Virality project (China): coronavirus conspiracy claims.* Freeman Spogli Institute for International Studies, Stanford University, 31 March. Available from: https://fsi.stanford.edu/news/china-covid19-origin-narrative.

Moynihan, D. and Porumbescu, G., 2020. Trump's "Chinese virus" slur makes some people blame Chinese Americans. But others blame Trump. *The Washington Post.* 16 September. Available from: https://www.washingtonpost.com/politics/2020/09/16/trumps-chinese-virus-slur-makes-some-people-blame-chinese-americans-others-blame-trump/.

Ong, J.C., 2009. The cosmopolitan continuum: locating cosmopolitanism in media and cultural studies. *Media, culture & society,* 31 (3), 449–466.

People's Daily Online, 2020a. Japanese TV report sparks speculations in China that COVID-19 may have originated in US. 23 February. Available from: http://en.people.cn/n3/2020/0223/c90000-9661026.html.

People's Daily Online, 2020b. 10 questions on COVID-19 that must be answered by U.S. politicians. 1 May. Available from: http://en.people.cn/n3/2020/0501/c90000-9686382.html.

Pinch, T.J. and Bijker, W., 1984. The social construction of facts and artefacts: or how the sociology of science and the sociology of technology might benefit each other. *Social studies of science,* 14, 399–441.

Poynter, 2020. *False: Japanese Asahi Shimbun TV: USA caught COVID-19 before Wuhan, according to American CDC.* 3 March. Available from: https://www.poynter.org/?ifcn_misinformation=japanese-asahi-shimbun-tv-usa-caught-covid-19-before-wuhan-according-to-american-cdc.

Silverstone, R., 2006. *Media and morality: on the rise of the mediapolis.* London: Polity.

Treichler, P.A., 1987. AIDS, homophobia and biomedical discourse: an epidemic of signification. *Cultural studies,* 1 (3), 263–305.

U.S. Department of State, 2020. Secretary Michael R. Pompeo with Martha Raddatz of ABC's This Week with George Stephanopoulos. 3 May. Available from: https://www.state.gov/secretary-michael-r-pompeo-with-martha-raddatz-of-abcs-this-week-with-george-stephanopoulos/.

Venuti, L., 2008. *The translator's invisibility: a history of translation.* London: Routledge.

Wang, F., 2020. 10 questions for the U.S.: Where did the noval coronavirus come from? CGTN. 19 March. Available from: https://news.cgtn.com/news/2020-03-19/10-questions-for-the-U-S-Where-did-the-novel-coronavirus-come-from--OZrgRTSZfa/index.html.

Zhang, C., 2020. Right-wing populism with Chinese characteristics? Identity, otherness and global imaginaries in debating world politics online. *European journal of international relations,* 26 (1), 88–115.

Religion and urban political eco/pathology: exploring communalized coronavirus in South Asia

Asif Mehmood ⓘ, Sajjad Hasnain ⓘ and Muhammad Azam ⓘ

ABSTRACT

wWe use the urban political ecology perspective to explore how communities of *homo religiosus* (re)configure politics of COVID-19 in India and Pakistan. This urban health crisis unfolds in five parallel registers of conflictualities: (i) where religious communities carve out a domain for self-governance of the pandemic with their own 'knowledge and truths', (ii) where embodied religious practices challenge or undermine state biopower and transform governmentalities, (iii) where the spatial dimension of conflict evolves into the crisis of technologies of governance, (iv) where religious identities are stigmatized and the minority groups are excluded and (v) where communalism organizes around international relations. It is argued that religious groups in South Asia influenced the urban political (eco)pathology with their disruptive potential which transformed biosecurity regimes and enhanced health risks on the one hand and on the other, they embraced and internalized discords of disease within their antagonistic communal and sectarian memories and histories and weaponized the pandemic to produce more cracks in the social fabric. This essay underscores the significance of unusual actors in the urban political ecology framework and calls for a renewed understanding of human–nature interface by incorporating religion and religious beliefs and how they view and shape the metabolic flows in the urban spaces for social sustainability of the city as a 'natural object'.

... Between fields, which are regions of force and conflict, there are blind fields ... The urban is defined as the place where people ... engender unexpected situations ... It has been this way ever since there have been cities, and ever since, alongside objects and actions, there have been situations, especially those involving people (individuals and groups) associated with divinity, power, or the imaginary ... Therefore, the urban [is] considered as a field ... [and] [b]lindness consists in the fact that we cannot see the shape of the urban, the vectors and tensions inherent in this field, its logic and dialectic movement, its immanent demands ...

(Henry Lefebvre, The Urban Revolution)

Introduction

Urban political ecology, pandemic and the blind fields of South Asia

Urban political ecology (UPE) analytic views city environments as a co-pro-duction of multiple natural–technical–social–cultural processes intercon-nected without demarcations. The 'urban' is 'cyborg' and there is no binary in urban–nature relationship. This association binds humans and nonhumans through fascinating as well as chaotic networks, flows and circulations of water, waste, energy, fat, chemicals and viruses or germs constantly reposi-tioning themselves along with capital, labour and technologies. The very transboundary characteristics reveal intrinsic frictions, conflicts, struggles and power relations on the questions of access–control, inclusion–exclusion, costs–benefits, gains–losses and redistribution of ecological resources (Castree 2000, Heynen, *et al.* 2006, Kaika and Swyngedouw 2014). The trans-boundary nature of urban dynamics is also multiscalar – operating and influencing various spatialities from local to global and global to local back and forth. While much attention is paid to the tensions on resources in the UPE discussions, 'absent actors' like viruses and other microbes that play an active role in our contested urban lived realities go unattended except when they reclaim their due space through pandemics (Braun 2008) and invite further investigation into the global governance of 'urban political pathology' (Keil 2011, p. 722).

Working along these lines, this essay seeks to focus on the metabolic flows and the circulation of coronavirus in South Asia during the COVID-19 pan-demic which transformed urban ecologies by generating disease. The resul-tant urban–nature interface (the sick hyphen between) is heavily politicized by the state biosecurity apparatus, the power of spirituality and the disease. And within these power geometries, the most unusual actors of the UPE framework – the religious communities – arguably, (i) introduced another version of 'Nature' to the existing power equation and by virtue of their disruptive potential approached the urban political (eco)pathology in such a way as to challenge, undermine or transform the biopower of the state, its technologies of governance and capabilities to manage the discords, (ii) enhanced health risks and inflicted slow violence (Nixon 2011) on society by sticking to orthodoxies of religious assemblies, (iii) embraced and interna-lized the conflictualities of pandemic within their antagonistic communal and sectarian memories and histories and weaponized the disease to produce more fissures than harmonies and (iv) simultaneously in their religio-public domain, acted as proponents of natural objects (e.g. water, herbs or animal waste) as cure in continuation of religious 'knowledges, truths and social order associated with governmentality and self-regulated governance' (Garmany 2010).

All this evolved in the blind fields. As in the past, Schillmeier noted about the spread of SARS, that ' ... [h]uman and social practices that dealt with SARS were organized precisely around not knowing what it was, why and how it acted as it did and what its future evolution could be' (Schillmeier 2008, p. 193). We take this licence of using the Lefebvrian metaphor of *blind field* (Lefebvre 2003) as first, the communal and sectarian urban politics of coronavirus appeared in the many unknowns, inadequacies, incapacities, failures and suspensions of beliefs and disbeliefs which reinforced path-dependent religious orderings in these countries. And secondly, we contend that these issues have not been addressed adequately in theory (of UPE) and in practice (of pandemic as a health concern). It is against this backdrop that we explore communalization/sectarianism of the coronavirus in the cityscapes of South Asia (India and Pakistan) by addressing some important questions like how the recent COVID-19 crisis unfolded vis-à-vis the religious communities in India and Pakistan and what major conflictualities of political pathology were involved? What does that mean for these societies as a whole and the minority groups especially? How the institutional power and the generic political actors emerged in engaging, negotiating, controlling or disciplining religious bodies in the urban spaces?

To address the propositions made and questions raised here, this analysis is divided into three subsequent parts. The next section will offer discussion on how the 'political' is formed within the urban political ecologies and how it transforms in the times of urban health calamities, especially in the contagious diseases. It would be followed by the third section (in the general order of this essay) that highlights the metamorphosis of the South Asian urban political (eco)pathology specifically answering the propositions of this essay. The last and concluding passages will offer more questions for further investigations.

It is noteworthy that this qualitative exploratory piece (based on web content analysis) positions itself in and contributes to the existing body of literature in response to various thematic invitations from scholars who encourage more critical engagements on religion and political ecology debates (Wilkins 2020) or religion and epidemiology analyses (Wildman *et al.* 2020); or stress on the need to have more rigorous treatment of the 'body as a material and political site' in the UPE debates within the postcolonial context (Doshi 2016, p. 1) and those who emphasize on broadening the range of urban experiences to guide the UPE theory on the dynamic construction of urban environments and their politicization through a grounded, situated and/or provincialized analyses from the global South (Zimmer 2010, Lawhon *et al.* 2014, Arboleda 2016, Izaninis, *et al.* 2020). We move on to the next section that offers the review of some of the discussions on the foundation of contested grounds of the 'political' within the urban political eco/pathology.

Formation of the 'political' in urban political eco/pathology

Donna Haraway asserts that social beings essentially produce nature which becomes a socio-physical process that carries political power and cultural meaning (Haraway 1991). The networks of socioecological relations that create uneven environments and geographical developments are those territories around which 'political action crystallises and social mobilisations take place' (Swyngedouw and Heynen, 2003, p. 902). In connection with environmental politics, Kenis and Lievens (2014) refer to various political thinkers like Lefort, Schmitt, Ranciere, Mouffe and Marchart who recognize the 'political' as 'a symbolic or discursive order that represents the social in a way ... that acknowledges the existence of conflict, power and division'. And (among them, for Carl Schmitt) politicization is a process of 'openly declaring and disclosing friends/enemy distinctions; only when conflict is acknowledged and given a place can it be fought in a more or less orderly way' (2014, p. 535).

Narrowing down to the 'political' of the UPE – the hosting space of the conflicts, contestations, differentiations, inequalities, inequities and imbalances – one finds it emerging from the conceptualization of the city in the UPE theory. The two pivotal phenomena associated with the formation of the political are *metabolism* and *circulation* or the flows of water, waste, fat, chemicals, energy, germs and viruses in and around the city spaces and regions through their networked infrastructure. The 'urban' is a metabolic circulatory enterprise built on the consumption of nature which accommodates the 'political' that is made within the socio-cultural and economic relations configured by the power dynamics (Swyngedouw 2006).

As the UPE is conceptually built on the Marxist geography, for Grove (2009), the 'political' can be located within the metabolic processes 'in which human capacities and nonhuman potentialities are combined in the production of new environmental forms' (p. 208) and as an outcome, struggles over the ecological changes emerge in three ways: first, the space of contestation where the metabolic interaction takes place and differential over the labour process is witnessed. Secondly, it is linked to the contestation on distribution between the interest groups for control over the environmental changes. Thirdly, the uneven distribution of metabolic processes and products is the creation of uneven distribution of wealth and power. Keil (2003) also emphasizes the distributional and systemic inequalities in the socio-economic order linked to social–nature relationship as generative of the ecological politics. Adding on to this, he puts forth two other factors: catalysing the 'political' i.e. thrust of democratization and the way environmental issues are being made part of the public deliberations. With that, he suggests that nonhuman actors must be part of this 'political universe' as the environments are co-produced in terms of their socio-physical construction.

Environmental transformations in cities cannot be 'socially or ecologically neutral'. The outcomes of these changes impact one group adversely and the other favourably which cause rifts and displacements – both literally and figuratively. The UPE pays special attention to the power relations that determine the winners or the losers of these conflicting sides within the urban environments (Heynen *et al.* 2006). The political pillar of the UPE approach also underscores the intersectionality of this uneven socio-cultural and bio-physical development in the urban spaces. The transformative processes in the cities work across class, gender, faith and ethnicities and produce different kinds of conditions for the weak and the powerful reflected in the positions of empowerment and/or disempowerment (Bond 2002).

Recalibration of the metabolic and circulatory flows to the transnational level reveals that a new global urbanism is delivered from the living bodies and technologies through which these interactions develop. The changes in this scenario especially during the pandemic risks (underscoring the need to focus on flows of viruses, the spread of disease and the sick bodies) are generative of a cosmopolitics (governing the transnational urban political pathology) that demands re-mapping of local–global, human–nonhuman, nature–culture assemblages and questioning the common modes of 'calculations, rationalities, values, perceptions, and practices' (Schillmeier 2008 p. 193, Keil 2011).

Deeper further, this re-mapping unfolds geographies of health and health-related risks in an interconnected biological and political essence which is both local and global. This essentially makes the city a biopolitical space. And viewing the 'urban' through viral diseases enables us to see how power penetrates bodies – social engineering of people and their habits – and how some are included, and others are excluded i.e. through the withdrawal of state protections/safeguards. Here, the biopolitics remains no longer concerned with the 'local' but it has the tendency of going 'global' in the garb of a global 'biosecurity' venture where 'states of emergence are translated into states of emergency'. This becomes a worldwide 'diagram of power' in which some are sheltered, and others are exposed to health risks – risks 'which are matters of concern and object of government' (Braun 2008, p. 252). But the analysis of health hazards needs to be done holistically keeping in view other socio-economic factors especially when we add newer dimensions to the UPE framework – i.e. transnational and nonhuman actors. It is reiterated that the upscaling of the UPE framework during the pandemic as transnational UPE may be read with its exposition of the power differential at local/global levels so that newer (re)articulations of transnational and human–nonhuman dynamics are better addressed both In theory and practice of the pandemic – the unattended *blind fields* as suggested earlier. For instance, for Caduff (2020) the knee-jerk policy reactions in the form of blanket lockdowns, closures and curfews exacerbated existing socio-economic inequalities and further excluded the poor, vulnerable and marginalized segments of societies around the world.

Reconnecting with the 'political' within the ecology of disease, we see that it emerges from its (perceived/actual) risks which are managed (solely) through the bio/necropolitical tools. This entails the control of populations and their environments which is achieved by a certain governmental rationality expressed through various institutional expressions, devices and techniques (Foucault 1980, 2013, Mbembe and Meintjes 2003). In this case, biosecurity comes to the fore as an organized way or the logic of state biopower or the formal expression of the bio/necropolitical governance to manage disease on the local to global scales (Collier and Lackoff 2006). As the state logics of biosecurity (as an ancient struggle against disease to separate illness from healthy lives) continue, its methods of spatial closures, monitored extensions or controlling life through power (Hinchliffe *et al.* 2012) are heavily contested. The contestations underscore that managing a pandemic in urban spaces is a dynamic and heterogeneous process where biosecurity cannot be a singular method. There can be multiple modes, and actors involved – mutually supporting, conflicting or indifferent (Hinchliffe and Bingham 2008).

The bio/necropolitics of COVID-19 reveals to us the socio-cultural fact that it is not always the state that makes decisions about life and death (Robertson and Travaglia 2020). We have seen that one of the most potent biosecurity challenges came from the communities of *homo religiosus* all around the world. Through this essay, we present an account of the religious communities from India and Pakistan offering a wealth of insights into the socio-spatial behaviour and embodied practices enabling us to answer our questions. We move on to explore in the next section those multiple sites of the urban conflict configured by the rationalities of religion.

The politics of COVID-19 in South Asia

The 'political' of urban pathology in South Asia is formed around five differential spatialities: (i) where the religious communities carve out a (contested) domain for self-governance of the pandemic with their own type of 'knowledge and truths' on disease, (ii) where embodied religious practices challenge or undermine state biopower and transform governmentalities, (iii) where the spatial dimension of conflict unfolds the crisis of technologies of governance, (iv) where religious identities are stigmatized and the minority groups are excluded by virtue of power imbalance and (v) where the communalism organizes around international relations. In the following passages, we offer glimpses into each one of these subfields that were in operation simultaneously in India and Pakistan.

Religious self-governance of disease

Infectious diseases are a biophysical phenomenon which are linked to the presence of certain social practices, conditions and circumstances. While the UPE of pandemics tends to introduce various unusual actors like animals, birds, virus, bacteria and other microbes in the urban spaces (Ali and Keil 2008, Braun 2008), adding a variable of religion brings a new complicated situation both in terms of theory and practice as the new type of 'Nature' enters the arena and completely transforms the dynamics of political pathology. While it is duly acknowledged that the public life of religion is political, arguably, its (re)positioning as 'Nature' being intangible, omnipotent and omniscient force came to the fore as an alternative to the apparently 'incapable' and 'inadequate' 'human' and the 'mundane'. This in turn necessitated a regime of self-governance in the voids of pandemic to offer its own solutions to the problem.

As the COVID-19 crisis originated in the many unknowns, the ensuing empty zones of existence confronting *homo religiosus* are filled with religious beliefs. In the South Asian milieus where spirituality has its own 'scientific logics', the (contested) self-regulatory space for the management of disease carved out by religious groups is built on the existing support from its constituencies within the state, society and even academia. For example, in Pakistan, a proposal to replace fossil and nuclear fuels with Djinn power was initiated by the Pakistan Atomic Energy Commission in 1970. In September 2016, a renowned university in Islamabad organized a public lecture/workshop of a 'spiritual cardiologist' on djinns and black magic. In other instances, a university in Karachi offered to its students the 'graphic glimpses into life in the next world'. The senior faculty member from an elite school in Lahore sent an email to his fellows claiming that 'reciting or listening to certain holy versus can control genes and metabolites' and suggesting 'that specially equipped audio-visual rooms be made in hospitals to treat terminally ill patients' (Hoodbhoy 2015). Likewise, in India, various 'scientists' were quoted as saying in a prestigious scientific conference held in June 2019, that the stem cell and test tube technologies existed in ancient India or the demon king had aircrafts or Lord Vishnu used guided missiles. The ruling Bharatiya Janata Party's Higher Education Minister said that Darwin's theory of evolution was wrong and he vowed to incorporate the same in the national curriculum. In 2015, the Prime Minister Modi stressed on the existence of plastic surgery in ancient India (France-Presse 2019).

Continuing with their 'truths', the Pakistani clerics in their sermons not only disregarded guidelines on health safety but also instilled in their followers a sense of 'fearlessness' against the virus. And this is not only the intangible protection through beliefs but also by using natural objects like water for ablution as a preventive mechanism against the virus. One of the believers is quoted as saying

> Our prayer leader told us that the virus can't infect us the way it does Western people. He said we wash our hands and we wash our face five times a day before we say our prayers, and the infidels don't, so we need not worry. God is with us. (Shahzad 2020)

The belief in 'healing properties' of water, which is associated with cleanliness and godliness, is said to be an integral part of the Islamic traditions since the seventh century (Gruber 2020). Similarly, a leading religious personality, Maulana Tariq Jameel advised his followers to use *Ajwa* dates for the treatment of coronavirus. Besides, a popularly known herb *Kalonji* (Cumin seeds) – 'cure-for-all-diseases' according to the Islamic medicine – has also been advised (Hoodbhoy 2020, Naya Daur 2020).

In India, various Hindu religious groups also proposed their versions of therapies. The President of the Akhil Bharti Hindu Mahasabha came up with the treatment which included burning of *Loban* (gum resin taken from the bdellium tree commonly known as *Gugal* or Mukul myrrh) that is placed on cow dung. The smoke should be spread in the entire house with the chants of '*Om Namah Shivay*' (Adoration to Lord Shiva). He also proposed that people should drink cow urine, perform *yagyas* (the fire ritual) and plaster their homes with cow dung (Awasthi 2020). Some of the members from the ruling BJP also propagated the same treatment (e.g. Suman Harpriya from Assam state), and the followers of the Hindutva groups organized a cow urine-drinking party to prevent the virus (Deutsche Welle 2020). Similarly, the BJP's Union Minister for alternative medicine 'celebrated' the success of Ayurvedic medicine on Prince Charles, the heir to the British throne. He advised that after this 'success', the treatment (herbal medicine, breathing exercises and meditation) should be made public for COVID-19 patients in India. The news was rejected by the British government though (Kumar 2020a). An NGO proposed to the Indian Water Ministry to conduct a study on the holy water of the Ganges River that contains a 'ninja virus' which could kill coronavirus. The proposal was duly forwarded to the Indian Council of Medical Research (ICMR). After considering the issue and citing other important matters to attend to, the Council conveyed that they would assist the ministry concerned if they decided to go ahead with the project (Sampal 2020).

On the one hand, the religious communities in a unique way take us back to the generic units of investigation in the UPE framework (i.e. the natural resources like water, waste and herbs) but not as resources for secular urban politics, instead, as a key element of religion versus science dialectics in the current pandemic. On the other hand, proposing therapies (which is opposed to the scientized efforts of the global institutions) or shaping up social behaviour of believers vis-à-vis the pandemic may also be seen in the light of Jeff Garmany's argument that religion and its institutions tend to 'produce and maintain the knowledges, truths, and social order associated with governmentality and self-regulated governance' (Garmany 2010). With this in context, we move on to the next part where we consider how these religious groups dealt with the biosecurity protocols in India and Pakistan.

Bending the biopower

In view of the massive new and unusually restrictive structures, rules governing the biosocial domains and norms emanating from constantly shifting state rationalities, the believers either defied the secular governmentalities of disease control and health risk management or forced the administrations to readjust to their versions. Perhaps, for them as postcolonial subjects, the curfews, lockdowns, check-posts and mass policing have been an occasional and localized affair and/or always meant for 'pure political' or the secular domains. This second parallel stream of the politics of pandemic in India and Pakistan runs in the defiance of the state institutions on the part of religious bodies.

The Indian Tablighi Jamaat (a conservative Sunni Muslim proselytizing group) was one religious entity singled out and stigmatized for the 'spread' of virus throughout India, but other groups that continued with their faith-based activities include the Hindus and Sikhs at various places with sheer disregard of the precautionary and prohibitory orders. Notably, in March 2020, several large religious assemblies were organized. For instance, BJP's Uttar Pradesh Chief Minister participated in a public gathering at Ram Temple, Ayodhya with several state officials in violation of his own government's protocols on social distancing (Rashid 2020). In Kerala state, a ten-day festival (*Attukal Pongala* at Thiruvanathapuram) was attended by thousands of devotees despite the outbreak warnings (Onmanorama 2020). A religious leader of the Sikh faith, Baldev Singh, organized and attended a six-day festival of *Hola Mohallah* in the Punjab state visited by thousands of devotees a day. The priest returned from his tour of Italy and Germany and refused to self-isolate himself. He died of coronavirus after the festival and subsequently 40,000 of his followers were quarantined (BBC 2020a). Similarly, in April 2020, large crowds of Hindu communities assembled to offer prayers at Burdwan town in West Bengal at the event of Ram Navmi (Times Now 2020). A chariot carrying procession was taken out as part of the *Siddalingeshwara* fair in the Kalaburagi district of Karnataka state (The Wire 2020).

In Pakistan, the Tablighi Jamaat set aside government advisories to cancel their annual event scheduled to take place in March 2020 in Raiwind, a sub-district of Lahore. The gathering hosted thousands of followers from Pakistan and abroad. Jamaat's leaders believed that the calls for cancellation were motivated by 'anti-religious bias'. One of the organizers said, 'Every other year, something or other happens which makes people afraid of getting together. We just focus on action, on deeds, and Allah protects' (Hadid 2020). The rationality for defiance is said to have multiple dimensions beyond adherence to beliefs. As this group relies on financial support from public donations, the closure of religious sites has been considered as an economic restraint on them. Moreover, biopolitical controls of the state are also viewed in the postcolonial context even if apparently this missionary group eschews politics. The Jamaat considered the state protocols as colonial governmentality (Chaudry 2020), therefore, they ignored repeated requests from the government officials constantly persuading them to cancel their annual session – otherwise reported to be a major cause in the spread of coronavirus in Pakistan (Chaudhry 2020).

But resistance to the government guidelines goes beyond the Tablighi Jamaat in Pakistan. Other religious leaders from different subsects of both the Sunni and Shia sects have been issuing statements that flouted state protocols on public health. At various occasions in their public congregations, they either clearly denounced the restrictions being contrary to the injunctions of the faith or if noticed by the state institutions or got informed on, they issued statements that readjusted to 'include' government instructions for safeguarding public health concerns as well (IBC-TV 2020). Interestingly, in March 2020, the President of Pakistan obtained a *Fatwa* (religious edict) from the council of Islamic scholars in Al-Azhar University of Egypt (a traditional seat of Islamic learning) in favour of banning group prayers in mosques during health emergencies. Despite that, the clerics refused to accept the *Fatwa* considering it an ancillary instrument of the existing prohibitory legal apparatus in place. A group of leading clerics went on to issue their own operating procedures that included stay-home instructions (for children, older people, the sick and people nursing them), cleanliness and installing sanitizers in mosques. But they resisted the ban on mass prayers five times a day, maintaining that they needed collective prayers for God's forgiveness in the times of pandemic (Tanzeem 2020).

This might appear as an appeasement policy towards the religious elite and proletariat by the government in Pakistan which did not want to lose the support of the religious right (Shahzad 2020, Siddiqa 2020). But, arguably, the refusal to comply with the standard operating procedures (SOPs) issued by the state on the part of religious groups might also be the result of their frustrated disbelief as to how could the government curb the same religious practices that otherwise constituted or consolidated the state power in the normal circumstances i.e. the religious ideology enshrined in its laws. In a way summarily, the religious power appeared to be acting in a visibly potent way if not superior in the times of COVID-19. This connects us to the spaces of believers as a subunit of analysis as they engendered intersectional tensions (disproportionate state action against religious/ethnic minorities and minorities versus other vulnerable groups e.g. women) on the one hand, and on the other delivered a crisis of inadequacy of health infrastructure. We explore this theme in the next subsection.

Religious spaces and technologies of governance

The spatial dimension of politics is critical as the pandemic generated inequalities, inequities and crises of inadequacies and confidence all along the technologies of governing the viral outbreak in urban spaces of control and management – health infrastructure (quarantine centres, medical wards, field hospitals and locked religious centres) and postcolonial apparatus (curfews, police actions, penal codes, security and epidemic prevention laws).

As the power differential acts in complicated intersectional ways, we note that in the middle of stigmatization on the spread of disease, in April 2020, some members of Tablighi Jamaat were reported to be misbehaving with the female nurses employed in a quarantine facility in Ghaziabad, Uttar Pradesh state, India – fanning the flames of anti-Muslim fire in the country. The state government booked them under the National Security Act, which is not usual for the violators of COVID-19 directives. The Act (allowing the authorities to detain a person for up to 12 months without a charge) had previously been used against the minorities and dissidents (journalists, Dalits and cow-slaughtering Muslims) and had been a frequently used instrument of the BJP Chief Minister Yogi Adityanath. Moreover, the government also decided not to deploy female staff at the quarantine centres where Tablighi Jamaat members were kept (India Today 2019, Outlook 2020).

Conversely, when the legal action against the Tablighi Jamaat was taken in Pakistan especially after their annual conference held in March 2020, in (Raiwind) Lahore, the most prominent voices in their support were from two ex-Chief Ministers of Punjab, Shahbaz Sharif and Pervez Ilahi (currently the opposition leader in the National Assembly and the Speaker of Punjab Assembly, respectively). Pervez Ilahi said that no oppression or excesses with the Tablighi Jamaat would be tolerated. The members of Jamaat arrested from the mosques should immediately be released and shifted to mosques or Tablighi centres declaring them as quarantines and providing them with ration and facilities (Dawn 2020a, The News 2020). Accordingly, their centres were declared as quarantines with the directions to provide all the facilities to the members of Jamaat (AFP 2020, Ali 2020). On the other hand, the Shia minority pilgrims returning from Iran had been agitating against the unfair treatment and insufficient facilities at their isolation wards in Balochistan and Sindh provinces where the mismanagement of isolation quarters also became a Twitter tiff between the Chief Ministers of these provinces as well (Asianlite 2020, Mandhro 2020). This takes us to the crisis of inadequacy of technologies of pandemic governance.

It is important to note that the religious spaces had been acting as a source of urban health risk and resultantly generative of the crisis of inadequacy of health infrastructure. Understandably, it is tough to handle a public health calamity where the religious sites are a great supplier of hazards to a wider scale with an increasing sensitivity for religiosity. The spiritual leaders in Pakistan called on the President of Pakistan in April 2020 for an agreement on the opening of mosques in the holy month of Ramadan. The two sides agreed on twenty SOPs mainly social distancing during prayers and the usage of disinfectants among other things (Hussain 2020a). In response to the agreement, top medical body, the Pakistan Medical Association (PMA) called in question the practicality of the SOPs agreed upon. The PMA requested the faith leaders to review their decision on opening the mosques as it would cause the exponential growth of infections and would burden the already insufficient medical infrastructure – ICUs, ventilators and personal protective equipment (Dawn 2020b). Though a non-governmental entity, the PMA is a nationally represented body of doctors in Pakistan constituted in 1948 in Dhaka, then East Pakistan (PMA 1948). Its counterpart in India is the Indian Medical Association established in 1928 (IMA, 2020).

Though not binding on the government or the religious authorities, the PMA advisories went unattended and the religious sites remained open for the congregational prayers in the month of Ramadan. It is perhaps against this backdrop that one of the top state officials showed the predicament by saying, 'This is a sensitive matter, we don't want to impose it using a stick. And even if we wanted to, there aren't enough sticks to implement it across Pakistan' (Shahzad 2020). While these religious entities continued to assert themselves in social orderings and to (re)negotiate their spaces with the state institutions, they were differentially weighed in the power equations in their respective societies. The next subsection will explore how the religious communities work around the differences in their religious identities.

Identities, stigmatization and exclusion

Viewing the urban spaces through infectious diseases enables us to consider the quotidian penetration of power into living bodies through the social engineering of spaces and commanding new social habits. It also allows us to see how certain bodies are excluded/included from/in the biopolitical spaces (Braun 2008). Maligning the religious identity of the minorities, stigmatization and their exclusion from the state and society networks is one set of events and processes through which urban politics of disease is revealed to us in the COVID-19 emergency in South Asia.

Coronavirus outbreak in Pakistan started with sectarian blaming of the Shia Muslim community (a minority in a Sunni dominated country) returning from their pilgrimage in Qom and Mashhad cities of Iran in February 2020 and calling it the *'Shia Virus'*. Though certain incidents of denying Hindus and Christians access to food and groceries by some of the charity groups were reported, the Shia community has been a focal point of this exclusionary blame game. In Balochistan province, which borders Iran, the precise target was the *Hazara* tribe among Shias. In March 2020, government organizations in the provincial capital Quetta (e.g. the police department and the Water and Sanitation Authority [WASA]) formally notified Shia employees belonging to the *Hazara* tribe to proceed on leave. And other entities like the State Bank of Pakistan and the Civil Hospital informally sent them on forced leave. The Chief Secretary of the province (the highest civil servant) ordered to segregate *Hazara* neighbourhoods from the rest of the Quetta city (Mirza 2020a).

As the international border crossing between Iran and Pakistan at Taftan town was closed, out of all the returnees from Iran, only Shias were quarantined. Their quarantine facilities were reported to be like prisons or unhygienic quarters without the necessary supplies for human consumption. The blame game was not limited to the common pilgrims. Maulana Ahmad Ludhyanvi (a Sunni cleric heading an anti-Shia organization, *Ahl-e-Sunnat Wal Jamaat*) also dragged into it a Federal Minister, Ali Zaidi, and Special Assistant to the Prime Minister, Zulfiqar Ali Bukhari, both Shias, alleging them to be complicit in the spread of virus through the Shia pilgrims. It was followed by Shia bashing on the social media (Mirza 2020b). During this massive anti-Shia tirade, Mr. Bukhari sued one of the prominent opposition leaders from the Pakistan Muslim League-Nawaz (PML-N) Khawaja Muhammad Asif for defamation on making the accusations. Responding to this, Mr. Asif (brazenly) said, 'The whole country is now saying this' (Hussain 2020b). The anti-Shia harangue abated only after one of the mainstream conservative Sunni groups – the Tablighi Jamaat – surfaced in the media as the new 'hotspot' at their annual gathering of thousands in Lahore – March 2020. While the dynamics of Tablighi Jamaat's 'connection' with the crisis in Pakistan evolved in their own way, they offer a political theatre of bigger conflictualities in India.

Across the border in India, the coronavirus eruption was called *'Tablighi Virus'*. This singled out the Tableeghi Jamaat – the Sunni Muslim proselytizing group – as the 'super-spreader' after their Delhi gathering in March 2020 which was attended by thousands of devotees from all around the country and abroad. With the allegations of being the 'starting point', it was feared that it would generate a new wave of anti-Muslim sentiments in India after the deadly communal violence in February 2020 in the wake of recent controversial citizenship law. The Citizenship (Amendment) Act, (CAA) 2019 (allegedly) excluded Muslim migrants from the fast-track citizenship scheme (Slater *et al.* 2020). Moreover, this legislation is argued to be a part of the ruling BJP's other policies like revoking the autonomous status of Kashmir (the only Muslim majority state in India) and building the controversial temple on the site of a razed mosque (Slater and Masih, 2020).

Later in April 2020, the leader of Tablighi Jamaat, Maulana Saad Khandalvi, was booked by Delhi police for manslaughter in connection with organizing the religious congregation in violation of the government orders which caused 1,023 cases of coronavirus in 17 states (BBC 2020b). The Union Minister for Minorities, Mukhtar Abbas Naqvi, labelled Tablighi Jamaat's assembly as a *'Talibani Crime'* and the social media called it the *'Corona Jihad'* (Trivedi 2020). The following incidents show a widespread anger against the Muslim community in India after the virus outbreak e.g. members of the ruling Bhartiya Janata Party (BJP) calling for the boycott of Muslim street vendors in Uttar Pradesh (Scroll 2020); government hospital in Ahmadabad (Gujarat state) segregating Muslim coronavirus patients from the Hindu patients (Jha 2020); the High Court of Gujarat blaming the Tablighi Jamaat for the epidemic in the country; arrests of Muslim dissidents (of citizenship legislation/CAA 2019) for violating lockdown regulations; incidents of beating Muslims in different cities or inviting others to shoot them or issuing them warnings or anti-Muslim media portrayals (Ayyub 2020, Frayer 2020, Kumar 2020b). The communal concern was raised by the opposition leader, Sonia Gandhi who said, '[T]he BJP continues to spread the virus of communal prejudice and hatred. Grave damage is being done to our social harmony' (Naqshbandi 2020). This communal/sectarian power imbalance and the resultant rifts also re-territorialized elsewhere. We proceed to the next subsection that highlights how the communalized South Asian pandemic is configured by international politics.

Religious bodies and the international relations

While other states had to manage a multidimensional global disease, India and Pakistan received it with added intricacies of religious influence in management and controls. In Pakistan, the often-repeated religious conspiracy theories were voiced in connection with the COVID-19 spread. On the closure of religious sites, a religious leader, Mufti Kafayatullah, was reported as saying, 'we will be forced to think that mosques are being deserted on America's instructions. We're ready to give our lives, but not ready to desert our mosques' (Shahzad 2020). According to a market research by Ipsos, 43 percent of Pakistanis thought that the coronavirus was a conspiracy by America or Israel to weaken Muslims (Tanzeem 2020).

In India, the contested spaces of faith are connected to hosting people from different countries. The foreign participants also bore the brunt of the communal wave. The Indian government blacklisted 960 foreign nationals (out of around 2100) who participated in Tablighi Jamaat's Delhi gathering in March 2020 on account of violation of tourist visa conditions. Since 2015, the government blacklisted (i.e. revocation of visa and ban on future travelling to India) more than four thousand Muslim foreigners on participating in Jamaat's activities (HT 2020). Conversely, it is also thought that the legal action against Jamaat is not enough, especially against its leader Maulana Saad Khandalvi. Some elements in the Indian 'establishment' considered the Tablighi Jamaat as a major 'asset' for India as the organization had a considerable following in many countries around the world especially some of the 'important' Muslim countries. It was an apolitical group confined to its missionary activities only. Resultantly, any penal action against its leader might strengthen religious groups in Pakistan (Kapoor 2020).

The communalization of the coronavirus and ensuing Islamophobia did not go unnoticed internationally, especially in the Middle East. Some of the notable voices from the Arab world like the Princess of UAE, Hend Al Qassemi, Saudi Scholar Abidi Zahrani, Kuwaiti lawyer Meibal Al Shakira, Kuwaiti activist Abdur Rahman Nassar and Bahraini lawmaker Jamal Bouhassan raised the issue by calling out the hate-spewing elements, seeking the lists of hard-liners working in the Arab countries or resolving to raise voice against Indian Islamophobia on international forums. The Organization of Islamic Conference (OIC) urged the Indian government to protect minority Muslims and take steps to stop Islamophobia (Pasha 2020). Beyond the Muslim countries, the United States Commission on International Religious Freedom (USCIRF) condemneds the incident of segregating Muslim coronavirus patients in a civil hospital of Ahmadabad in Gujarat state, maintaining that such activities would increase the stigmatization of Muslims in India (USCIRF 2020). The Commission, in its annual report, recommended that India should be placed in the list of 'countries of particular concern' that would be subject to sanctions if they do not improve their credentials on religious freedoms. The countries on 'particular concern' list include Pakistan, China, Iran, Myanmar, North Korea, Saudi Arabia, Tajikistan and Turkmenistan (Aljazeera 2020). Similarly, the UN Under-Secretary General, Adam Dieng, also showed apprehensions on the discrimination and hate crimes against Muslims in India and called for unity and solidarity in the times of the COVID-19 crisis (Grewal 2020).

Conclusion

COVID-19 and beyond

This exploratory analysis has taken up (evolving) forms of the pandemic politics being shaped by the religious actors in the Indian subcontinent using the UPE framework. It has shown five parallel theatres of political contestations – i.e. contested self-governance of coronavirus by religious actors, embodied defiance to the institutional biosecurity; religious spaces generating the crisis of technologies of governing the disease; the intercommunal shades of disparities and showcasing of communalism in international relations. It has been argued that religious communities in India and Pakistan approached the UPE of COVID-19 with their disruptive potential which altered biosecurity regimes and enhanced health hazards for their respective societies. Moreover, they embraced and internalized ensuing disputes within their hostile communal and sectarian memories and histories and weaponized the pandemic which damaged the already weakening social coherence.

The dynamics of South Asian religious communities as one of the key challenges in the management of the pandemic are in a way similar to various other cases in different countries. For example, in South Korea around five thousand cases were traced to the 'Patient 31' belonging to Shincheonji Church of Jesus in Daegu city. The Church propagated in-person meetings, praying while touching and banning face masks. In Trinidad (West Indies), a church was found to be bullying the members to show up in the prayer sessions and confronting the government officials. In Baton Rouge (USA), a pastor of Life Tabernacle Church defied Governor's orders and was quoted as saying, 'The virus, we believe, is politically motivated. We hold our religious rights dear and we are going to assemble no matter what someone says' (Wildman *et al.* 2020). Likewise, orthodox Jewish group *Haredis* also saw it difficult to adjust to the public health policies because of the religious instructions in which prayer and recitation gatherings are supreme considerations than anything else. One of the Rabbis said, 'Canceling Torah study is more dangerous than the coronavirus. Without Torah, the world falls' (Dalsheim 2020). Beside their adherence to the religious assemblies in defiance of the state directives, religious leaders have also shown similarities in advancing their varieties of 'knowledge and truth' on COVID-19 treatment. Roman Catholic archbishop Samuel Kleda's herbal oil in Cameroon (Kindzeka 2020); perfume, flower oil or from Iran's clerics (Alijani 2020) or healing through TV screens by Evangelical preacher Kenneth Copeland in Texas, USA (Niemietz 2020) are a few examples in this regard.

What differentiates the South Asian groups is the scale on which their communal and sectarian hostilities operated and also the historicized metamorphosis of the pandemic as an instrument of exclusion cutting across various spaces. The COVID-19 and its tensions constitute one exclusive zone of urban emergency, whereas outside of that, in the city regions the two countries faced another ecological calamity threatening their food security – the locust attack in May 2020. In Pakistan, the desert locust devoured massive agricultural produce in 60 districts in all the four provinces – a loss estimated to be around $3.72 billion. The armies of grasshoppers also invaded the crops in Indian states of Rajasthan, Maharashtra and Gujarat (Latif and Kapoor 2020). In view of this, there are questions that go beyond the coronavirus pandemic. How do these countries look at such urban and regional disasters where nonhumans play a central role in disrupting the equilibrium of urban life? And how do they prepare themselves to respond when the (essential) religious actors add more challenges to the crisis management by influencing belief systems and state governmentalities especially where they are co-constitutive of the state power? How the city and regional design and institutions are going to be reformed incorporating these actors? How effective are the traditional and/or religious ways of thinking in the broader problem-solving efforts in urban and regional development? How the power geometries would look like after that and what would be new rules of business and engagement for both the state and religious communities?

With these and other similar challenges at hand, it is important to take a holistic view of the urban political eco/pathology by returning to the constitution of the 'urban' as a metabolic circulatory enterprise where 'capital, labour, technologies, and germs reposition themselves in and through urban life' (Keil 2011, p. 722). This approach calls for the recognition of the centrality of socio-cultural and religious values and beliefs related to the urban processes in traditional societies like the Indian subcontinent by broadening the policy and planning horizon to incorporate these aspirations and actors. Giving due space to the social aspects of public calamities would enable us to see who is left out when we opt for myopic biosecurity methods as the single solution to deal with these crises. The revised understanding of a comprehensive pandemic planning also requires an appropriate incubator. And we contend that this should be taken to the public arena to take its roots instead of the cloisters of marketized technocracy.

Acknowledgments

The authors are grateful to the reviewers/editors for their valuable comments/feedback on the manuscript.

Disclosure statement

No potential conflict of interest was reported by the author(s).

Further information

This Special Issue article has been comprehensively reviewed by the Special Issue editors, Associate Professor Ted Striphas and Professor John Nguyet Erni.

ORCID

Asif Mehmood 🔟 http://orcid.org/0000-0002-2101-4116
Sajjad Hasnain 🔟 http://orcid.org/0000-0002-6796-5988
Muhammad Azam 🔟 http://orcid.org/0000-0001-5405-8628

References

AFP. 2020. *COVID-19: 20,000 quarantined in Pakistan after gathering.* [Online] Available from: https://gulfnews.com/world/asia/pakistan/covid-19-20000-quarantined-in-pakistan-after-gathering-1.1586100853639 [Accessed 15 April 2020].

Ali, I. 2020. *IGP Sindh directs Tableeghi Jamaat members to stay in marakiz, consider them as quarantine centres.* [Online] Available from: https://www.dawn.com/news/1545268 [Accessed 15 April 2020].

Ali, S.H., and Keil, R., 2008. Introduction: networked disease. In: S.H. Ali, and R Keil, ed. *Networked disease: emerging infections in the global city.* Oxford: Blackwell Publishing Ltd, 1–7.

Alijani, E. 2020. *Prophet's perfume and flower oil: how Islamic medicine has made Iran's Covid-19 outbreak worse.* [Online] Available from: https://observers.france24.com/en/20200330-iran-coronavirus-islamic-medicine-covid-19-worse [Accessed 15 April].

Aljazeera. 2020. *India should be placed on religious freedom blacklist: US panel.* [Online] Available from: https://www.aljazeera.com/news/2020/04/watchdog-india-religious-freedom-blacklist-200429030352021.html?utm_source=website&utm_medium=article_page&utm_campaign=read_more_links [Accessed 16 April 2020].

Arboleda, M., 2016. In the nature of the non-city: expanded infrastructural networks and the political ecology of planetary urbanisation. *Antipode,* 48 (2), 233–251.

Asianlite, T.V. 2020. *Shia cleric blames imran for plight of pilgrims,* [Online] Available from: https://www.youtube.com/watch?v=wGQdUGMlPzM [Accessed 16 April 2020].

Awasthi, P. 2020. *Cow dung, cow urine and yagya to combat coronavirus says Hindutva group chief.* [Online] Available from: https://www.theweek.in/news/india/2020/02/04/cow-dung-cow-urine-and-yagya-to-combat-coronavirus-says-hindutva-group-chief.html [Accessed 16 April 2020].

Ayyub, R. 2020. *Islamophobia taints India's response to the coronavirus.* [Online] Available from: https://www.washingtonpost.com/opinions/2020/04/06/islamophobia-taints-indias-response-coronavirus/ [Accessed 17 April 2020].

BBC. 2020a. *Coronavirus: India 'super spreader' quarantines 40,000 people.* [Online] Available from: https://www.bbc.com/news/world-asia-india-52061915 [Accessed 17 April 2020].

BBC. 2020b. https://www.bbc.com/news/world-asia-india-52306879. [Online] Available from: https://www.bbc.com/news/world-asia-india-52306879 [Accessed 18 April 2020].

Bond, P., 2002. *Unsustainable South Africa: Environment, development and social protest.* Pietermaritzburg: University of Kwazulu Natal Press.

Braun, B., 2008. Thinking the city through SARS: bodies, topologies, politics. In: S. H. A. a, and R. Keil, ed. *Networked disease: emerging infections in the global city.* Oxford: Blackwell Publishing Ltd, 250–266.

Caduff, C., 2020. What went wrong: corona and the world after the full stop. *Medical athropology quarterly,* 4 (34), 467–487.

Castree, N., 2000. Marxism and the production of nature. *Capital and class,* 24 (3), 5–36.

Chaudhry, A. 2020. *Tableeghi Jamaat in hot water in Pakistan too for Covid-19 spread.* [Online] Available from: https://www.dawn.com/news/1547354 [Accessed 18 April 2020].

Chaudry, S. 2020. *Coronavirus: Pakistan quarantines Tablighi Jamaat missionaries.* [Online] Available from: https://www.middleeasteye.net/news/coronavirus-pakistan-tablighi-jamaat-missionaries-quarantined [Accessed 16 April 2020].

Collier, S.J., and Lackoff, A. 2006. *Vital systems security.* [Online] Available from: https://core.ac.uk/download/pdf/5015692.pdf ARC Working Paper [Accessed 16 April 2020].

Dalsheim, J. 2020. *Jewish history explains why some ultra-Orthodox communities defy coronavirus restrictions.* [Online] Available from: https://theconversation.com/jewish-history-explains-why-some-ultra-orthodox-communities-defy-coronavirus-restrictions-135292 [Accessed April 28 2020].

Dawn. 2020a. *Doctors demand strict lockdown, urge religious scholars to review decision to open mosques.* [Online] Available from: https://www.dawn.com/news/1551370 [Accessed 23 April 2020].

Dawn. 2020b. *Tableegi Jamaat finds supporters in Elahi and Shahbaz.* [Online] Available from: https://epaper.dawn.com/DetailImage.php?StoryImage=02_04_2020_176_008 [Accessed 23 April 2020].

Deutsche Welle. 2020. *Hindu group hosts cow urine drinking party to ward off coronavirus.* [Online] Available from: https://www.dw.com/en/hindu-group-hosts-cow-urine-drinking-party-to-ward-off-coronavirus/a-52773262 [Accessed 16 April 2020].

Doshi, S., 2016. Embodied urban political ecology: five propositions. *Area,* 49 (1), 125–128.

Foucault, M., 1980. *Power/knowledge: selected interviews and other writings 1972–1977.* Sussex: Harvester Press.

Foucault, M., 2013. Society must be defended, lecture at the colege de France, March 17, 1976. *In:* Timothy Campbell and Adam Sitze, eds. *Biopolitics: a reader.* Durham and London: Duke University Press, pp. 61-81.

France-Presse, A. 2019. *India outcry after scientists claim ancient Hindus invented stem cell research.* [Online] Available from: https://www.theguardian.com/world/2019/jan/07/india-scientists-claim-ancient-hindus-invented-stem-cell-research-dismiss-einstein [Accessed 16 April 2020].

Frayer, L. 2020. *Blamed for coronavirus outbreak, muslims in India come under attack.* [Online] Available from: https://www.npr.org/2020/04/23/839980029/blamed-for-coronavirus-outbreak-muslims-in-india-come-under-attack [Accessed 14 April 2020].

Garmany, J., 2010. Religion and governmentality: understanding governance in urban Brazil. *Geoforum,* 41 (6), 908–918.

Grewal, K. 2020. *UN official raises concerns over hate speech in India, cites Subramanian Swamy's comments.* [Online] Available from: https://theprint.in/india/un-official-raises-concerns-over-hate-speech-in-india-cites-subramanian-swamys-comments/425337/ [Accessed 21 May 2020].

Grove, K., 2009. Rethinking the nature of urban environmental politics: security, subjectivity, and the non-human. *Geoforum*, 40 (2), 207–206.

Gruber, C. 2020. *Long before face masks, Islamic healers tried to ward off disease with their version of PPE*. [Online] Available from: https://theconversation.com/long-before-face-masks-islamic-healers-tried-to-ward-off-disease-with-their-version-of-ppe-138409 [Accessed 22 May 2020].

Hadid, D. 2020. *Mass religious gathering in Pakistan leads to fresh concerns over COVID-19 spread*. [Online] Available from: https://www.npr.org/sections/coronavirus-live-updates/2020/03/23/820043866/mass-religious-gathering-in-pakistan-leads-to-fresh-concerns-over-covid-19-sprea [Accessed 28 March 2020].

Haraway, D., 1991. *Simians, cyborgs and women – the reinvention of nature*. London: Free Association Books.

Heynen, N., Kaika, M. & Swyngedouw, E., 2006. Urban political ecology: politicizing the production of urban natures. In: Nik Heynen, Maria Kaika, and Erik Swyngedouw, eds, *In the nature of cities urban political ecology and the politics of urban metabolism*. London and New York: Routledge, pp. 1-19.

Hinchliffe, S., *et al.*, 2012. Biosecurity and the topologies of infected life: from borderlines to borderlands. *Transactions of the institute of British geographers*, 38 (4), 531–543.

Hinchliffe, S. & Bingham, N., 2008. People, animals and biosecurity in and through cities. *In*: Roger Keil, and S. Harris Ali, eds, *Networked disease: emerging infections in the global city*. Oxford: Wiley Blackwell, pp. 214–227.

Hoodbhoy, P. 2015. *Jinns invade campuses*. [Online] Available from: https://www.dawn.com/news/1212051 [Accessed 24 May 2020].

Hoodbhoy, P. 2020. *Coronavirus is Pakistan's debt for lifelong rejection of Darwin*. [Online] Available from: https://theprint.in/opinion/coronavirus-is-pakistans-debt-for-lifelong-rejection-of-darwin/395478/ [Accessed 24 May 2020].

HT. 2020. *Foreigners from at least 41 countries among those blacklisted for Nizamuddin Markaz*. [Online] Available from: https://www.hindustantimes.com/india-news/foreigners-from-at-least-41-countries-among-those-blacklisted-for-nizamuddin-markaz/story-coLtMyWVqJePiya9eEbQaL.html [Accessed 15 April 2020].

Hussain, J. 2020a. *President Alvi outlines plan agreed with ulema on congregational prayers during Ramazan*. [Online] Available from: https://www.dawn.com/news/1550265 [Accessed 20 April 2020].

Hussain, J. 2020b. *Zulfi Bukhari sends Rs1 billion defamation notice to PML-N's Khawaja Asif over Taftan allegations*. [Online] Available from: https://www.dawn.com/news/1544983 [Accessed 20 April 2020].

IBC-TV. 2020. *#CORONAVIRUS & Religious Leaders of Pakistan, Funny Statements* [Online] Available from: https://www.youtube.com/watch?v=qZFtBaCiCYU [Accessed 15 April 2020].

IMA. 2020. *What is IMA? And it's history*. [Online] Available from: https://www.ima-india.org/ima/left-side-bar.php?pid=299 [Accessed 30 November 2020].

India Today. 2019. *What is the national security act: all you need to know*. [Online] Available from: https://www.indiatoday.in/fyi/story/what-is-national-security-act-india-1449395-2019-02-06 [Accessed 16 May 2020].

Jha, S. 2020. *Govt hospital in Ahmedabad allegedly separates Hindu, Muslim coronavirus patients; govt denies*. [Online] Available from: https://www.deccanherald.com/national/west/govt-hospital-in-ahmedabad-allegedly-separates-hindu-muslim-coronavirus-patients-govt-denies-825586.html [Accessed 17 May 2020].

Kaika, M., and Swyngedouw, E. 2014. *Radical urban political-ecological imaginaries.* [Online] Available from: https://www.eurozine.com/radical-urban-political-ecological-imaginaries/ [Accessed 1 May 2020].

Kapoor, C. 2020. *Inside track: double speak on dealing with Tablighi Jamaat.* [Online] Available from: https://indianexpress.com/article/opinion/columns/pk-mishra-ajit-doval-tablighi-jamaat-covid-19-coomi-kapoor-6424384/ [Accessed 30 May 2020].

Keil, R., 2003. Urban political ecology. *Urban geography*, 24 (8), 723–738.

Keil, R., 2011. Transnational urban political ecology: health and infrastructure in the unbounded city. In: G. B. Watson, ed. *The new Blackwell companion to the city.* Oxford: Blackwell Publishing Ltd, 713–725.

Kenis, A., and Lievens, M., 2014. Searching for 'the political' in environmental politics. *Environmental politics*, 23 (4), 531–548.

Kindzeka, M.E. 2020. *Hundreds rush for popular cleric's herbal COVID 'cure' in Cameroon.* [Online] Available from: https://www.voanews.com/covid-19-pandemic/hundreds-rush-popular-clerics-herbal-covid-cure-cameroon [Accessed 13 May 2020].

Kumar, R. 2020a. *Face it: the Indian government is peddling pseudoscience.* [Online] Available from: https://science.thewire.in/health/indian-government-pseudoscienc e-covid-19/ [Accessed 16 April 2020].

Kumar, S. 2020b. *BJP is using Covid-19 as a weapon to crackdown against democratic dissent.* [Online] Available from: https://www.dawn.com/news/1558260/bjp-is-using-covid-19-as-a-weapon-to-crackdown-against-democratic-dissent [Accessed 22 May 2020].

Latif, A., and Kapoor, C. 2020. *Amid COVID-19, locust attack risks famine in Pakistan, India.* [Online] Available from: https://www.aa.com.tr/en/asia-pacific/amid-covid-19-locust-attack-risks-famine-in-pakistan-india-/1856085 [Accessed 30 May 2020].

Lawhon, M., Ernstson, H., and Silver, J., 2014. Provincializing urban political ecology: towards a situated UPE through african urbanism. *Antipode*, 46 (2), 497–516.

Lefebvre, H., 2003. *The urban revolution.* Minneapolis, MN, US: University of Minnesota Press.

Mandhro, S. 2020. *Quarantined pilgrims highlight 'inhumane' experience at Taftan border.* [Online] Available from: https://tribune.com.pk/story/2176319/1-quarantined-pilgrims-highlight-inhumane-experience-taftan-border/ [Accessed 16 April 2020].

Mbembe, A., and Meintjes, L., 2003. Necropolitics. *Public culture*, 15 (1), 11–40.

Mirza, J.A. 2020a. *COVID-19 fans religious discrimination in Pakistan.* [Online] Available from: https://thediplomat.com/2020/04/covid-19-fans-religious-discrimination-in-pakistan/ [Accessed 20 April 2020].

Mirza, J.A. 2020b. *Pakistan's Hazara Shia minority blamed for spread of Covid-19.* [Online] Available from: https://www.ids.ac.uk/opinions/pakistans-hazara-shia-minority-blamed-for-spread-of-covid-19/ [Accessed 20 April 2020].

Naqshbandi, A. 2020. *BJP continues to spread virus of communal prejudice, hatred: Sonia Gandhi.* [Online] Available from: https://www.hindustantimes.com/india-news/test-trace-quarantine-model-has-no-alternative-sonia-gandhi-on-covid-19/story-U1QfumxreB2n5VUWwdqNVK.html [Accessed 30 April 2020].

Naya Daur. 2020. *Singer Salman Ahmed Comes up with absurd theory about recovery from COVID-19.* [Online] Available from: https://nayadaur.tv/2020/04/singer-salman-ahmed-comes-up-with-absurd-theory-about-recovery-from-covid-19/ [Accessed 30 April 2020].

The News. 2020. *Pervaiz for stopping negative propaganda against Tableeghi Jamaat.* [Online] Available from: https://www.thenews.com.pk/print/638248-pervaiz-for-stopping-negative-propaganda-against-tableeghi-jamaat [Accessed 16 April 2020].

Niemietz, B. 2020. *SEE IT: Televangelist claims to cure coronavirus through television sets.* [Online] Available from: https://www.nydailynews.com/news/national/ny-televangelist-cure-coronavirus-television-sets-20200313-wvkb2aqkwzfvzgu3lzwhw6223u-story.html [Accessed 2 April 2020].

Nixon, R., 2011. *Slow violence and the environmentalism of the poor.* Cambridge: Harvard University Press.

Onmanorama. 2020. *Lakhs celebrate Attukal Pongala amid coronavirus fears; 6 foreigners sent back.* [Online] Available from: https://www.theweek.in/news/india/2020/03/09/lakhs-celebrate-attukal-pongala-amid-coronavirus-fears-6-foreigners-sent-back.html [Accessed 2 April 2020].

Outlook. 2020. *Tablighi Jamaat members face NSA for misbehaving with nurses in UP hospital.* [Online] Available from: https://www.outlookindia.com/website/story/india-news-tablighi-jamaat-members-face-nsa-for-misbehaving-with-nurses-in-up-hospital/349989 [Accessed 10 April 2020].

Pasha, S. 2020. *India's coronavirus-related Islamophobia has the arab world up in arms.* [Online] Available from: https://thewire.in/communalism/indias-coronavirus-related-islamophobia-has-the-arab-world-up-in-arms [Accessed 1 May 2020].

PMA. 1948. *Pakistan Medical Association.* [Online] Available from: https://www.pmacentre.org.pk/ [Accessed 30 Naovember 2020].

Rashid, O. 2020. *U.P. Chief Minister Adityanath shifts Ram idol amid lockdown.* [Online] Available from: https://www.thehindu.com/news/national/other-states/up-chief-minister-adityanath-shifts-ram-idol-amid-lockdown/article31160225.ece [Accessed 1 April 2020].

Robertson, H., and Travaglia, J. 2020. *The necropolitics of COVID-19: will the COVID-19 pandemic reshape national healthcare systems?.* [Online] Available from: https://blogs.lse.ac.uk/impactofsocialsciences/2020/05/18/the-necropolitics-of-covid-19-will-the-covid-19-pandemic-reshape-national-healthcare-systems/ [Accessed 20 December 2020].

Sampal, R. 2020. *Can Gangajal treat Covid-19? Modi govt wants a study, ICMR says no.* [Online] Available from: https://theprint.in/health/can-gangajal-treat-covid-19-modi-govt-wants-a-study-icmr-says-no/415365/ [Accessed 8 May 2020].

Schillmeier, M., 2008. Globalizing risks – The cosmo-politics of SARS and its impact on Globalizing sociology. *Mobilities*, 3 (2), 179–199.

Scroll. 2020. *Caught on camera: UP BJP MLA Brij Bhushan Rajput threatens to beat up Muslim vegetable vendor.* [Online] Available from: https://scroll.in/video/960643/caught-on-camera-up-bjp-mla-threatens-to-beat-up-muslim-vegetable-vendor [Accessed 4 May 2020].

Shahzad, A. 2020. *God is with us: Many Muslims in Pakistan flout the coronavirus ban in mosques.* [Online] Available from: https://www.reuters.com/article/us-health-coronavirus-pakistan-congregat/god-is-with-us-many-muslims-in-pakistan-flout-the-coronavirus-ban-in-mosques-idUSKCN21V0T4 [Accessed 20 April 2020].

Siddiqa, A. 2020. *Like India, Pakistan has a Tablighi Jamaat Covid-19 problem too. But blame Imran Khan as well.* [Online] Available from: https://theprint.in/opinion/pakistan-tablighi-jamaat-covid-19-problem-blame-imran-khan-as-well/394229/ [Accessed 15 April 2020].

Slater, J., and Masih, N. 2020. *What Delhi's worst communal violence in decades means for Modi's India.* [Online] Available from: https://www.washingtonpost.com/world/

asia_pacific/what-days-of-communal-violence-mean-for-modi-and-for-india/2020/
03/01/3d649c18-5a68-11ea-8efd-0f904bdd8057_story.html   [Accessed   30
December 2020].

Slater, J., Masih, N., and Irfan, S. 2020. *India confronts its first coronavirus 'super-spreader'
– a Muslim missionary group with more than 400 members infected.* [Online]
Available from: https://www.washingtonpost.com/world/asia_pacific/india-corona
virus-tablighi-jamaat-delhi/2020/04/02/abdc5af0-7386-11ea-ad9b-254ec99993bc_
story.html [Accessed 30 December 2020].

Swyngedouw, E., 2006. Metabolic urbanization: the making of cyborg cities. In: Erik
Swyngedouw, Nik Heynen, and Maria Kaika, ed. *In the Nature of Cities: urban political
ecology and the politics of urban metabolism.* London, New York: Routledge, 20–39.

Swyngedouw, E., and Heynen, N.C., 2003. Urban political ecology, justice and the politics of scale. *Antipode*, 35 (5), 898–918.

Tanzeem, A. 2020. *Pakistani clerics insist on keeping mosques open.* [Online] Available
from: https://www.voanews.com/science-health/coronavirus-outbreak/pakistani-
clerics-insist-keeping-mosques-open [Accessed 6 May 2020].

Times Now. 2020. *Despite lockdown, crowd gathers at temples in Bengal for Ram
Navami.* [Online] Available from: https://economictimes.indiatimes.com/news/
politics-and-nation/gujarat-fire-breaks-out-at-chemical-factory-in-surat-12-fire-ten
ders-rushed-to-spot/videoshow/75926201.cms [Accessed 13 April 2020].

Trivedi, D. 2020. *Targeting a community.* [Online] Available from: https://frontline.
thehindu.com/cover-story/article31374077.ece [Accessed 18 May 2020].

Tzaninis, Y., et al., 2020. Moving urban political ecologybeyond the 'urbanization of
nature. *Progress in human geography*, 1–24. doi:10.1177/0309132520903350.

USCIRF. 2020. *USCIRF is concerned with reports of Hindu & Muslim patients separated*
[Online] Available from: https://twitter.com/USCIRF/status/1250444587795189761
[Accessed 20 April 2020].

Wildman, W.J., et al., 2020. Religion and the COVID-19 pandemic. *Religion, brain &
behavior*, 10 (2), 115–117.

Wilkins, D., 2020. Where is religion in political ecology? *Progress in human geography*,
1–22. Available from: https://doi.org/10.1177/0309132520901772.

The Wire. 2020. *Karnataka: Chariot pulling ritual held in violation of lockdown, police
register case.* [Online] Available from: https://thewire.in/government/kalaburagi-
chariot-pulling-covid-19-lockdown-violation [Accessed 20 April 2020].

Zimmer, A., 2010. Urban political ecology: theoretical concepts, challenges and
suggested future directions. *Erdkunde*, 64 (4), 343–354.

Doing cultural studies in rough seas: the COVID-19 ocean multiple

Elspeth Probyn

ABSTRACT

This article seeks to demonstrate what a conjunctural analysis of the oceanic manifestation of COVID-19 might look like. While the ocean has seemingly remained on the periphery during the ongoing pandemic, the marine has nevertheless been deeply affected as a space of more-than-human connection. As we know, it was at a seafood market (The Huanan Seafood Market) that the first signs of the virus allegedly emerged – an event that propelled the circulation of disgust and racism that was to follow. I take three sites: Botany Bay, Sydney; the Ruby Princess cruise ship; and the effect of COVID-19 on fish supply chains and the lives and livelihoods of fishers especially in the global south. I draw on John Clarke's argument that 'tracing the different dynamics and forces that come together to constitute the conjuncture is a substantial challenge', and Meaghan Morris' call for site-specific thinking in cultural studies. This is, I argue, a time for messy digging in the swamp of the pandemic if we are to find thin threads of hope for our more-than-human world, and our discipline.

Trying to do cultural studies in lockdown

Trying to do anything in the lockdown is hard. Trying to think and plan for even the near future is tough – but necessary, if we are to keep on going on. There is a careful balancing act between using analytical skills to understand the present conjuncture in which we differentially find ourselves, and rushing to pronounce about it from on high. In April 2020, Warwick Anderson noted the ways in which 'Within weeks of its emergence, SARS-CoV-2 was galvanizing celebrity European philosophers and social theorists, most of them men in a vulnerable age demographic, to reflect publicly and plentifully on the meaning of the pandemic' (2020). He concluded that 'in the haste to manufacture mental personal protective equipment against the Coronascene, it is all too easy to make mistakes, to mass produce instead fatuity, guesswork, and irrelevance' (2020).

It depends on what cultural studies project one is trying to do in lockdown. For many years my own practice tended to use conceptual framings to understand various everyday conjunctures of sexuality and gender. It is feasible that had I continued in this vein, I could have gone on doing a certain form of cultural studies. However, several years ago I veered towards a more grounded form of cultural studies that needs a solid ethnographic basis in and from which to think. And thus, it was at the beginning of 2020 that I found myself with a new project funded by the Australian Research Council called *Selling the Sea: a comparative study of the cultural, economic, and environmental roles of urban fish markets in the global north and south*. This project would/will push my ethnographic involvement further in requiring fieldwork at fish markets in Manila, the Philippines, and Dakar, Senegal, as well as Sydney, Australia. Before I could even think about organizing it, my university – and the world – shut down, with no international travel permitted for the foreseeable future.

So in lieu of actually observing people's practices and talking to them, I find myself back to words and texts. In this article, I want to use the manifestations of COVID-19 in and on the ocean to think through what a conjunctural analysis of the human-marine present might look like. What might it add to other cultural studies analyses? Is there a place for the ocean in cultural studies' present and future? What might a non-terrestrial perspective contribute?

In her new book on *Wild Policy*, Tess Lea argues that 'Familiar tools of scrutiny can blind us to what might also be there, hidden in plain sight, if we care to look askance' (Lea 2020, p. 9). The ocean has not been a familiar object of scrutiny in cultural studies, notwithstanding Steven Mentz' (2009a, 2009b) nomenclature of 'blue cultural studies', whose fascinating project is a poetic history of the ocean. However, my project involves using familiar concepts in cultural studies while 'looking askance' at the ocean's own materialities and at its material entanglement in human life.

A perspective whereby the methodological is inseparable from the epistemological guides my thinking and my turn to the ocean, fisheries, and fish over the last several years (Striphas 2013). Of necessity, this move exceeds the discursive even while it attends to the material effects of colonial history, international law, and the particular systems which bind humans and the marine. The ocean is fundamental as a means of communication: think, for instance, that ocean-going cargo ships transport something like 99 percent of our consumer goods, and that since the 1850s 300 cable systems cover 550,000 miles of the sea floor. In these and many other ways, the ocean is a lively and fluid medium that connects the human and the more-than-human (Probyn 2020). As one of the last although highly vexed commons (Probyn 2016), and as a medium itself the ocean is central to modes of transmitting, sharing, and 'making common to many' (Williams 1976, p. 73).

If the ocean is 'cultural', it is also most certainly economic. Geographer Phillip Steinberg writes that 'the history of the modern world economy can be read as a history of the simultaneous "opening" and "closing" of the ocean frontier' (Steinberg 2001). 'The formation of mercantilist empires that claimed exclusive rights to maritime trade routes formed the foundation for modern capitalism' (Steinberg 2018, p. 327). 'Even today, the ocean's primary economic function remains as a transportation surface whose value is dependent on the absence of boundaries' (2018, p. 338). Steinberg's work on the ocean is extensive, and his first book, *The social construction of the ocean* (2001), is widely cited as one of the early social science forays into the marine. His wide-ranging publications consider many aspects of the oceanic, including his work with Kimberly Peters, which considers the ocean's 'three-dimensional and turbulent materiality' in what they call

> a wet ontology not merely to endorse the perspective of a world of flows, connections, liquidities, and becomings, but also to propose a means by which the sea's material and phenomenological distinctiveness can facilitate the reimagining and reenlivening of a world ever on the move. (2015, p. 278)

However, their sea is often devoid of life-traces. In more bluntly political terms, Elizabeth Havice and Anna Zalik argue that 'The narrative of an empty ocean has deliberately excluded human activity in it, notably the transatlantic slave trade and Black history' (2018, p. 225).

While these analyses suggest rich ground, they take us away from a cultural studies understanding of how the ocean substantiates and communicates, forms and informs. Anyone trained in cultural studies in Canada or touched by the work of James Carey (1989), will know of Harold Innis' insistence on the history and economics of communication as the movement of people and ideas, perhaps most notably expressed in *The Cod Fisheries: The history of an international economy* (1940). For Innis, staples shaped societies in a profound way. They allowed, to paraphrase Williams, whole ways of life. As Herbert Heaton wrote in a review shortly after the publication of *The Cod Fisheries*, Innis fundamentally changed Western notions about the ocean as movement, presenting, for instance, the Atlantic 'as a network of waterways uniting two sides, four continents, and six regions of an international and intercontinental economy' (1941, p. 60). Heaton continues:

> Put those six points–Newfoundland, New England and the Maritimes, the West Indies, West Africa, western Continental Europe, and the British Isles–on a blackboard; then trace all the possible journeys of ships and transfers of goods–direct, triangular, quadrilateral, or hexagonal–and note the part played by fish cargoes (1941, p. 60)

As Heaton emphasizes, Innis 'neglected no approach, economic, political, technological, geographical, historical, or ichthyological, and tries to reveal the interplay of factors, changing or constant, which produce the "cycles of disturbance" that have spelled weal or woe to this or that region' (1941, p. 60).[1]

In our time of fast scholarship, the breadth of Innis' (at times idiosyncratic) scholarship is hard to find in cultural studies – or anywhere. However, as Meaghan Morris – herself a proudly slow scholar – recently argued, it is precisely 'the thick medium of Cultural Studies work and the complexity of the problems that confront us' (2020, p. 149). This is, I think, especially important in these dizzying times. Morris' point here, and across much of her career, is to focus 'on the arts of making things happen', and cultural studies' potential in helping this process along. On her way to demonstrating this via Kung Fu, she is stopped by two images by the artist Dawn Moore of the reality and the imagined future of the seemingly endless construction of the Sydney Light Rail through the centre of Sydney. This project began in 2014. At the time of writing, these 'trams' (actual trams were ripped out to make way for cars in 1961) now whizz along empty of passengers, who are confused by the differing messages from different levels of authority about the safety of public transport during the crisis.

For Morris, part of the tragicomic tale of the delays in the completion of the project is due to the fact that 'before an old tarmac is lifted no-one really has a clue what is under there or how the historically layered utilities systems (which might, or might not, have been mapped) are tangled together with tree roots and unpredictably intersect' (2020, p. 149). From this 'muddy image', Morris questions:

> How do all the material forces at work in a situation — environmental, political, social, and economic as well as whatever we decide to call "cultural" — connect and affect each other? What disparate sites do they come from, what changes do they mark, what traces of history do they carry, where are they heading beyond these boundaries … ? Making things happen requires this kind of site-specific thinking, and this necessity to work in the mud distinguishes Cultural Studies from the clean lines, big vistas and glossy visions of "Cultural Theory," with which our field is sometimes confused (2020, p. 149)

In what follows, I describe three muddy sites (a beach, a ship, and a fish market) to ask what they can tell us about the conjuncture of COVID-19. Looking at the present from the athwart position of the human-marine may shake up common sense notions about the terrestrial as the ground of cultural change. In moving cultural studies away from its own blind spots, and reenergize the desire 'to make things happen'.

Botany Bay

In late March (southern hemisphere late summer), the weather was still warm and the ocean balmy. The summer of 2019/2020 had been a doozy. Bushfires raged for months creating some of the most polluted air in the world. It was hard to venture out when you couldn't see the other side of the street because of smoke, and ash rained down.

Under clear skies, and feeling momentarily buoyed (maybe the crisis wouldn't be too bad?), I went swimming in Botany Bay, more properly known as Kamay in the Dharawal language. One of the reasons we were at Botany Bay was that across the city at Bondi Beach the warm weather had resulted in huge crowds. On 21 March it was like New Year's Day weather-wise (36 degrees Celsius), and crowd-wise, with thousands blanketing the beach. Social distancing disappeared as beer and sunscreen and the scent of coconut oil bonded people's bodies. The councils immediately closed all the beaches of the Eastern suburbs as the affluent area became one of the hot spots for the transmission of the virus: wealthy residents had gone skiing in Aspen (they couldn't head down the South Coast to their beach houses because of the bush fire crisis). They returned from swanky snow resorts and mixed with overseas backpackers who are also a large part of the population in the area – all in all, a perfect cocktail for virus-transmission.

So, there we were on the other side of Sydney getting away from the petri-dish of Bondi on a beach infamous for being Cook's first arrival spot on 29 April, 1770. Cook was struck by the number of stingrays and it was at first renamed Stingray Bay, until being renamed again as Botany Bay because of the amount of plant specimens collected by the botanists onboard. In his journal, Cook recalls 'that his landing party encountered two men and that a rock that was thrown by one of the men. He then goes on to describe the firing of a warning shot, followed by two other shots, noting that one man was wounded' (Williams n.d., np). As Dr Shayne T. Williams, an Indigen-ous scholar and cultural consultant, writes:

> Cook saw a group of two Gweagal men (who) were assiduously carrying out their spiritual duty to Country by protecting Country from the presence of persons not authorised to be there. In our cultures it is not permissible to enter another culture's Country without due consent. (Williams n.d.)

As a descendent of two grandmothers who were proud Dharawal women, Williams thinks back to that moment of contact with Cook and the saltwater peoples of Kamay (Botany Bay). 'It was on Gweagal Country that Lieutenant Cook, and his landing party, first encountered the Gweagal warriors' (Williams n.d.).

2020 marked the 250 years since Cook's arrival but because of the mount-ing sense of crisis, the celebrations for the Sestercentennial were muted. The event had been tagged by various government bodies as 'the view from the ship and the view from the shore'. However, as Maria Nugent argues 'it's a wrong-headed idea. It suggests each party remained – and can remain still – suspended in their own separate worlds: on the ship or on the shore'

(Nugent 2020, np). She reminds us that this meeting happened 'on "the beach" – the literal and metaphorical space where cross-cultural encounters, misunderstandings and, too often, violence has taken place' (2020).

That first contact initiated the devastation to Indigenous populations that continues 250 years later, even as the celebration of Cook was overtaken by COVID-19. The coincidence didn't go unremarked. On April 30, 2020 Victoria's deputy Chief Health Officer Annaliese van Diemen published a post on her personal Twitter account noting this coincidence: 'Sudden arrival of an invader from another land, decimating populations, creating terror. Forces the population to make enormous sacrifices & completely change how they live in order to survive. COVID-19 or Cook 1770?' (in Towell and Coleangelo 2020, np). Her comments unleased fury that she was indulging in 'cultural wars' during the pandemic.

But of course, the arrival of the Europeans in Australia did bring immense death and suffering to Indigenous people. Judy Campbell writes that:

> The epidemic of smallpox among Aborigines in eastern Australia between 1829 and 1831 was the second of three smallpox epidemics seen in Aboriginal Australia between 1788 and 1870. The first was seen on the east coast at Port Jackson, Botany Bay, Broken Bay and on the Hawkesbury in 1789 (Campbell 1983, p. 536)

As Tess Lea argues, the point is not the arrival but how that moment reverberates through social policy that continues to haunt. She cites Eve Tuck and K. Wayne Yang's crucial observation: 'the disruption of Indigenous relationships to land represents a profound epistemic, ontological, cosmological violence. This violence is not temporarily contained in the arrival of the settler but is reasserted each day of occupation' (in Lea 2020, p. 141; 2017, p. 5).

Back on the beach that warm day the water looked clear and inviting. Usually it is murky, not only with history but with the pollution from the infrastructure that is central to global and regional trade. Botany is home to the Sydney (Kingsford Smith) Airport, the longest-running airport in the world since its inception in 1920. However, that day the skies were empty of planes. As I write, it is still very quiet. Australia is seemingly the only country which will not let its citizens leave. Next to the ever-sprawling airport, the cargo container precinct Port Botany was established in the 1970s. There doesn't seem much movement there, but I later learned that it has continued to be busy with the largest container ship ever to visit stopping by a few days ago – at 980 feet, and as high as a 15-storey building, the vessel is twice the size of normal container ships. The Ural (named after the mountains in Russia) is owned by China International Marine Containers Group, based in Shenzhen, China, and flies under the flag of Malta.

As Brett Neilson and Ned Rossiter write, 'the conditions of work at sea are caught in a game of evasion and control' (2011, p. 63). Evasion and control also seem to sum up the history and present of Botany Bay. The world keeps coming to us, commodities come and go. As do Covid's masks, gloves and test kits, washed up on shores around the world. Contaminated waste is burned, and the toxins seep into the ocean to be carried by currents. According to one reporter, 'We tried to be eco. Now plastic is back' (Rumbelow 2020). Beaches may be closed to humans but our bodies and environments are porous to the toxic realities of the COVID-19 world.

A ship called Ruby

After the fiasco of the British-registered Diamond Princess, which was quarantined at Yokohama, Japan from 4 February 2020 for approximately one month, and resulted in the deaths of 14 people, on 8/9 March the Ruby Princess embarked from Sydney on a cruise to New Zealand. The ship carried 2,700 passengers who had not quarantined. On 14 March, the Australian government ordered that everyone arriving into Australia, including cruise passengers, would need to self-isolate for 14 days. The following day, the government announced the closing of ports. By that time the Ruby Princess was in Wellington, and quickly made her way back to Sydney. On 19 March, the ship slunk into Sydney Harbour in the early morning with over 660 infected people on board. Passengers disembarked although there were no results from the very few swab tests conducted. Amy Dale writes that 'the cruise cluster, which is believed to have originated from an infected crew member distributing food and drinks, has been responsible for at least 20 deaths' (Dale 2020). Twenty of the overall 908 deaths recorded in Australia came from one ship.

While different levels of government, State, Commonwealth, and assorted agencies all passed the buck, the Ruby Princess was shunted off to Port Kembla, south of Wollongong on 19 March. After 14 days of quarantine, most of the passengers boarded flights to their home destinations. However, the majority of the crew remained. In the news at the time, the attention was mainly on the passengers but the plight of the crew was much more horrific. Unpaid, squashed in inner cabins, and sick, they were invisible victims. As one crew member put it, 'Some nationalities like myself have been left totally in the dark. There is even a repatriation flight leaving to South Africa on the 28th of April but we have been given no option to leave. We have to stay onboard and the company have not even told us where we are sailing to' (Zhou 2020). NSW Police Commissioner Mick Fuller had a stern message to all cruise ship operators: 'They don't pay taxes in Australia, they don't park their boats in Australia … time to go home' (in Reddie 2020).

However, where is home? Freya Higgins-Desbiolles notes that, 'As the cruise ships became stranded around the world as ports closed to them, the question of exactly where home for them was, as they operated under FOC, began to be discussed' (Higgins-Desbiolles 2020, p. 7). As Natalie

Klein writes, 'In early April 2020, it was estimated that 15,000 crew were stranded on 18 cruise ships around the Australian coast with concerns that coronavirus would take hold and spread' (2020, p. 2). On 23 April 23, the Ruby Princess left for the Philippines where it joined a huge stilled flotilla: mid-year, Manila Bay was the world's biggest 'parking lot' for cruise ships, with many thousands of crew still on board (Sutton 2020).

The question of 'home' is tricky because of the complicated system of vessel flags, especially 'open registry' versus 'closed registry'. Under the *UN Convention on the Law of the Sea* (UNCLOS), the latter represents a 'genuine link' between the ship and the flag under which it sails. The former, more often referred to as 'Flags of Convenience' (FOC). As set out under Article 90 of 1982 UNCLOS: every State, whether coastal or land locked, has the right to sail ships flying its flag on the high seas. This then can lead to weak claims:

> it may be that a ship has no physical connection with its flag State. Indeed, it may never visit its notional "home port", or even find it possible to do so, given that some open registries, such as those of Mongolia or Bolivia, are based in land-locked States. (Kaye 2020, p. 1)

This leads to a strange situation whereby the regulation of the ship is under the exclusive jurisdiction of the flag State, which may have no means (e.g. access to the seas) to exercise any control. Equally, they may have little interest in ensuring that the ship follows protocol about labour conditions or environmental ones. As Higgins-Desbiolles states: 'Cruise companies choose to use a FOC as part of their economic model, helping their business gain profits by helping them avoid stringent economic, social and environmental regulations' (Higgins-Desbiolles 2020, p. 6). At the end of April 2020, it was reported that 'Around the world, more than 100,000 crew workers are still trapped on cruise ships, at least 50 of which have COVID-19 infections .... They have in effect become a nation of floating castaways, marooned on boats from the Galapagos Islands to Dubai port' (McCormick and Greenfield 2020). This is the haunting reality of stranded boats and people rebuffed from port to port. A tangle of land-based laws allows land-locked countries such as Mongolia (the largest land-locked country in the world) to sell cheap and worthless flags with underpaid crew mostly from the Global South. As one sailor put it, these ships 'roam the world, unsuspected, leaking, polluting time bombs for the sailors aboard' (cited in Brooke 2004). In the time of COVID-19, they became a marine vector fuelling the virus' world-wide spread.

Down at the fish market

As is well known, on 1 January 2020, Chinese authorities closed down a wet market in Wuhan, which may have been the spark that lit the coronavirus fires. It was somewhat overlooked that the market was a seafood market.

The Huanan Seafood Market sold 'wild life' along with live seafood, and 'chickens, donkeys, sheep, pigs, foxes, badgers, bamboo rats, hedgehogs, and snakes' (Woodward 2020). Images of caged animals were splashed across newspapers across the world, and debate raged about whether or not the market was responsible for the outbreak. While wet markets have sometimes been proven to enable zoonotic diseases that leap between and among humans and non-human animals, to western readers these images are framed to trigger disgust.

However, as Christos Lynteris and Lyle Fearnley (2020) argue, 'shutting down Chinese "wet markets" could be a terrible mistake' because it would simply send the mainly small producers of these animals onto the unregulated black market. Their argument raises the complex debates about how '[t]hese images communicate a sense of disgust toward the eating habits of the Chinese and at the same time reflect a fear of the interconnectedness of two types of "emergence" in China: viral emergence and economic emergence.' Published on 31 January 2020, their argument about the intertwined fear of the virus and China's economic power was prescient. For instance, the tariff wars that China unleashed on Australia were seen to be in retaliation to the Australian Foreign Minister's call on 19 April 19 for an independent inquiry into the origin of the virus. In the Prime Minister, Scott Morrison's words: WHO (the World Health Organization) needs 'tough new "weapons inspector" powers to investigate what caused the outbreak' (cited in Dziedzic 2020). On 18 May, China imposed an 80 percent tariff on Australian barley, one of Australia's three top exports. Then on 6 June, the Chinese Ministry of Culture and Tourism warned its citizens not to travel to Australia for education or tourism because of racial discrimination against Chinese. In China's foreign ministry spokesman Zhao Lijian's words: 'To be candid, we don't think it is in Australia's best long-term interests when certain people, acting out of their own political interests, choose to turn away from facts and engage in politicising the pandemic and sabotaging relevant international cooperation' (ABC News 2020).

That there have been racist attacks against Chinese in Australia is undeniable, and the recent ones thrown up by COVID-19 rest upon centuries of white Australian racism against the Chinese. Friends, students and colleagues have been shaken by the blatant racist abuse that confronts them on the streets of Sydney if they 'look Chinese' and if they dare to wear a mask.

The effects of COVID-19 on seafood have been little remarked upon outside of fisheries' circles. Seafood is a delicate commodity, always rendered precarious by the dependence on the state of the seas, and by the markets that connect fish, fisher, and consumer. I visited and continue to visit the Sydney Fish Market (the second largest by species in the world) throughout the ongoing crisis. I wander through the empty halls. Where once buses, filled with mainland Chinese tourists, jostled to find a park, the pelicans were sombre – no fish and chips to scavenge from tourists and consumers. When on 4 February 2020 China put a halt to live animal trade over coronavirus fears, individual sectors within the industry were, and continue to be, differentially hit. The high-value ones immediately suffered. South Australia's rock lobster industry, which exports 95 percent of its stock to China, was devastated. Most of Queensland's live coral trout market (99 percent), normally bound for China, came to a screeching halt. A hand-written sign at the empty entrance to the Sydney Fish Market touting two for one abalone was a poignant sign of the times.

Just as things seemed to calm down, an outbreak of COVID-19 was associated with a Beijing fish market, with worries that imports of salmon from Norway were infected by the virus. Xinfadi market supplies about 70 percent of Beijing's fruit, vegetables and seafood. While fear that actual salmon were infected was soon denied by scientists, the news triggered a consumer boycott of salmon throughout China. The fear that live seafood could carry the virus resulted in lobster exporters from Canada having to sign a declaration that the lobsters were Covid-free, and the lobsters were swabbed and tested. Given that tests can take up to 36 h to process, there would have been a lot of sad lobsters. Then, in mid-July 2020, China detected the virus inside the containers and on the outside of the packaging of Ecuadorian shrimp, sending the depressed markets ever downward (Craze 2020). In Dalian, a port city processing hub in China, a man working for a seafood processor tested positive in July for COVID-19, the first reported case in the city for over three months. The 58-year old man, named 'patient Shi', tested positive for the virus after suffering from fever and fatigue. He presented himself at Dalian Central Hospital on 21 July (Harknell 2020). He apparently worked at Dalian Kaiyang Seafood. The chief epidemiologist of China's Center of Disease Control (CDC) was reported as saying the recent outbreak of COVID-19 in Dalian was 'likely caused by imported, contaminated seafood', dealing another blow to Chinese consumer confidence in seafood products (Harkell 2020).

Across the Global South the 'pandemic has also locked down coastal fishing communities and seriously impacted livelihoods. … Earnings have dropped because of lack of fish, market access, traditional credit sources and clear government policy enabling relief'(Jamwal 2020). This has particularly hit women fishers and fish workers hard as they are often not recognized as such (Frangoudes and Gerrard 2019, p. 128), and therefore have not been entitled to receive government relief where it has been made available. Of the roughly 120 million people employed in the fisheries industry globally, more than 90 percent work in small-scale fisheries and 97 percent live in developing countries (Pille-Schneider 2020). Following the broken supply chains and the devastation on fishers and processors is part of my ongoing research. Given the limits of space, suffice to say it is a messy and often deadly state of affairs.

Covid conjunctures

These descriptions only scratch the surface of what is going on. Of course, within cultural studies to ask 'what's going on' is to interrogate the conjuncture. In Lawrence Grossberg's elaboration of this concept/method/mode of analysis:

> A conjuncture is a description of a social formation as fractured and conflictual, along multiple axes, planes, and scales, constantly in search of temporary balance or structural stabilities through a variety of practice and processes of struggle and negotiation .... Yet a conjuncture has to be constructed, narrated, fabricated (2010, pp. 40–41)

In John Clarke's understanding, the narrating and fabricating of a particular conjuncture can only be 'no more than a sketch, since tracing the different dynamics and forces that come together to constitute the conjuncture is a substantial challenge and one unlikely to be accomplished by a single author within the confines of a journal article' (2018, np). And one of the dangers of this form of slow documentation of a conjuncture is that one can disappear into the minutia of detail – of international law of the seas, of human-made disasters that allowed passengers from a cruise ship to return to their homes across the world while the crew and boats remained at sea, of the multitude of ways that show 'we are *not* all in this together'. While the affirmative and the negative phrasings of this statement abound, I wonder if there is a way of conjoining affective solidarity and material difference.

To return to Morris' argument that I cited at the outset, we need 'site-specific thinking' that locates 'the material forces at work in a situation' (2020, p. 149). As Clarke has argued, this brings to the fore multiple temporalities, which are 'central to this view of a conjuncture as a site in which they become condensed, entangled and co-constitutive of crisis' (Clarke 2010, p. 341). In the words of the authors of *Policing the Crisis*, still one of the most exemplary conjunctural accounts: 'The depth of the crisis, in this sense, is to be seen in the accumulation of contradictions and breaks' (Hall *et al.* 1978, p. 219).

To conclude, what do my descriptions of the oceanic COVID-19 – painfully researched but still undercooked – add to a specifically cultural studies understanding of our present conjuncture? Writing in the time of the conjuncture, I have attempted to sketch how understanding the depths of the ocean's temporalities and spatialities deepens the breadth of cultural studies' potential to grasp the uneven flows of the virus. Yes certainly, COVID-19 is 'about' globalization but in a very different key. I could have followed more deeply the ways in which colonization (the arrival of Cook), cruising (the catastrophe of the Ruby Princess), and fishing (the upending of supply chains and livelihoods) display the uneven movement of COVID-19. But I hope it is clear that the maritime has enabled what we inhabit today. And the framing of the ocean as multiple reveals the eddies of specificities that make COVID-19 the manifestation of 'contradictions and breaks', as well as of continuity. That some are free to travel with the virus, and others are confined to stasis, whether as crew on stateless ships or locked down in homes or rendered homeless, reveals one painful vector of the material difference of this crisis. It is up to us to think across these stark differences about where affective solidarity might emerge. We are in rough seas, bound together and divided by how history haunts us in this painful present.

Note

1. While Innis's approach was foundational in Canada, his influence also spread to Australia where, as Ian Angus and Brian Shoesmith argued in 1993 a revived interest in Innis could intervene in what they termed 'cultural studies ... endless oscillation between text and audience which effaces questions of power, or deflects them into spurious claims of resistance' (1993, p. 6).

Disclosure statement

No potential conflict of interest was reported by the author(s).

Further information

This Special Issue article has been comprehensively reviewed by the Special Issue editors, Associate Professor Ted Striphas and Professor John Nguyet Erni.

Funding

This work was supported by ARC Discovery Project [grant number DP200100447].

References

ABC News, 2020. China accuses Australia of disinformation and 'political manipulation' in foreign ministry rebuke. 18 June. Available from: https://www.abc.net.au/news/2020-06-18/china-says-australia-spreads-disinformation-marise-payne/12366948.

Anderson, W., 2020. Epidemic philosophy, *Somatosphere*, 8 April. Available from: http://somatosphere.net/2020/epidemic-philosophy.html/.

Angus, I. and Shoesmith, B., 1993. Dependency/space/policy: an introduction to a dialogue with Harold Innis. *Continuum*, 7 (1), 5–15.

Brooke, J., 2004. Landlocked Mongolia's seafaring tradition. *The New York Times*, 4 July. Available from: https://www.nytimes.com/2004/07/02/business/landlocked-mongolia-s-seafaring-tradition.html.

Campbell, J., 1983. Smallpox in aboriginal Australia, 1829–31. *Historical studies*, 20 (81), 536–556.

Carey, J.W., 1989. *Communication as culture: essays on media and society*. London: Routledge.

Clarke, J., 2010. Of crises and conjunctures: the problem of the present. *Journal of communication inquiry*, 34 (4), 337–354.

Clarke, J., 2018. A sense of loss? Unsettled attachments in the current conjuncture. *New formations*, 96-97, 132–146.

Craze, M., 2020. Ecuador's president requests Xi Jinping intervention in COVID-19 shrimp dispute, 14 July. Available from: https://www.undercurrentnews.com/2020/07/14/ecuadors-president-requests-xi-jinping-intervention-in-covid-19-shrimp-dispute/.

Dale, A., 2020. COVID-19: all out to sea, *LSJ: Law Society of NSW Journal*, No. 66, May, 40–43.

Dziedzic, S., 2020. Australia started a fight with China over an investigation into COVID-19 — did it go too hard? 5 May. Available from: https://www.abc.net.au/news/2020-05-20/wha-passes-coronavirus-investigation-australia-what-cost/12265896.

Frangoudes, K. and Gerrard, S., 2019. Gender perspective in fisheries: examples from the South and the North. In: R. Chuenpagdee and S. Jentoft, eds. *Transdisciplinarity for small-scale fisheries governance*. New York: Springer, 119–140.

Grossberg, L., 2010. *Cultural studies in the future tense*. Durham, NC: Duke University Press.

Hall, S., *et al.*, 1978. *Policing the crisis: mugging, the state and law and order*. London: Macmillan.

Harkell, L., 2020. More cases of COVID-19 linked to employee at Dalian seafood processor. *Undercurrent News*, 23 July. Available from: https://www.undercurrentnews.com/2020/07/23/more-cases-of-covid-19-linked-to-employee-at-dalian-seafood-processor/.

Havice, E. and Zalik, A., 2018. Ocean frontiers: epistemologies, jurisdictions, commodifications. *International social science journal*, 68 (229-230), 219–235.

Heaton, H., 1941. The cod fisheries: the history of an international economy by Harold A. Innis. *The Canadian historical review*, 22 (1), 60–63.

Higgins-Desbiolles, F., 2020. Socialising tourism for social and ecological justice after COVID-19. *Tourism geographies*, 22 (3), 610–623.

Innis, H., 1940. *Cod fisheries: the history of an international economy*. Toronto: University of Toronto Press.

Jamwal, N., 2020. Left in the lurch. As a result of the coronavirus pandemic and nation-wide lockdown, fisherwomen in Maharashtra, India, have few fallback options. *Yemaya* No. 60, May. Available from: https://www.icsf.net/images/yemaya/pdf/english/issue_60/355_Yemaya%2060_ICSF_May2020.pdf.

Kaye, S., 2020. Port access and assistance to cruise ships during the COVID-19 pandemic. *Australian law journal*, 94 (6), 420–426.

Lea, T., 2020. *Wild policy: indigeneity and the unruly logics of intervention*. Stanford: Stanford University Press.

Lynteris, C., and Fearnley, L., 2020. Why shutting down Chinese 'wet markets' could be a terrible mistake. *The Conversation*, 31.

McCormick, E. and Greenfield, P., 2020. Revealed: 100,000 crew never made it off cruise ships amid coronavirus crisis. *The Guardian*. 30 April. Available from https://www.theguardian.com/environment/series/seascape-the-state-of-our-oceans.

Mentz, S., 2009a. Toward a blue cultural studies: the sea, maritime culture, and early modern English literature. *Literature compass*, 6 (5), 997–1013.

Mentz, S., 2009b. *At the bottom of Shakespeare's ocean*. London: A&C Black.

Morris, M., 2020. Institutional kung fu: on the arts of making things happen. *Inter-Asia cultural studies*, 21 (1), 145–163.

Neilson, B. and Rossiter, N., 2011. Still waiting, still moving. In: D. Bissell, ed. *Stillness in a mobile world*. New York: Routledge, 51–68.

Nugent, M., 2020. A failure to say hello: how captain cook blundered his first impression with indigenous people. *The Conversation*, 29 April. Available from: https://theconversation.com/a-failure-to-say-hello-how-captain-cook-blundered-his-first-impression-with-indigenous-people-126673.

Pille-Schneider, L., 2020. Small-scale fishers in West Africa hit hard by COVID-19 pandemic. *GRID-Arendal*, July 15. Available from: https://news.grida.no/smallscale-fishers-in-west-africa-hit-hard-by-covid19-pandemic.

Probyn, E., 2016. *Eating the ocean*. Durham, NC: Duke University Press.

Probyn, E., 2020. Wasting seas: oceanic time and temporalities. In: F. Allon, R. Barcan, and K. Eddison-Kogan, eds. *The temporalities of waste: out of sight, out of time*. London: Routledge, 179–191.

Reddie, M., 2020. First Ruby Princess crew members disembark after coronavirus isolation, hundreds still left on board. *ABC News*, 22 April. Available from: www.abc.net.au/news/2020-04-21/some-crew-on-coronavirus-cruise-ship-ruby-princess-taken-off/12167856.

Rumbelow, H., 2020. We tried to be eco. Now plastic is back. *The Times*, 17 August. Available from: https://www.thetimes.co.uk/article/we-tried-to-be-eco-now-plastic-is-back-n50f5kxd6?shareToken=779c7fdd3ce7eeef8f9d24d1030206b6.

Steinberg, P.E., 2001. *The social construction of the ocean*. Vol. 78. Cambridge: Cambridge University Press.

Steinberg, P.E., 2018. The ocean as frontier. *International social science journal*, 68 (229-230), 237–240.

Steinberg, P. and Peters, K., 2015. Wet ontologies, fluid spaces: giving depth to volume through oceanic thinking. *Environment and planning D: society and space*, 33 (2), 247–264.

Striphas, T., 2013. Keyword: critical. *Communication and critical/cultural studies*, 10 (2-3), 324–328.

Sutton, C., 2020. Cruise ship staff still adrift after 110 days and counting. *News Com*, 2 July. Available from: https://www.news.com.au/travel/travel-updates/health-safety/

cruise-ship-staff-still-adrift-after-110-days-and-counting/news-story/fb7b81b83c78
07420133096c2088feca.

Towell, N. and Colangelo, A., 2020. Calls for deputy CHO to resign over Captain Cook
virus tweet. *The Age*, 30 April. Available from: https://www.theage.com.au/national/
victoria/calls-for-sutton-s-deputy-to-resign-over-captain-cook-virus-tweet-2020043
0-p54opy.html.

Tuck, E. and Wayne Yang, K., 2017. Decolonization is not a metaphor. *Decolonization:
indigeneity, education & society*, 1 (1), 1–40.

Williams, R., 1976. *Keywords: a vocabulary of society and culture*. London: Fontana/
Croom Helm.

Williams, S.T., n.d. An indigenous Australian perspective on Cook's arrival. British
Library Available from: https://www.bl.uk/the-voyages-of-captain-james-cook/
articles/an-indigenous-australian-perspective-on-cooks-arrival#authorBlock1.

Woodward, A., 2020. Both the new coronavirus and SARS outbreaks likely started in
Chinese wet markets. Photos show what the markets look like, 23 January.
Available from: https://www.businessinsider.com.au/wuhan-coronavirus-chinese-
wet-market-photos-2020-1?r=US&IR=T.

Zhou, N., 2020. Ruby Princess crew fear for their health as ship leaves Australia. *The
Guardian*, 23 April. Available from: http://www.ruby-princess-crew-fear-for-their-
health-as-ship-leaves-australia.

COVID-19 at sea: 'the world as you know it no longer exists'

Christiaan De Beukelaer [ID]

ABSTRACT

The 2020 COVID-19 pandemic has impacted virtually everyone on the planet. But the impacts have been diverse and uneven. In this article, I reflect on the plight of seafarers during the pandemic. I suggest that being 'locked in' is intrinsic to life at sea, as one can't simply leave a ship. What makes the experience of the pandemic so challenging at sea is being 'locked out' of land. With border closures prohibiting 'crew change', many seafarers have been forced to extend their contracts, stay aboard, and postpone going home for long and often undefined periods of time. My article combines a reflexive personal narrative of being confined to a ship at sea for five months, while being excluded from land, with the question of how spending the pandemic at sea could be understood in relation to maritime labour.

The sound was deafening. At noon, on May 2020, all ships' horns blasted. The horn of our ship, the *Avontuur*, did too. But we couldn't even hear it on our own deck. It is not the most confident of horns at the best of times. But that day it felt like it was failing us.

Our horn wasn't audible above those of much larger vessels such as the *Great Intelligence* and the *Ithaca Riga* that shared the dock with us in the port of Veracruz, Mexico. We were moored in the sleepless and dirty commercial port, opposite the colonial fortress of San Juan de Ulúa, to load green coffee destined for Germany (Figure 1).

I was not supposed to have been aboard any longer. I was supposed to have disembarked on Marie Galante, a tiny island just south of Guadeloupe in the French Antilles, by the end of March. But I was not allowed to. And neither were the captain and several other crew who were scheduled to leave the ship. This caused me to experience the first half of 2020 in a unique way: While people ashore were confined to their houses, we were confined to our ship, as many seafarers were – and remain – to theirs (De Beukelaer 2020c).

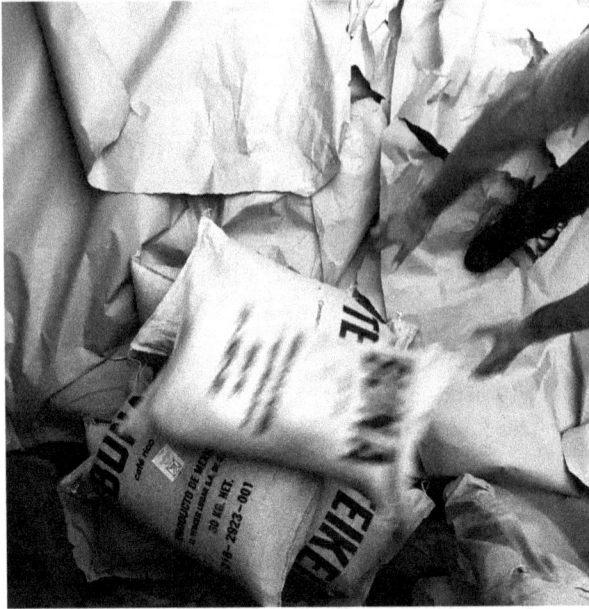

Figure 1. Loading a cargo of green coffee in Veracruz, Mexico (CC BY-NC-ND Christiaan De Beukelaer https://ocean-archive.org/collection/45).

The government of the Australian state of Victoria, where I live, argues that 'staying apart keeps us together' and many countries have urged their inhabitants to strictly observe 'contact bubbles' to reduce 'community transmission' of COVID-19. Our ship, like other cargo vessels, was a very closely-knit bubble of fifteen. Staying at sea was safe for us, and others. But it was also owing to the strict confinement of seafarers to their vessels, that countries have been able to maintain essential supplies since lockdowns started.

Here, I reflect on my personal experience of being confined to the sea – or rather our exclusion from land – for five months. To advance this inquiry, I build on Foucault's distinction between *exclusion* and *containment* as biopolitical responses to infectious disease, respectively leprosy and the plague (Foucault 1995), by questioning how they are both used to suppress (or in some cases eliminate) COVID-19. In linking these interconnected biopolitical regimes to the political economy of cargo shipping, I suggest that the current response to the pandemic exacerbates inequalities in the political economy of the global shipping industry.

Sea blind

Few people have documented the social, economic, and environmental impact of the maritime industry with greater analytical precision than the late American photographer Allan Sekula (1995, 2017). In *The Forgotten Space*, a 'film essay' he created with Noël Burch shortly before his death, Sekula interrogates life in twenty-first century maritime logistics. He argues that shipping has become as predictable and monotonous as industrial production, while factories are now traversing the world in search of cheaper labour. In this reversal of functions, and through the uniform box that is the shipping container, the sea of 'exploit and adventure' has turned into a 'lake of invisible drudgery' (Sekula and Burch 2010). Labour at sea is challenging at the best of times. A pandemic merely exacerbates this. While this can be said of labour in general, there is no possibility to walk away from the job when at sea, making the position of seafarers structurally precarious.

Seafarers tend to spend a long time aboard the vessels on which they work. Depending on rank and country of origin, contracts commonly range from four to seven months. The maximum that is allowed under the *ILO Maritime Labour Convention* of 2006 is eleven months (Baumler 2020). *Force majeure* like the COVID-19 pandemic trumps such regulations (ILO 2020), leaving hundreds of thousands of seafarers stranded at sea – or unable to return to work from their place of residence – every month. As crew change is now possible in many – but not all – ports, criticism has mounted. The initial force majeure is no longer at play, as crew change is possible, though often complex and expensive (De Beukelaer 2020d). In response to these difficulties, charterers aim to secure the scheduled delivery of their cargo by including 'no crew change' clauses in their contracts with shipping companies; a move that faces strong criticism from IMO Secretary-General Kitack Lim (IMO 2020e).

Over one and a half million seafarers work on cargo ships on any given day of the year, commonly labouring ten to twelve-hour shifts, seven days a week. The scheduled time of rest in between stints at sea punctuates contracts and lives, making contact with family and friends much anticipated and necessary breaks from shipboard life. During the COVID-19 pandemic, seafarers are not only stuck at sea beyond their contracts – resulting in sea time in excess of 18 months (Cotton 2020, ITF 2020b) – they are also unsure how long these extensions will be. This insecurity means they do not know when they might return home. This makes the unexpectedly long time at sea even more difficult for many (Ha *et al.* 2020), because the lives of their families on land have changed in their absence.

This uncertainty also affected us, aboard the *Avontuur*, though our situation differed from seafarers employed on 'conventional' shipping vessels.

The *Avontuur*

We, fifteen people aboard the *Avontuur*, play but a modest part in the global seaborne trade. But we are neither a large bulk carrier (like the *Ithaca Riga* and the *Great Intelligence*) nor a massive containership. We are a hundred-year old, 43.5-meter long, two-masted schooner that transports coffee and cacao from Honduras, Belize, and Mexico to Hamburg, Germany (De Beuke-laer 2018, 2020a).

Six of us are professional seafarers (master, chief mate, second mate, bo'sun, and two deckhands) to comply with manning regulations of its German flag. The only other paid crew aboard is the cook. The remaining eight crew (including myself) have joined as paying trainees ('shipmates'). This means that we have paid for the privilege of working to sail the vessel across the ocean. This arrange-ment is common on 'sail training' vessels (that rarely carry cargo), as it helps novice or amateur sailors gain experience on traditional sailing vessels, while tra-velling to see the world – or the sea at least (Figures 2 & 3). Unlike large contain-erships, we live in really close quarters: ten of us share the fo'c's'le, before the mast. No matter how cramped our shipborne living conditions may seem, on shore we live far more privileged lives than most 'ordinary seamen' ever will.

The *Avontuur* completed its fifth Atlantic round-trip for Timbercoast, upon arriving in Hamburg on July 23rd 2020. She sailed from her home port of Elsfleth, on the Weser estuary in northern Germany, on 17th January. The first officer and I joined the vessel on 24th February, in Santa Cruz de Tenerife, while carnival was in full swing there. The rest of the crew have been on board

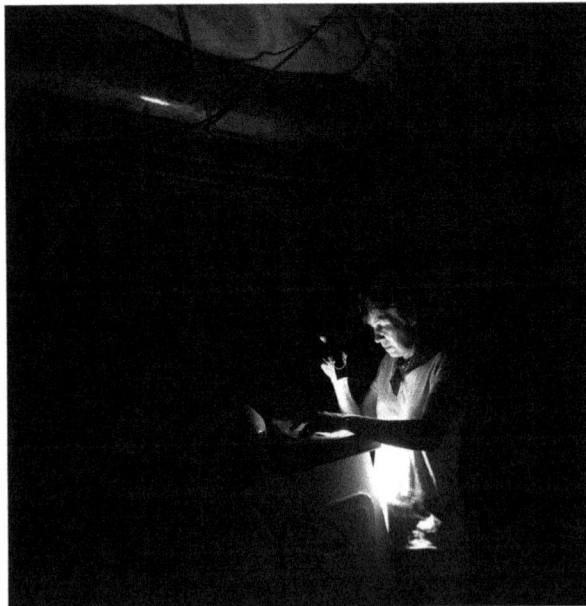

Figure 2. Anchor watch in Puerto Cortés, Honduras (CC BY-NC-ND Christiaan De Beuke-laer https://ocean-archive.org/collection/45).

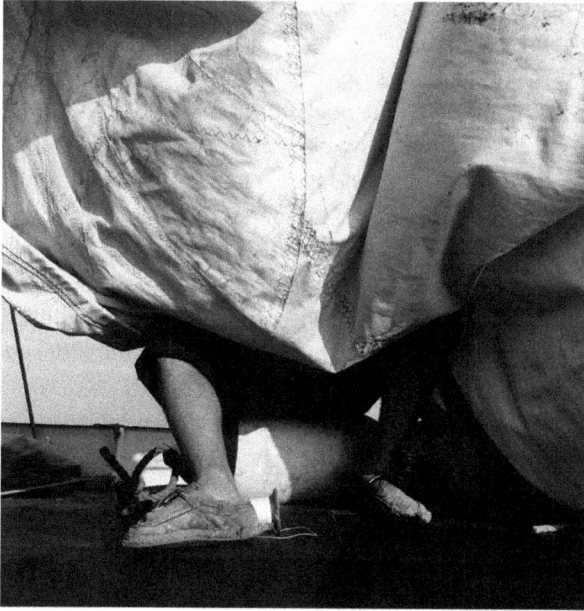

Figure 3. While anchored off the Belize coast over Easter, we spent our time mending sails and maintaining the ship (CC BY-NC-ND Christiaan De Beukelaer https://ocean-archive.org/collection/45).

since early January, as they lived on the ship while finalizing preparations for the voyage.

Few people on the planet will have lived through the 2020 COVID-19 pandemic as disconnected from news and restrictions as we have. We have been in perpetual motion at sea, living in a group, not having to practice social distancing, and not being bombarded with a never-ending stream of news and pandemic speculation (De Beukelaer and Corcoran 2020). My experience was, at face value, comparable to that of other seafarers. But beyond the extended time at sea lies a long history of exploitation of maritime labour I was not confronted with.

Labour day

At face value, the sounding of our ships' horns was a sign of worker solidarity. In that sense, there was little unusual about sounding horns on Labour Day. It could have happened in any port, on any Labour Day – in any port with strong union labour, at least. But May 1st 2020 was different.

The day prior, on 30th of April, the captains of all vessels in port received a message from Gabriel Ángel Carréon Pérez, the harbourmaster of the *Puerto Regional de Veracruz*. In this letter, on the official *Secretaria de Marina* letterhead, he asked all vessels to sound their *silbatos* (horns) for thirty to sixty seconds at 12:00 local time.

The horns were meant as a sign of solidarity with the 1.6 million seafarers in the merchant marine. At that point in time, very few countries classified seafarers as 'key' or 'essential' workers, which would allow them to fly internationally to and from work, instead they had been confined to their places of work. Ironically, the confinement of seafarers to their ships is necessary because shipping is a key industry; their work is crucial to global supply chains and, as a result, security of food, fuel, and medical supplies (Cowen 2014). A year on, the crew change crisis that resulted from border closures continues to impact hundreds of thousands of seafarers, despite repeated calls from the United Nations to resolve the issue (IMO 2020d).

Ships must keep running, for shipping is the handmaiden of trade. Seafarers are, Pérez states, the forgotten heroes that support global trade, which secure countries' supplies of food, fuel, and other important goods such as life-saving medical equipment. They do so not only during the COVID-19 pandemic, but as a matter of course.

Labour Day, and the fight for good working conditions is vital to improving the livelihoods of seafarers. While, since 1919, the International Labour Organization (ILO) has sanctioned an 8-hour working day and a 48-hour working week, seafarers work well in excess of such hours. Days of 14 working hours and weeks of up to 98 working hours are sanctioned by the ILO Maritime Labour Convention and the IMO International Convention on Standards of Training, Certification and Watchkeeping for Seafarers (STCW), respectively: 'While undeniable success has been achieved onshore, the 8-hour norm has not been implemented at sea,' Raphael Baumler (2020, 11) argues, because 'the nineteenth century construction of a 'special nature' of shipping and fishing detached sea workers from other sectors and facilitated their isolation. Consequently, the sea workers' standards of work attached to the nature of the sector more than to their human nature.' The COVID-19 pandemic has thus exacerbated – rather than created – seafarers' challenging working conditions, which have always been regulated and understood as existing in a world entirely disconnected from shore-based life.

While entire populations are confined to their houses, cities, and countries, seafarers are excluded from returning to land. This is, ostensibly, to both stop ships turning into vectors of viral spread from port to port and to limit risk of entire crews contracting the virus while at sea. However, the logistics infrastructure maintained by seafarers is critical to the security and economic activity of countries, while the workers that make this happen are forgotten. Or, conveniently ignored.

Seafarers, one could argue with Foucault (1995), pose a biopolitical 'risk to society', as the mobility of ships maintains connection between places and bodies at a time when human contact is deemed risky. While they are at sea, it is possible to exclude seafarers by keeping them out of sight and out of contact, like lepers, while maintaining a regime of confinement on land. An invisible fast-spreading virus cannot be halted, after all, by excluding solely those with symptoms. But seafarers are also among the most vulnerable, as cruise liners have shown that ships are environments, like plague villages, in which viral spread is difficult to contain. There are, after all, no knock-on effects from the cruise-line industry coming to a halt. Surely, jobs were lost, and companies ended up in difficulties, but unlike cargo ships, cruise-liners are not a precondition for keeping global trade flows to remain intact. Though the greater visibility of cruise ships – they have rich people on board, after all – means that ships in general were quickly identified as viral vectors early in the pandemic. This grounded such ships, as cruise passengers wanted to avoid the risk of infection, initially leaving many crew stranded aboard (McCormic and Greenfield 2020). Eventually the industry suspended operations (McMahon 2020) which meant that many cruise ships ended up sold for scrap (Saunders 2021).

The risk, inherent in maritime crew mobility, is not only to shore-based communities, but also to those aboard. Despite seafarers' invisibility, and unlike their counterparts working aboard cruise ships, they are indispensable to maintaining 'good mobility' (of cargo, and therefore capital). But in order to continue trade while halting the virus, seafarers become collateral victims of ad-hoc biopolitical regimes erected in response to the sudden COVID-19 pandemic: their work facilitates good mobility that keeps economies and populations on land alive, but their bodies need to be kept safely at sea in order to maintain the integrity of supply chains. This reduction to the economic role, more than their being potential vectors of transmission, is what keeps seafarers at sea well beyond their labour contracts.

When confined to one's ship, making noise is the only thing seafarers can do to make their presence known, especially when moored in a securitized port that is inaccessible for anyone who does not work there. Most commercial ports around the world now operate in compliance with the *International Ship and Port Facility Security* (ISPS) code administered by the *International Maritime Organization*, which came into force – after pressure from the USA – in 2004 as a post-9/11 measure to increase security in 'critical' logistics infrastructure (see Cowen 2014).

Ashore, pandemic response measures are put in place to save lives. At sea, measures are put in place in function of the purpose bodies aboard ships serve: the circulation of goods that gives life to the economy – and thereby lives on land. The primary aim of COVID-19 regulations is the integrity of global supply chains. Seafarer well-being is a secondary concern.

Harbormaster Pérez echoes the messages conveyed by the *International Maritime Organization*, the *International Chamber of Shipping*, and the *International Labor Organization*. They stress that seafarers are 'key workers' that should be exempt from travel restrictions, so they can travel between work and home, and thus ship and shore without limitation (ICS 2020, ILO 2020, IMO 2020c, 2020a). The *International Maritime Organization* has worked with member states to facilitate crew change and repatriation throughout lockdowns, but as of July 2020, more than 200,000 crew 'are still waiting to be repatriated, many having stayed on long beyond the end of their original contracts' (IMO 2020b). As 2020 progressed, the number of seafarers stuck at sea steadily grew, up to some 400,000 people by September (De Beukelaer 2020c, IMO 2020c).

Lockdown or lock-out?

Making sense of a double lockdown, being excluded from land while confined to our ship, comes with a major challenge: While at sea we did not live through the lockdown experience that nearly everyone on land went through. As a result, my framework of reference is the world as we knew it, not the world as it has become.

At times, when trying to understand the predicament I was in, I felt like the inverse of Kimmy Schmidt, the protagonist of the Netflix series *The Unbreakable Kimmy Schmidt*. In this show (2015–2019), created by Tina Fey and Robert Carlock, Kimmy Schmidt finds freedom after having been held in captivity by doomsday cult leader Reverend Richard Wayne Gary Wayne for fifteen years. He had kidnapped Kimmy when she was a teenager and convinced her and three other women that they are the sole survivors of a nuclear apocalypse. Upon being set free from her time locked away in the (fictitious) town of Durnsville, Indiana, she settles in New York to enjoy the freedom she has never known.

The eighteenth century English author Samuel Johnson once likened being at sea to being in jail, but 'with the chance of being drowned'. While it may not be possible to leave the ship, the open ocean hardly feels like confinement.

To me, the penitentiary analogy only makes sense now, after having been not simply confined to the ship when at sea but also excluded from shore leave when in port. In the 1962 film *Mutiny on the Bounty*, master's mate Fletcher Christian retorts to the claim of one of his fellow mutineers that their choice was between prison or mutiny, by saying that: 'You're in prison now, Mills. With one difference. We are not locked in; we are locked out.'

We are of course no mutineers, and we will not forever be locked out. But we have been locked out, along with other seafarers. Fortunately, I have reason to disagree with Samuel Johnson when he says that 'a man in a jail has more room, better food, and commonly better company'.

Our ship, for all its superficial discomforts, would reach Germany where we would be allowed ashore. So, any comparison between our lives and those of a racialized class of under-paid seafarers is difficult to uphold: our discomfort and uncertainty is temporary and exceptional, theirs is permanent and normal. More worryingly, we were free to speak up about the difficulties we faced without fear for repercussion, while many professional seafarers risk being blacklisted when doing so.

Upon disembarking at Hamburg, we were no longer be locked out. But unlike Kimmy Schmidt, we didn't find a world that promises freedom and nigh-endless possibility. We found a world of restrictions, facemasks, virus-swabs, and social distancing. Most importantly, we found a world in which social mores had changed in our absence. Kimmy struggled to find ways to adapt to her newly found freedoms, but we now have to deal with restrictions that everyone else has gradually socialized into. But much like Kimmy, we have a hard time behaving according to the 'new normal' of social – and often legal – norms. Even so, in Hamburg, we returned from a temporary sus-pension of some freedoms and privileges to a world in which we became invisible, yet welcome.

We were no longer confined, nor excluded. The conditions of the pan-demic had not changed; the context had. We were no longer sailors in foreign ports. We were home. But the globalized shipping industry, with its international labour force, knows no 'home' ports where neither ship nor crew are strangers.

Much like Kimmy during her confinement, our understanding of the outside world relied largely on information we obtained through a single person. While we were on the high seas, the ship's owner kept our captain updated on changes to shore life. Despite their genuine efforts, we received precious little information, in large part because ship's emails are sent through a – prohibitively expensive – *Inmarsat-C* satellite connection. This meant that, whenever at sea, the only information we obtained from the outside world was through the correspondence between captain and ship-owner. We did not have personal access to phone or internet networks, except when in port.

Sailing to a new world

One of the messages we received from the shipowner while at sea suggested that the world had changed to the extent that 'the world as you know it no longer exists'. We were sailing to a New World. Not a colonial fantasy of unknown shores – even though we sailed a colonial trans-Atlantic trade route, and carried goods from tropical former colonies, but a world that had changed in our absence. Much like the world had changed during Julian West's century-long sleep, as described in Edward Bellamy's 1888 novel *Looking Backward*. In this story, Bellamy describes the techno-socialist America of the year 2000, told from the perspective of a nineteenth century Bostonian, who had spent the preceding 113 years in a hypnosis-induced sleep. It takes the entire book for West to properly understand how his world has changed in his absence.

When we embarked the *Avontuur*, the strict quarantine of millions in Wuhan by Chinese authorities was still deemed an unprecedented measure that was possible only because China is an authoritarian state. Democracies, the argument went, would never be able to impose similar limitations on people. Until they did.

While at sea, it remained near impossible to know or imagine whether and how things might have changed on land. We knew of lockdowns but could not quite imagine what they were like. At times it felt like a surreal, or rather hyperreal, theatre that had been put on show to fool us. Unlike Julian West or Kimmy Schmidt, we were able to anticipate and speculate the change that awaited us.

Much like a ship sounding its horn in the fog, unable to see beyond a few shiplengths, we were steering blind. We relied on short and imprecise contacts with the world to make sense of how the pandemic had changed our surroundings.

I had hoped that by the time we finally stepped off in Hamburg, nothing would feel much different. Mostly because the situation in Germany seemed to be returning to 'normal' while we were on our way there. My hope, which now seems utterly naïve, was that we'd only know the 2020 pandemic lockdown through stories and accounts of others.

Within days from disembarking the *Avontuur*, I flew from Frankfurt to Sydney via Singapore. As if by miracle, I was able to get on the first flight out to Australia. During the voyage, I realized that the world had really changed. Changi was deserted, planes nearly empty.

As I spent fourteen days in a designated quarantine hotel in Sydney, Melbourne – where I live – faced ever-tightening restrictions in a bid to curb the 'second wave', resulting in one of the world's strictest lockdowns that would last 112 days.

I have returned home – and to my position at the university. But for over a million seafarers, extended time at sea will remain the norm. Global passenger travel has slowed down, but demand for cargo transport has remained comparatively strong (UNCTAD 2020). While being *confined* is integral to life at sea, being *excluded* from land for undefined periods creates makes lockdowns at sea particularly challenging (De Beukelaer 2020b).

What had changed most, it seemed, was the 'security pact' between citizens and their governments (Hannah, Hutta, and Schemann 2020). People accepted severe limits on their liberties, in exchange for the protection of the common good. Whether people accepted this wilfully, begrudgingly, or forcefully, a new power balance between state and citizen had emerged.

Initially, this new 'security pact' included firmly closed borders, including to key workers like seafarers, which they and their unions duly accepted as 'force majeure' (ITF 2020a). But as the International Labour Organization stressed that crew changes could only be held off until borders would open again (ILO 2020), the number of seafarers stranded at sea has continued to grow even though most countries now allow crew change – though often under strict rules. Crew change is now possible, but at greater effort and cost than prior to the COVID-19 pandemic.

Without a clear view of society ashore, and out of sight of those on land, seafarers sounded their ship's horn on May 1st to give them a voice in a world that relies on shipping. As the pandemic continues, unequal and evolving regimes of biopolitical regulation continue to impact seafarers more severely than most people. Meanwhile, their proverbial horns continue to sound. But the 'sea blind' world would rather, conveniently, forget that the 'life' of the economy, and the consumer habits of people on land, relies on the many people stuck at sea.

Seafarers may be invisible; they are also indispensable. But rather than recognize their importance, the COVID-19 pandemic has further eroded the rights of these precariously employed workers. Despite the changes caused by the COVID-19 pandemic, it is thanks to seafarers that the life as we know it still mostly exists.

Acknowledgements

I would like to thank Ted Striphas and John Erni for editing this special issue on the COVID-19 pandemic, as well as their constructive comments that have helped to improve my argument. I would also like to thank all participants of the (virtual) *COVID-19 and Theory* seminar on 5th August 2020, organized by the *English and Theatre Studies* program at the University of Melbourne; with special thanks to speakers Justin Clemens and Joe Hughes, and convener Sarah Balkin. Many thanks to Robbie Fordyce for helpful conversations on the topic.

Disclosure statement

No potential conflict of interest was reported by the author(s).

Further information

This Special Issue article has been comprehensively reviewed by the Special Issue editors, Associate Professor Ted Striphas and Professor John Nguyet Erni.

ORCID

Christiaan De Beukelaer ⓘ http://orcid.org/0000-0002-9045-9979

References

Baumler, R. 2020. Working time limits at sea, a hundred-year construction. *Marine Policy*, August, 104101. Available from: https://doi.org/10.1016/j.marpol.2020. 104101.

Cotton, S. 2020. Beyond the limit of safe shipping – ITF general secretary's UN address. *International Transport Workers' Federation*, 24 September. Available from: https:// www.itfglobal.org/en/news/beyond-limit-safe-shipping-itf-general-secretarys-un-address.

Cowen, D., 2014. *The deadly life of logistics: mapping violence in global trade*. Minneapolis: University of Minnesota Press.

De Beukelaer, C. 2018. Plain sailing: how traditional methods could deliver zero-emission shipping. *The Conversation*, 28 May. Available from: https://theconversation. com/plain-sailing-how-traditional-methods-could-deliver-zero-emission-shipping-97180.

De Beukelaer, C., 2020a. Sail cargo: charting a new path for emission-free shipping. *UNCTAD transport and trade facilitation newsletter* 87 (65).

De Beukelaer, C. 2020b. From locked out to locked in. *The Monthly*, September.

De Beukelaer, C. 2020c. The hundreds of thousands of stranded maritime workers are the invisible victims of the pandemic. *Jacobin*, October.

De Beukelaer, C. 2020d. Stranded at sea: the humanitarian crisis that's left 400,000 seafarers stuck oncargo ships. *The Conversation*, 8 December.

De Beukelaer, C. and Corcoran, J. 2020. In the stillness between two waves of the sea. *Ocean Archive*, 7 May. Available from: https://ocean-archive.org/collection/45.

Foucault, M., 1995. *Discipline and punish: the birth of the prison*. 2nd ed. New York, NY: Vintage Books.

Ha, K.O., *et al.* 2020. Worst shipping crisis in decades puts lives and trade at risk. *Bloomberg*, 18 September. Available from: https://www.bloomberg.com/features/ 2020-pandemic-shipping-labor-violations/.

Hannah, M.G., Hutta, J.S., and Schemann, C. 2020. Thinking through covid-19 responses with foucault – an initial overview. *Antipode Online*, 5 May. Available from: https:// antipodeonline.org/2020/05/05/thinking-through-covid-19-responses-with-foucault/.

ICS. 2020. Global shipping fleet to sound horns on 8 July to remind governments over need for urgent crew change. *International Chamber of Shipping*, 30 June. Available from: https://www.ics-shipping.org/news/press-releases/2020/06/30/global-shipping-fleet-to-sound-horns-on-8-july-to-remind-governments-over-need-for-urgent-crew-change.

ILO. 2020. Information note on maritime labour issues and coronavirus (COVID-19). *International Labour Organization*. Available from: https://www.ilo.org/global/ about-the-ilo/newsroom/news/WCMS_747293/lang–en/index.htm.

IMO. 2020a. Governments pledge action for seafarers at crucial crew change summit. *International Maritime Organization*, 8 July. Available from: https://www.imo.org/en/MediaCentre/PressBriefings/Pages/22-crew-change-summit.aspx.

IMO. 2020b. Coronavirus (COVID-19) – outcome of the international maritime virtual summit on crew changes organized by the United Kingdom. *International Maritime Organization*. Available from: https://www.imo.org/en/MediaCentre/HotTopics/Documents/COVID%20CL%204204%20adds/Circular%20Letter%20No.4204-Add.24%20-%20Coronavirus%20(Covid-19)%20-%20Outcome%20Of%20The%20International%20MaritimeVirtual%20Summit%20On%20Crew%20Change.pdf.

IMO. 2020c. 400,000 seafarers stuck at sea as crew change crisis deepens. *International Maritime Organization*. 24 September. Available from: https://www.imo.org/en/MediaCentre/PressBriefings/Pages/32-crew-change-UNGA.aspx.

IMO. 2020d. IMO welcomes UN resolution on keyworker seafarers. *International Maritime Organization*. 1 December. Available from: https://www.imo.org/en/MediaCentre/PressBriefings/pages/44-seafarers-UNGA-resolution.aspx.

IMO. 2020e. IMO secretary-general denounces 'no crew change' clauses. *International Maritime Organization*. 21 December. Available from: https://www.imo.org/en/MediaCentre/PressBriefings/pages/46-no-crew-change-clause-.aspx.

ITF. 2020a. ITF agrees to crew contract extensions. *International transport workers' federation*, 19 March. Available from: https://www.itfglobal.org/en/news/itf-agrees-crew-contract-extensions.

ITF. 2020b. Crew change crisis risks becoming forced labour epidemic as tragedy hits six-month mark on world maritime day. *International Transport Workers' Federation*, 24 September. Available from: https://www.itfglobal.org/en/news/crew-change-crisis-risks-becoming-forced-labour-epidemic-tragedy-hits-six-month-mark-world.

McCormic, E. and Greenfield, P. 2020. Revealed: 100,000 crew never made it off cruise ships amid coronavirus crisis. *The Guardian*, 30 April. Available from: https://www.theguardian.com/environment/2020/apr/30/no-end-in-sight-100000-crew-on-cruise-ships-stranded-at-sea-coronavirus.

McMahon, S. 2020. Cruising won't resume in U.S. waters until 2021, with lines renewing a voluntary suspension. *Washington Post*, 3 November. Available from: https://www.washingtonpost.com/travel/2020/11/03/cruises-2021-voluntary-suspension/.

Saunders, A. 2021. Which cruise ships will be scrapped or taken out of service because of the COVID-19 pandemic? *Cruise Critic*, 16 January. Available from: https://www.cruisecritic.com.au/news/5423/.

Sekula, Allan. 1995. *Fish story*. Düsseldorf: Richter.

Sekula, Allan. 2017. *OKEANOS*. Ed. Daniela Zyman and Cory Scozzari. Berlin: Sternberg Press.

Sekula, A. and Burch, N. 2010. *The forgotten space*. Available from: https://www.theforgottenspace.net/.

UNCTAD, 2020. *Review of maritime transport*. Geneva: UNCTAD.

Back to the future: lessons of a SARS hysteria for the COVID-19 pandemic

Allen Chun

ABSTRACT

During the COVID-19 global pandemic, Taiwan has been universally praised for its policy actions in preventing its initial outbreak there from Wuhan and for its strict measures in containing its communal spread locally. Memory of the SARS crisis played a major role, but people in Taiwan forget that SARS was initially considered a problem confined mostly to Hong Kong. Taiwanese did not seem urgently aware, until infections multiplied locally. Taiwan's health authorities eventually adopted a draconian quarantine policy, but mainly as a political tactic to contain the widespread panic, as though the dam had suddenly burst. In retrospect, the extremity and internal contradictions of the policy are remarkable, but they are instructive. The initial reaction of unprepared governments, most notably in the US, during COVID-19 mirrors this same ineptitude. Enabling hysteria and resorting to scapegoating were in turn diversions to cover up their inability to prevent a crisis. In the US, racism emerged, China and the WHO were blamed, people were even urged not to wear masks to avoid a run on short supplies. This is the tip of the political iceberg, if one adds tightened immigration and economic effects on the U.S. elections.

The fog of panic in the making of a mass media hysteria

Panic is the result of 'losing control'. In this regard, hysteria can create the existence of a 'mass', which is not, strictly speaking, the sum of individual agitations. It is instead created or orchestrated, simply by casting the existence of crisis as a social problem. Panic and hysteria are imaginative facades for political repression that necessitate urgent re-imposition of control.

The origins and causes of SARS were initially unclear. By the time doctors in different venues verified the existence of a new coronavirus, SARS had begun to spread globally. In March 2003, SARS in Hong Kong grew to epidemic proportions. In Taiwan, the outbreak at Heping Hospital in Taipei on 24 April 2003 caused health officials to order all staff to return there for mandatory quarantine. Dr. Zhou Jingkai, who had already returned home by this time, opted to remain at home to self-quarantine, citing WHO guidelines to this effect. In light of current understandings of virus prevention, this would have been deemed appropriate behaviour. But in the early days of SARS, panic caused by uncertainty influenced the need for stringent policy.

Dr. Zhou was eventually forcibly taken from his house to the hospital. In the two weeks of the Heping Hospital lockdown, 57 staff members were infected, and 7 died; 97 other people trapped within the hospital became infected, 24 died (1 by suicide), and this incident incited an even wider epidemic throughout the island.[1] As a result of Dr. Zhou's refusal to comply, he was docked 3 months without pay and fined 240,000NT (US$8000). After he was fired, a year short of retirement, no hospital would hire him. He also spent 7 years unsuccessfully suing the government for wrongful termination. His career was completely destroyed in the aftermath.

Dr. Zhou's downfall was perhaps the most newsworthy incident that took place during the SARS crisis. However, the plight of a research academic at Academia Sinica, Dr. Chen Yilin, illustrated the extent to which SARS policy was in fact a strategy of extreme containment that was haphazardly conceived and forcibly put into practice more to control a chaotic, hysterical public than to medically contain the spread of the virus. Like Dr. Zhou, the government went to great lengths to punish Dr. Chen, if anything, as an example to show official determination.

Chen Yilin was less a victim of quarantine policy than its ongoing social chaos. The press alleged that he 'escaped' SARS quarantine and was potentially spreading the virus overseas. His case made headline news in Taiwan, because Lee Yuan-tse, the President of Academia Sinica (where he was a Research Fellow), was the chief architect of the quarantine policy. The public endangerment that officials alleged he caused became a source of moral indignation.

Chen was invited to give a series of talks at Hong Kong City University, and he had been planning to do library research afterward. His trip was delayed twice in view of the seriousness of SARS there, but, after his hosts thought that it was fine to proceed with his talks, he decided to take personal leave, out of an abundance of caution. To minimize health hazards, he decided to abbreviate his total stay, then, instead of taking a continuous three-week trip to Hong Kong, Australia and the US (leave for the latter venues was approved), he decided to make separate trips. The day after he departed for Hong Kong on 26 April, the Taiwan government imposed a ten-day quarantine on all travellers arriving from SARS affected areas. Needing to return to Taiwan to retrieve necessary papers for his upcoming two-week trip (which eventually would be extended another six weeks for participation at two conferences and other library research), he returned from Hong Kong to Taipei, knowing that a mandatory quarantine would threaten to cancel talks in Melbourne and Santa Cruz. He called Health Bureau officials, who said that it was fine to leave, as long as he did not show symptoms of illness. He left Taipei on 6 May.

What happened later was beyond comprehension. *The China Times* published on 22 May a full page of featured articles, reporting that a Research Fellow at Academia Sinica escaped quarantine and left the country.[2] According to the reports, this researcher returned from Hong Kong, a SARS affected area, and was supposed to be quarantined for 10 days. Academia Sinica President Lee Yuan-tse, in responding to an inquiry at the Legislative Yuan, said that this Chen surnamed academic did indeed escape the country for the US and that 'on his return to Taiwan, he would be severely punished'.[3] One legislator, Qiu Zhuangjin, argued, 'such academics of questionable character who present a threat to society should be summarily fired'.[4] Liu Dexun, Vice-Chairman of the Mainland Affairs Council, remarked, 'he should be shot'.[5] Academia Sinica officials noted that Chen was a US citizen, thus legally it was not possible to prevent him from leaving the country. *The China Times* surmised that he had dual nationality and that, according to Wu Xueyan, Vice-Director of the Exit and Entry Customs Control, he probably used a Taiwan passport to enter and a U.S. passport to exit the country, which explains why he could leave Taiwan undetected.[6] His whereabouts in Taiwan and elsewhere were a mystery. He was a menace that had to be punished. One could not ignore the gravity of this situation.

When the news broke, Chen was in the US, near the end of his two-week trip. Prior to leaving Taiwan, he filed for a month extension of his leave, which included participation at a conference and funded library research. After he was told of the news, his Institute revoked the remainder of his research trip, essentially forcing him to return. First of all, certain people decided that he had indeed broken a law, and secondly they thought that the crime was serious enough to warrant cancellation of his leave, forcing him to return, threatening also to fire him.

What was the fuss all about? Why did the President of Academia Sinica go out of his way to reprimand him, without bothering to seek his explanation or defense of these alleged actions? As it turned out, policymakers did not realize that there was a gap between official policy and policy as practiced. Chen did not doubt the content of what his local Health Bureau told him. If the Customs officer allowed him to leave, in full knowledge of those facts, then it was legal. Below the surface of events, there was another reason why this story provoked intense reaction to the point of provoking official concern. Lee was the chief architect of the quarantine policy. The fact that one of his own employees violated his quarantine policy was clearly embarrassing. But if this was really about politics, then Chen was a useful scapegoat for these purposes.

The SARS panic in Taiwan did not start with SARS per se. It started with the *perception* of crisis, engendered not by the implementation of the new quarantine policy, strictly speaking, but rather the exaggerated emphasis placed on the source of the epidemic coming from affected areas, namely Hong Kong and PRC. The media played a role in exacerbating the panic, which contributed now to a kind of mass hysteria. The strict quarantine of passengers from affected areas gave the misleading impression that disease was still coming from the outside instead of spreading from within. The mysterious whereabouts of this academic who seemed to evade all sorts of controls added to a growing threat, not only to the health of people but to society. The newspapers proudly displayed a photo of him, subtitled with a caption 'Criminal G027857'.

In piecing together his whereabouts two weeks after the fact, the media painted a picture of him running 'all over the island' like a fugitive from justice:[7] first of all it noted that, on his Health Bureau entry form, he failed to tick Hong Kong as his port of embarkation, hinting that he was deliberately evasive.[8] He also cited his office address as his home quarantine address, which suggested that he had no intention of going home at all. He supposedly 'broke into' the side entrance then forced his way into the building, which was recorded by CCT video.[9] During his brief presence there, many people saw him, causing great consternation. The Director's secretary, then the Vice-Director and the Director, called or visited to persuade him to leave the premises and go home but were met with obstinate refusals.[10] After repeated warnings, he reluctantly went home late that night. The secretary then reported him to the Health Bureau.

News then reported that his Institute notified National Chiao Tung University the next day that he would be going there to teach classes, at which point the department promptly cancelled his classes. After he went to the University, he tried to check into the University hostel, but this too was met by stiff refusal by the University. As a result, he had nowhere else to go but home. Few days later, he surreptitiously left the country, exact whereabouts unknown.[11] The Nankang office of the Health Bureau, where he should have reported, based on the quarantine address he supplied on arrival at Taoyuan airport on May 1, stated that it had no record of him.

Not long after *The China Times* articles appeared, he received dozens of hate messages from unknown people, most of which castigated his reckless behaviour, for example: (1) 'You shitty motherf***r, stop traveling around the world'; (2) 'F*** you, human junk'; (3) 'You are really a shame of Taiwan'; (4) 'What is in your water brain? You do not respect Taiwan; you abuse Taiwanese, our system and our government ... F*** out of here'. These feelings were not necessarily endorsed by official policy, but they were empowered by a policy that implicitly attributed the primary cause of disease transmission to threats from the outside, which became exaggerated by media hype.

Colleagues who heard about his entry into the Institute demanded that the building be thoroughly disinfected. Others called for immediate disciplinary action. A former Director of his Institute contributed further to character assassination, saying that he often made improper overseas calls, signed library entry ledgers as Mao Zedong and did not get along with colleagues, as if to suggest that he was prone to deviant criminal behaviour.[12]

In the midst of this hysteria, no one bothered to point out that we were all set up for this crisis by the overconfidence displayed by health authorities who consistently maintained that they were 'in control'. Panic was a consequence of ignorance and uncertainty. Fingering the blame on people who bring disease from the outside was the easy way to alleviate all fears and anxieties. Ironically, it was safer in Hong Kong. More than 80 percent of people there wore masks in public, and public facilities were rigorously disinfected. In contrast, less than 20 percent of people in Taiwan wore masks in public, and the only health measures that his Institute put into effect were to close the annex entrances to the building and shut down the elevator. People who saw Chen wearing a mask laughed, as if they had seen an alien being. Things changed much later.

There was no need for the media to exaggerate his mysterious whereabouts. He observed home quarantine until the time he left Taiwan. Many people initially believed that AIDS was a homosexual disease. We now know in fact not to blame homosexuals for the spread of AIDS. We just tell people now to wear condoms. We also did not ban travel to and from Africa just because AIDS was a lethal disease that could spread easily. What made SARS any different?

The root of the crisis in Taiwan had to do with the failure of health authorities to control the spread of disease that had already been there and their lax quarantining of all people having direct contact with affected patients. Lax control and gross medical incompetence exacerbated the spread of disease, leading to the closure of two hospitals as a last resort. Such developments gave birth to the urgency of strict quarantine measures. In contrast, all of Hong Kong's SARS cases originated from a single doctor from Guangdong. Thousands continued to pass between Hong Kong and Guangdong, yet there were no new cases of SARS spreading across borders. Macau also suffered no instances of SARS. The quarantine was thus an act of *desperation*.

The policing of an extremist health policy as cultural corrective

COVID-19 has apparently turned out to be much more infectious than SARS or MERS. Outside Asia, cases of SARS were successfully isolated and treated without strict quarantine and travel bans, which can be questioned on health grounds. As for Taiwan, quarantine policy was less the outcome of rational planning than the result of its initial failure to implement the necessary health measures to contain the problem. SARS infected only .02 percent of the population in these affected countries. It was most urgent to quarantine people afflicted by the virus. For all else, wearing a mask, public disinfection and social distancing were sufficiently preventive.

The adoption of a draconian quarantine policy was really a politically expedient response to a chaotic social situation, and its implementation reflected ignorance of the facts, uncertainty of strategy and institutional disorganization. During the initial crisis, when the main outbreak was confined mostly to Hong Kong, authorities took no action. Things began to worsen, when a massive outbreak of SARS cases occurred at Heping Hospital in Taipei on 22 April. This spike led to the closure of the hospital on 24 April and forced quarantine of all people present there. Another outbreak occurred at nearby Renji Hospital, leading to its closure on 29 April.[13] On 26 April, Taiwan recorded its first death, a 56-year-old male who was infected by his brother visiting from Hong Kong. The latter was a resident of Amoy Gardens, which was the site of Hong Kong's first localized quarantine. This rapid turn of events precipitated the government's decision on 27 April to institute a policy of containment to quarantine all travellers from SARS affected areas. Events surrounding the closure of Heping Hospital caused much controversy.[14] All medical staff working at the hospital, regardless of whether they had any contact with the SARS unit, were ordered to return there and be quarantined. There were also reports at Heping of numerous incidents of misdiagnosis of SARS as well as cases of non-SARS patients being put together with SARS patients, which exacerbated spread of disease. The subsequent chaos and misadventure caused the government to adopt hard line measures to force compliance with official policy. This climate of chaos, fear and retribution became rampant in ensuing weeks.

This atmosphere of general panic bordering on mass hysteria provided the background for media sensationalization of Chen's case. On 21 May, when Lee Yuan-tse delivered his SARS progress report to the Legislative Yuan, Chen had been out of Taiwan for two weeks. Lee was already informed of his having left the country early, and administrators had already requested documents in relation to him from airport customs control. They were certain of the facts and were prepared to answer any suspicions about his case, if so queried. The media lynching also diverted attention away from the disorganized implementation of a flawed policy. Rules were instituted on the fly, and many directives were not disseminated to the media and governing agencies until two to five days after policy proclamations. Some rules proved to be impractical, if not excessively draconian, prompting criticism from various quarters. In the meantime, the perception of crisis increased in proportion with the growing number of total infections and deaths. During the first week of the new quarantine policy, less than 20 percent of people wore masks on the street or public transport. The government eventually ordered all transit passengers to wear face masks and issued laws against spitting to control transmission of infectious fluids. By mid-May, infections had been reported throughout the island, causing some hospitals to close temporarily. Uncertainty and chaos had turned into panic and fear reproduced en masse.

By the latter half of May, when Chen's case appeared on headline news, repression from above combined with the everyday terror of an invisible, ubiquitous disease did not necessarily contribute to a more enlightened or manageable containment of the problem. On the contrary, it just contributed to a heightened sense of vigilance and collective paranoia. This was precisely the kind of raw reactions that was provoked, when news about him broke. Although he had left Taiwan two weeks earlier, many people believed that he was still potentially spreading the virus, when there was no evidence of him having any disease. The *thought* or possibility that he *risked* spreading SARS was morally repugnant. Thus, the issues that concerned the media most about his case had to with whether and how he managed to escape quarantine before the expiration of the ten-day period. Press accounts seem to have taken the liberty to elaborate on comments made by colleagues about his anti-social personality traits and eccentric thinking, as though to emphasize their direct relevance to his inherently perverse 'criminal' actions. Like Dr. Zhou Jingkai, the surgeon at Heping Hospital who insisted on quarantining safely at home and resisted returning to the hospital, Chen was legally charged with public endangerment.

What flaws in policy and legal loopholes were being covered up by the media distraction? Travellers arriving from an affected area had to deal with paperwork that was rarely followed up on, given the incoming hordes. They were not permitted to take public transportation, and no alternative means were provided, forcing people to fend for themselves. They had to report to a local Health Bureau personally within 24 h, again without being allowed to take public transportation. They could not go out in public, except for exercise and buying takeout meals. Despite these strict health rules, the government granted businessmen needing to travel to the PRC special exemptions to bypass quarantine. Some things took precedence over health (sic). Last but not least, foreigners could always break quarantine prematurely, simply by leaving the country, because there was nothing legal to prevent them from so doing, unless held for crimes.

At another level, the necessity of a strict quarantine policy fit the fear and ignorance that gripped the public mindset at the time. When Chen entered his Institute, he saw the Director's secretary, who was so shaken by this passing at a distance that she decided to quarantine herself for 10 days by living in her office and not going home, to avoid infecting her family members. Her husband, a Research Fellow at another Institute, flew to the US without letting her come home. To deter further visits to his office after his initial entry, the Vice-Director ordered IT technicians to lock Chen's office PC to prevent any access to it. Other colleagues insisted that the whole building be disinfected as a result of his entry. Academia Sinica was more disturbed by the internal complaints about his behaviour than his breaking of quarantine law per se. No news media was willing to publish his rebuttal of these events or appeals by other colleagues.[15]

COVID-19 redux: the politics of distraction in the US' mismanagement of a 'Wuhan Virus'

> His egregious and arguably intentional mishandling of the current (COVID) catastrophe has led to a level of pushback and scrutiny that he's never experienced before, increasing his belligerence and need for petty revenge as he withholds vital funding, personal protective equipment, and ventilators that your tax dollars have paid for from states whose governors don't kiss his ass sufficiently.
> —Mary L. Trump, Too Much and Never Enough:
> How My Family Created the World's Most Dangerous Man

Cronies first: this might be the rationale that drove President Trump to tap Jared Kushner, his son-in-law and White House advisor, to coordinate redistribution by the Federal Emergency Management Agency (FEMA) of personal protective equipment (PPE) in the early phase of its COVID-19 pandemic, which was in short supply and the object of intense competition between states. Crony capitalism has been an explicit hallmark of Trump's guiding political principles, thus the degradation of the coronavirus crisis into a battle over political survival divorced from considerations of health should come as little surprise. Trump's systematic downplaying of the emerging health crisis set the scene for a glaring lack of preparedness and an epic shortage of all manner of basic medical equipment from PPE, masks and testing supplies to ventilators. The cultural dimension of the crisis involved the way in which the administration attempted to rationalize its actions and promote its media message by practicing what Jeffrey D. Sachs aptly termed 'the politics of distraction'.[16] In the midst of the chaos and confusion that resulted out of an uncontrollable spike of infections, hospitalization and deaths, government policy not only had to affirm its sense of control but more importantly prevent public uncertainty and ignorance from exacerbating rampant shortages of essential material and overwhelming medical services.

The history of missteps that plagued American response to the global coronavirus spread has been well documented.[17] Trump dismantled the Global Health Security Unit that President Obama assembled in 2014, which included a 69pp. playbook to deal with potential pandemics. He ignored intelligence reports as early as November 2019 about the virus situation in Wuhan. He continued to marginalize warnings from various health officials throughout January about a looming health crisis. On January 20, South Korea and the US experienced their first case of coronavirus. From that point on, the policies and practices that developed in these respective countries to cope with the pandemic have irrevocably diverged. Korea immediately put into place a testing and contact tracing regime that localized in the long run further outbreaks and minimized deaths. In the US, the failure to provide reliable tests combined with government ineffectiveness in securing medical equipment and supplies for an overburdened hospital staff overlapped with other failures to exacerbate contradictions in changing policies and practices.

The failure to confront the health problem can be viewed as flaws in its scientific decision making and as a result of the government's relative prioritization of its political and economic agendas. Trump dismantled Obama's pandemic response team in order to divert its resources elsewhere. He was more concerned with global economic forums and the state of Wall Street, which led to a downplaying of the health issue until it exploded spectacularly.[18] The federal government was unable to address shortages experienced by medical workers everywhere in masks, PPE and ventilators. The lack of sufficient testing escalated the crisis exponentially by making an uncertain situation even more incomprehensible and uncontrollable. Lack of testing materials tightened practical restrictions, which prevented real prospects for disease discovery, not to mention serious contact tracing. PPE was reused, increasing endangerment. This created a widening gap between reality and the need to rationalize it to an even more confused public.

The most perplexing medical advice arising from this initial chaos was the stern rebuke against the wearing of masks. US Surgeon General Jerome Adams in a tweet on 29 February entitled 'Seriously people – STOP BUYING MASKS!' exhorted, 'they are NOT effective in preventing general public from catching #Coronavirus,' then later in an interview explained,

> folks who don't know how to wear them properly tend to touch their faces a lot, and actually can increase the spread of coronavirus. You can increase your risk of getting it by wearing a mask if you are not a healthcare provider.[19]

He added that his recommendation corresponded with WHO guidelines in March and April, which stated that a person should only wear a mask if caring for those with COVID-19 or suffering from symptoms. Reading below the surface, it was obvious that the more serious problem involved shortage of supplies for medical providers. A run on masks sparked by panic buying would have exacerbated the crisis and created hysteria among the general public. By that time, stores had already experienced a run on toilet paper, disinfectant and other goods. Mass hysteria and disorder were not inconceivable possibilities.

The state of the public during the initial outbreak of COVID-19 mirrored the disorder that reflected the early crisis caused by SARS in Asia. While mandatory quarantine and isolatable lockdowns were preferred policy strategies in Asia, Americans were generally resistant to the imposition of such nationwide restrictions on freedom of behaviour and movement. The politics in this context served as an elaborate coverup for the failure of government health policy purely as a medical endeavour, hence politics of distraction.[20] Trump began to refer to COVID-19 as the Wuhan virus, thus highlighting its alien origins and shifting the blame to China's failure of transparency as the main cause for its global spread. He then faulted WHO and threatened to defund it by proposing to abolish support. He also did little to dampen anti-Asian backlash by the general public. His subsequent emphasis on accelerating the development of a vaccine was also an effort to appeal to popular aspirations for a magic pill solution for the crisis that would at the same time deflect news of growing infections, intubations and deaths. Needless to say, a successful vaccine would eradicate the virus in a way that bypassed the pain of lockdown and quarantine measures. In an atmosphere of popular uncertainty and ignorance, it was thus more important to create a message and implement measures to alleviate cultural fears rather than to directly tackle the health epidemic per se, which had already overwhelmed policy capabilities.

In retrospect, it is necessary to ask, what exactly is the politics of health here? It has been too easy to attribute the position of the Trump administration and President Jair Bolsonaro in Brazil to political ideology, namely their prioritization of the economy over health, as well as the tactical gamble that economic success would guarantee continued electoral victory. At the same time, what is the relevance of cultural messaging in relation to politics? The virus played to different cultural audiences in Taiwan and the US, but the politics in both venues relied on maintaining control. During SARS in Taiwan, the government had already lost control thus had to enforce discipline. In the US, that loss of control involved a different cultural strategy.

Is health separable from politics? How did politics of the mass inevitably invoke culture?

When Sachs criticized Trump's politics of distraction that was at the root of his failure to contain the COVID-19 pandemic, his emphasis that the health crisis could only be resolved in its own terms was correct in principle. One can contrast Trump's policy with Governor Andrew Cuomo's handling of the crisis at its apex in New York. Based on epidemiological advice from health advisers, Cuomo opted for a strict lockdown to combat infectious spread, combined with social distancing and the wearing of masks. Despite severe shortages, it successfully reduced the number of infections and deaths. The highly contagious nature of COVID-19, whose actual causes were still undetermined, may also have led governments everywhere to impose harsh restrictions on international travel, which included outright bans on foreign visitors and 14-day quarantine on incoming passengers. The high proportion of asymptomatic persons and the long incubation period of the virus made it difficult to ascertain cases of cross-border transmission, but community infection was still a separate phenomenon that warranted a different strategy.

In situations marked by low incidence, the principle of social distancing and mask wearing should have been enough to prevent massive outbreaks. In Asia, where the virus was contained early on, it was not necessary to mandate universal stay-at-home lockdown or business closure. Yet in cases of extreme lockdown and travel quarantine, there were always exceptions. To say the least, medical frontline staff and other essential workers were exempt. Airline flight staff were also exempt from 14-day quarantine, and exceptions could always be made for high level personages. This was not to say that such people were immune from observing proper health restrictions. To the contrary, proper functioning of the system relied on such people following strict guidelines. On the other hand, it was more difficult to enforce such rules on the general public as a matter of social order, especially if there was resistance for whatever reason. Those areas where people did not respect the necessity of social distancing and the ethics of wearing masks not surprisingly produced new outbreaks. From a policy perspective, the need for social order clearly required something more than just observance of health restrictions. In Taiwan during the early SARS crisis, ignorance and uncertainty caused such panic and fear that it was deemed more expedient to opt for extreme repression, even fearmongering, to force the public to toe the line. In the US, the inability or unwillingness of the Trump regime to administer the required bitter medicine to contain the outbreak caused it to use diversionary tactics, by force opening the economy to counteract any health setback, scapegoating to deflect their own faults and otherwise denying the seriousness of the crisis to minimize the sense of panic and fear.

In sum, both SARS and COVID-19 were by nature health crises that required scientifically based solutions. However, especially in a situation where insufficient objective understanding of the phenomenon created uncertainty and fear, it created problems that involved in practice societal strategies. Politics was less a function of ideology than the fact that different slices of the population impacted differently to the crisis. *Disorder* was mostly a problem of the *mass*. Culture was a medium within which politics negotiated local reality. The current 'success' of Taiwan's COVID-19 policy seems to reflect its adherence to science, but it still fails to admit the flaws of its SARS policy and the lessons of panic and chaos that allowed it to make amends.

Notes

1. See Zhang Ziwu's (2020) retrospective of SARS.
2. News first appeared on the evening of 21 May in newspapers and on TV, followed by investigative reporting on the following day. *The China Times* devoted much higher attention to this case than the other major newspapers.
3. See the article by Lin Zhizheng and Jiang Zhaojing (2003, p. A3).
4. Lin and Jiang (2003, p. A3).
5. Quoted in Cai Huizhen and Huang Minyi (2003, p. A3).
6. Cai and Huang (2003, p. A3).
7. The following composite narrative is based on news reports that were published on 22 May in *The China Times* and *United Daily News*. Reporters relied on information from anonymous sources at Academia Sinica.
8. From Li Mingyang (2003, p. A5).
9. In Wu Dianrong and Chen Zhixian (2003, p. A3).
10. See Lin et al. (2003, p. A3).
11. From Lin Zhizheng and Jiang Zhaojing (2003, p. A3).
12. In Cao Mingcong (2003, p. A5).
13. The above incidents were extensively covered by most local newspapers in Taiwan.
14. Public awareness of the scandal erupting at Heping Hospital was amplified by news coverage of investigative reporters at Hong Kong's *Next Magazine* (*Yizhou kan*), who exposed numerous sloppy practices at the hospital.
15. The only essay sympathetic to Chen was an editorial in the English language *Taiwan News*, on 9 June 2003.
16. From Sach's (2020) opinion piece in CNN on 26 May.
17. See "Timeline: Trump's Coronavirus Response | NowThis" (2020), reproduced on youtube.
18. A Public Broadcasting Service Frontline documentary on 21 April 2020 entitled "Coronavirus Pandemic" contrasted policy differences between the two Washingtons (the state and federal government in DC) that reflected conflicts at the state and national level.
19. See the article by Nur Ibrahim (2020), which documents his later flip-flop.
20. In a position paper, Timothy W. Luke (2020) construes the politics of fear differently.

Disclosure statement

No potential conflict of interest was reported by the author(s).

Further information

This Special Issue article has been comprehensively reviewed by the Special Issue editors, Associate Professor Ted Striphas and Professor John Nguyet Erni.

References

Cai, H., and Huang, M. 2003. Having escaped quarantine, Academia Sinica researcher Chen Yilin incites public anger (Part 2). *The China Times*, 22 May, p. A3.

Cao, M. 2003. Having drawn a beard and moustache on his website photo, he calls himself a criminal. *United Daily News*, 22 May, p. A5.

Coronavirus Pandemic, 21 April 2020. Available from: https://www.pbs.org/wgbh/frontline/film/coronavirus-pandemic/.

Ibrahim, N. 2020, May 13. Did the US surgeon general recommend the public not wear masks? Available from: https://www.snopes.com/fact-check/surgeon-general-against-masks/.

Li, M. 2003. Academia Sinica researcher, flaunting quarantine, slips out of the country. *United Daily News*, 22 May, p. A5.

Lin, Z., and Jiang, Z. 2003. An enraged Lee Yuan-tse exclaims, 'he will definitely be punished'. *The China Times*, 22 May, p. A3.

Lin, Z., Shi, W., and Zhang, Z. 2003. Having escaped quarantine, Academia Sinica researcher Chen Yilin incites public anger (Part 1). *The China Times*, 22 May, p. A3.

Luke, T.W., 2020. The Dawn of the COVID-19 pandemic: the administration of fear and fear of administration in the United States. *Telos*, 191, 187–191.

Sachs, J.D. 2020 May 26. The one vital message of nearing 100,000 US deaths. Available from: https://us.cnn.com/2020/05/24/opinions/covid-politics-hundred-thousand-deaths-sachs/index.html.

Timeline: Trump's Coronavirus Response NowThis, 8 May 2020. Available from: https://www.youtube.com/watch?v=PD9XWTbbSGA.

Wu, D., and Chen, Z. 2003. He usually acts without regard to others, colleagues included; he often leaves the country without requesting leave, has been under supervisory probation, and on the day he was quarantined broke into the Institute building ... *The China Times*, 22 May, p. A3.

Zhang, Z. 2020, March 13. Return to Heping: indelible memories of the SARS quarantine black hole. Available from: https://www.twreporter.org/a/sars-memories-life-under-quarantine-in-heping-hospital.

Beyond the crisis: transitioning to a better world?

Ien Ang ⓘ

ABSTRACT

The COVID-19 crisis of 2020 is not just a short-term public health emergency. Instead, it has laid bare a broader and deeper organic crisis, produced by the intrinsic tensions and contradictions of the hegemonic neoliberal capitalist order. I discuss this organic crisis in terms of its active amplification of human divisiveness at various levels – class, racial, national, cultural – which impedes the generation of solidarity and cooperation in the name of a 'common humanity', required if humans are to live in harmony among each other and with the planet. By reflecting on a diverse range of barriers to such a desirable future, from the erosive role of human passions to the escalating new cold war between China and the West and the fundamental divisions exposed by the existential challenge of climate change, I argue that to have a chance of a liveable and equitable common future, we need to maintain a critical cosmopolitan horizon against the grain of self-interested closures and exclusions which underpin the organic crisis.

2020 was dominated by the Covid-19 crisis, an infectious disease pandemic caused by a coronavirus which was first identified in December 2019 in Wuhan, China, and has since spread throughout the world, killing almost two million people worldwide by the end of the year. However, the year also saw multiple other crises. In Australia, for example, from where I write this essay, the year began with unprecedented bushfires brought about by record-breaking temperatures and months of severe drought, burning down more than 18 million hectares of bush, forest and parks across the country, killing dozens of people and destroying thousands of dwellings and townships. In the United States, similar unprecedented fires also raged for weeks in the summer across the West Coast. A few months earlier, a crisis situation emerged with the eruption of the Black Lives Matter movement after the murder of George Floyd, an African American man who lost his life after a white police officer violently knelt on his neck for eight minutes, preventing him to breathe. The movement quickly spread the world over, inspiring many subaltern racialized groups to protest against continued racism in their local contexts. Towards the end of the year, the US experienced another unprecedented crisis when President Trump refused to concede his loss of the presidential elections to Joe Biden, endangering the system of democracy as such. These globally significant phenomena are among the multiplicity of other social, political and environmental crises erupting around the world, large and small, giving many people a sense that 'the world is falling apart' – a more profound sense of global crisis.

In this paper, I explore this deeper sense of crisis as the social experience of an epochal present that, punctuated by the Covid pandemic, articulates the untenability of the current global order, while at the same time highlighting the difficulty we have in imagining, let alone enacting the transformation of that order in politically desirable ways. This is a political crisis affecting the world at large, but it is experienced on the ground at the level of the every-day, where prospects of a shared, liveable and equitable future for all are fast receding, amplifying a cultural paralysis which is hard to overcome. I discuss this epochal sense of crisis by referring to Gramsci's concept of organic crisis, pointing to the intrinsic tensions and contradictions of the hegemonic neo-liberal capitalist order – tensions and contradictions which morbidly entrench multidimensional social divisions, at local and global levels, impeding the generation of an expansive perspective of solidarity and cooperation, required if we are to work towards a future humankind living in harmony among each other and with the planet. This is a big topic, and needless to say I can hardly do justice to the full complexities of our current predicament here. Instead, in the spirit of what Gramsci (1971) called 'the pessimism of the intellect', I will focus on a select few of the trickiest ways in which human divi-siveness is not just ingrained, but actively amplified today by the workings of the neoliberal capitalist order, making the envisioning of a 'common human-ity' virtually impossible. I will end with an attempt to sketch some avenues for an 'optimism of the will', which, however, will be necessarily modest and limited, starting at the level of the everyday, based on the understanding that, to have a chance of a common future, we need to maintain a critical cos-mopolitan horizon against the grain of the self-interested closures and exclu-sions underpinning the organic crisis.

Crisis, what crisis?

A 'crisis' tends to be constructed as an extraordinary event that interrupts a routine state of affairs. Wikipedia describes a crisis as an 'event or period that will lead, or may lead, to an unstable and dangerous situation affecting an individual, group, or all of society' (https://en.wikipedia.org/wiki/Crisis). Crises are deemed to be negative disruptions in 'normal' human affairs, especially when they occur abruptly, with little or no warning. They signify a 'testing time', caused by an 'emergency event'.

There are three problems with this narrow way of defining a 'crisis' as an abrupt, temporary and negative upheaval of normal affairs, caused by a singular emergency. First, this emphasis on the 'suddenness' of a crisis is problematic in relation to the three aforementioned crises. Many have sufficiently pointed out that the bushfires in Australia and elsewhere could have been anticipated, not just because of the drought, but more importantly, by the impacts of human-induced climate change. In this regard, the bushfires were not a sudden, extraordinary crisis, but a symptom of a longer term, more slow-burn crisis: what is now often called the 'climate crisis' (Baldwin and Ross 2020). The Black Lives Matter protests, while instantiated by the immediate outrage of Floyd's murder, were clearly intensified by the structural anti-black racism that has characterized US society for decades, if not centuries. In this sense, BLM does not signify a momentary crisis event, but represents the coming into play of what Anderson *et al.* (2019) call a 'slow emergency', a situation of 'attritional lethality' where racialized harm and damage suffered by black people are intrinsic to everyday life, not an exception to it. The Covid-19 crisis too should not be seen as a 'sudden' event, given that scientists have warned for years that a pandemic of this nature was not a question of if, but when. They suggest that viruses that have caused Sars, Mers and Covid-19 are just the vanguard of thousands of potential pathogens in animal reservoirs, and the risk of new outbreaks in future is increasing as a consequence of human intrusions into wild animal habitats, for example through massive deforestation and expansion of farmland to feed more and more humans, as well as human infrastructures such as globe-spanning transport networks and densely populated mega-cities (McCarthy 2020). In this regard, the Covid crisis too can be seen as part of a longer-term planetary crisis, a crisis signified by the concept of the Anthropocene (Duru 2020). It is not just a crisis of the changing climate, but a broader ecological crisis caused by the ways in which human societies are encroaching into the lifeworlds of animal populations. Disease ecologist Peter Daszak (2020) suggests that we now live in a 'pandemic era', in which humans may have to adjust to a new reality where new viral outbreaks are a regular part of life, just as we will be forced to adjust to a much warmer world in the decades to come.

The second problem of a narrow definition of crisis, therefore, pertains to seeing it as a *temporary* disruption of life as we know it. But as the pandemic has dragged on, it has become increasingly unlikely that we will just 'snap back' to 'business as usual' in the post-pandemic world. While how things would turn out to be is uncertain, history tells us that times of upheaval often generate transformative change. For example, the Great Depression and the second world war set the stage for the modern welfare state in Europe and the decolonization of much of Asia. Of course, change in response to crises is not always for the better, but can also have a much darker quality. For example, the US's War on Terror in response to the

September 11 attacks led to the decade-long destructive wars in Iraq and Afghanistan, and the global financial crisis in 2008 led to the massive propping up of banks and financial institutions and austerity politics in the broader society at great public cost (Öniş and Güven 2011). What qualitative changes might emerge as a result of this year of crisis (or crises), and what kind of 'new normal' could we expect to emerge? This question relates to the third problem with a narrow definition of crisis: the assumption that crisis always involves a *negative* disruption in human affairs. Of course, the loss of lives and livelihoods because of the pandemic is irrevocably a negative, tragic event. From a more long-view perspective, however, this crisis can also serve as a wake-up call, throwing light on what is wrong with the way the world has been operating, and possibly shaping political desires for drastic social change.

The organic crisis of neoliberalism

Joseph Masco (2017) has pointed to the conservative effect of the dominant way of talking about 'crisis'. As he puts it, '[c]risis talk today seeks to stabilize an institution, practice, or reality rather than interrogate the historical conditions of possibility for that endangerment to occur'. It evokes 'the need for an emergency response to the potential loss of a status quo' (Masco 2017, S73). Rather than seeing the pandemic as just a singular, transitory crisis then, one that will eventually pass, it is more illuminating to see it, as a range of critical observers have done (e.g. Anastasi 2020, Levenson 2020), as a symptom of a different, more historically protracted kind of crisis: a more long-term, much broader and deeper *organic* crisis (to use Gramsci's term) that permeates all levels of society, including economic structures, political institutions, social arrangements, longstanding ideologies and cultural values. From a Gramscian perspective, an organic crisis has to be understood not as a singular event, but as a much more protracted *process*: a multidimensional, transformative process of unravelling that originates in intrinsic contradictions and tensions within the prevailing social order (Babic 2020). An organic crisis like this cannot be resolved simply by medical, scientific or technological solutions (such as the track and trace app embraced by governments as a tool to manage infection rates, or even the development of a vaccine, on which so much faith and hope has been placed), because it points to a deeper societal impasse, one that requires more fundamental effort to overcome it.

   This impasse has already been quite clear in the intractable challenges, or so-called 'wicked problems', that have accumulated in the past few decades, which characterize our world today. It is difficult to ignore the seriousness of problems such as entrenched and worsening social inequality, institutional and political stagnation, chronic lack of investment in public infrastructures, and the degeneration of actually existing democratic systems into cynical marketing exercises dominated by short-term self-interest and greed. Under-pinning this multidimensional organic crisis is the supremacy of the preda-tory system of global neoliberal capitalism, which has gradually come to dominate the world in the past forty years or so (Duménil and Lévy 2011, Piketty 2020). Put simply, this is a system that ruthlessly prioritizes ceaseless economic growth, profit maximization and private interests at the expense of the public good and collective human wellbeing.

Contestations around the search for a vaccine against the coronavirus provide a good example. Vaccine production, just as medicines in general, in the current global system is in the hands of just a handful big pharma companies (Hira 2009). But these companies have for years been reluctant to invest in vaccine research and development, because it is so expensive and risky, and so difficult to make it profitable. In the course of 2020, as the world was in desperate search for a vaccine to tame the coronavirus, many governments, pharmaceutical companies and research teams have risen to the challenge of finding a vaccine. At the same time, there have been calls for a free 'people's vaccine'. Here, a vaccine is conceived as a 'global public good' that must be distributed equitably and free of charge to the whole world, based on the pooling of intellectual property so that there can be widespread, low-cost manufacturing of any vaccine that is developed – an idea that has equality and solidarity at its core. A resolution to this effect was campaigned for by many NGOs and world leaders in Europe, Asia and the developing world, and adopted at a World Health Assembly meeting in May 2020 (Oxfam International 2020). It is telling to note however that pushback was expressed especially by the United States, arguably the most unfettered neoliberal capitalist society in the world, on the argument that stripping the pharmaceutical industry of their patent rights would cut into their profits and discourage development of new products (Boseley 2020). What is being promulgated here, of course, is the neoliberal idea that profit maximization is the quintessential motive for the pursuit of knowledge and 'innovation', trumping any regard for the common human interest.

The disjuncture between corporate capitalist pursuits on the one hand, and the needs and interests of ordinary people and communities, on the other, as highlighted by the pandemic, exposes the dysfunctions of the pre-vailing economic system, which actively impedes efforts of human cooperation and the search for collective solutions. Indeed, neoliberal capit-alism also stands in the way of effective climate action, so increasingly urgently called for by hundreds of millions of citizens around the world, as the predominance of short-term economic thinking advances the vested cor-porate interests of the fossil fuel industry, making the slow emergency of climate change ever more difficult to tackle (Klein 2014, Parr 2014).

There is no shortage of powerful critiques of the systemic failures of neo-liberal capitalism, not just as an economic paradigm but also as a comprehensive social and cultural formation. Couze Venn (2018), for example, has synthesized how the confluence of crises affecting economic exploitation, environmental destruction, resource depletion and increasing social inequalities are inherent to capitalism as we know it. Some commentators have expressed the hope that the massive disruptions caused by the pandemic might be 'just the first heralds of a historic transformation in political and societal norms' (Lent 2020), and that this crisis might spell the end of neoliberalism. In this context, it was interesting to note (though no reason for celebration) how Margaret Thatcher's infamous neoliberal proposition that 'there is no such thing as a society' was explicitly discarded by Boris Johnson's admission that 'there really *is* such a thing as society' (*The Guardian*, 30 Mar 2020). Even before the pandemic, we have seen a proliferation of publications on post-capitalist futures (Gibson-Graham 2006, Mason 2015, Srnicek and Williams 2016), which challenge the neoliberal fundamentals on which the contemporary modern world is built and describe new avenues for a more humane future for all, a future beyond capitalism based on social justice, solidarity, and shared humanity, living in harmony with nature and the planet. Venn (2018), for example, imagines a world 'after capital' governed by a rejection of neoliberal values and a revaluation of 'commons': a 'postcapitalist life in common' ruled by generosity, welcoming of the other, and indebtedness (to nature and to other humans).

What is insufficiently considered in such imaginings of a radically different, postcapitalist future, however, are the hard logistics of realizing such fundamental change. How do we get to this wonderful new world? At issue here is the prosaic question of *transition* – a period of intense transformation towards a new world order, a new civilization. It would be misleading to consider such a period of transition as just a quick changeover from one order to the next. Nor is it realistic to think that any systemic 'revolution' would be on the cards, especially as – since the collapse of socialism in 1989 – no new vision for a political alternative exists that is compelling enough to simply replace neoliberal capitalism, no matter how much the latter is in crisis (Streeck 2017). In this regard, it is illuminating to remember the warning Gramsci made about organic crises: 'The crisis consists precisely in the fact that the old is dying and the new cannot yet be born; in this interregnum a great variety of morbid symptoms appear' (Gramsci 1971, p. 276).

In other words, we need to recognize the stretched-out temporality of this transition, or 'interregnum' as Gramsci put it – an indecisive, long drawn-out period, likely lasting decades or even longer, characterized by 'morbid symptoms' from which no stable new system or order will emerge. In his book *How Will Capitalism End?*, German political economist Wolfgang Streeck (2017) suggests that this interregnum will be an age of entropy, a disorderly, stale-mated (post)capitalist world of extended instability and uncertainty where constant crisis management may be 'the new normal', 'a crisis that is neither transformative nor adaptive, and unable either to restore capitalism to equilibrium or to replace it with something better' (Streeck 2017, p. 37). Thus, if it is indeed the case that the current organic crisis is leading us into such an interregnum, we should not anticipate it to be an easy one. Streeck provides a very bleak image of what we can expect on our road to a postcapitalist future, which will likely last for at least the rest of the twenty-first century:

> Before capitalism will go to hell, it will for the foreseeable future hang in limbo, dead or about to die from an overdose of itself but still very much around, as nobody will have the power to move its decaying body out of the way. (Streeck 2017, p. 36)

One reason why the interregnum might last longer than we'd want, according to Streeck, is precisely the continuing stranglehold of deeply entrenched neoliberal cultural values on people's efforts of survival, as they are encouraged to rely on individualized 'resilience' to make do, not on collective action and solidarity in quest of a shared better future. As Streeck (2017, p. 46) warns: 'It is only when the manufacturing of ideological enthusiasm for a neoliberal everybody-for-themselves existence will no longer work (...) that the post-capitalist interregnum may come to an end and a new order may emerge'. However, as Wendy Brown (2015) argues, three decades of neoliberal governmentality have eroded basic elements of democracy on which the generation of a common civic culture depends, as neoliberalism, as a peculiar form of reason, 'configures all aspects of existence in economic terms', including 'vocabularies, principles of justice, political cultures, habits of citizenship, practices of rule and, above all, democratic imaginaries' (Brown 2015, p. 17). As neoliberalism itself has severely weakened the social potential for democratic practice, which allows societies to overcome diversity and division towards negotiated shared goals, how can we mobilize people to join the collective struggle required to move beyond the organic crisis we are stuck in?

Passionate hostilities

To be sure, collective mobilization in the name of shared humanity and mutual solidarity is especially challenging in a societal environment dominated by neoliberal value orientations such as competitive individualism, pursuit of self-interest and veneration of personal freedom. The persistence of such values even in times of crisis can be seen as a morbid symptom in itself, and is reflected in the complex and contradictory impacts of human passions, affect and emotion on the social experience of crisis. During the pandemic, for example, we have seen widespread fury against physical distancing, self-isolation measures and the use of face masks, as people preferred to claim their personal liberty over a regard for public health, especially in the United States. We can see this as an expression of the selfish, possessive hyper-individualism so strongly promoted by the culture of neoliberalism, which is based on an ideology of 'the exaltation of a life in uncertainty as a life in liberty' (Streeck 2017, p. 46). The widely reported so-called Covid parties, in which young people defy protective measures deliberately to contract the virus, come to mind here (The New Daily 2020). Such practices are manifestations of what Lauren Berlant (2011) has called cruel optimism, where attachment to an object of desire – here, a warped sense of freedom – actually impedes the flourishing of the subject and the wider society. One can surmise that where such optimism, however cruel, is thwarted, anger and rage may ensue.

More broadly, rage and anger are pervasive today as a consequence of the profound social inequalities that the neoliberal capitalist regime has intensified. In the US, for example, neoliberal privatization of neighbourhoods, schools, and social welfare marginalized the poor and people of colour who are increasingly excluded from the right of citizenship (Hohle 2018). The explosion of the Black Lives Matter movement was strongly motivated by the sense of anger and frustration against persistent structural racism despite decades of struggle for racial equality, not just in the United States but throughout the Western and postcolonial world. While this struggle is one instilled by a desire for social justice and human solidarity, however, its reactionary counterpoint is the huge upsurge of the white supremacist far-right in the US and Europe in recent times, associated with the rise of nationalist populisms in so many Western countries. These movements too are mobilized by impassioned anger and resentment, whipped up by a fear of loss of white privilege or national identity, lashing out against a range of others including migrants and minorities, but also against what they see as 'elites' (which would include, I presume, intellectual communities such as Cultural Studies). How do we deal with such reactionary movements, who after all are also part of our common humanity?

The seemingly unstoppable rise of social media, instigated by primarily American corporate giants such as Facebook and Twitter, tends only to reinforce these divisions. Data-driven algorithms fragment society into individualized networks of users, who can seclude themselves from democratic mingling with diverse other voices. Predicated on the metrics of 'engagement', social media platforms incentivize content that is emotive and controversial, rewarding polarizing expressions of anger and outrage at the expense of 'rational' public discourse (Munn 2020). Can we ever heal such passionately-held divides? Or should we understand this deeply divisive, technologically enabled affective friction as part and parcel of the very organic crisis we are living through today – this long, protracted interregnum towards an uncertain future? In a time when we arguably need global solidarity more than ever, we see the empowerment of a cacophony of discordant, self-interested fractions, with little vision of a common future in sight.

New cold war into race war

Deep-seated, racially-tinged divisiveness is also on the rise on a global scale. In this regard, the escalating new cold war between China and the West is particularly concerning. The blame game against China as the origin of the pandemic was highlighted by President Trump's insistence on calling the pathogen the 'Chinese virus', and was bolstered by anti-China attitudes that have already been spiralling upwards in the past few years. Notwithstanding the necessity for international criticism of China's authoritarian regime when required, for example in relation to the repression of Uighurs in Xinjiang and China's imposition of a national security law on Hong Kong, it is important to stress that this anti-China stance is not just a strategic matter of protecting 'our' national interest, but is nourished *culturally* by a deeper and more persistent Sinophobia, which has run through Western societies for centuries, exemplified by the enduring trope of the Yellow Peril (Billé and Urbansky 2018). Visceral disgust of the so-called 'wet markets' today echoes the prejudiced association of disease with Chinese spaces, bodies and culture. This prejudice was prevalent more than one hundred years ago during the plague outbreaks in cities such as Vancouver, San Francisco and Honolulu, which resulted in the burning down or quarantining of whole Chinatowns (Lynteris 2018). Then as now, racist xenophobia against Chinese migrants was easily whipped up, as we have seen during this pandemic (Haynes 2020). The difference between then and now, however, is that China is no longer the 'degenerate' 'sick man of Asia' it was once dismissed to be, but an emerging global superpower.

China's sheer size and ancient civilization, routinely visualized as a terrifying dragon, reinforces a sense of dread for what it might do to the world, especially now that the dragon has well and truly awoken. However, as critical international relations theorists such as Michael Barr (2011) and Chengxin Pan (2012) argue, even though China is the object of legions of so-called China-watchers in the West, Western knowledge production on China tends to display an inability to see the country on its own terms, and this very 'lack of imagination contributes to the fear of China' (Barr 2011, p. 132). One reason why China is feared today, Barr observes, is not because China is so different, but because it has joined in the West's own neoliberal path of economic and technological modernization. Its apparent success in the neoliberal competitive game 'draws unwelcome attention to the West's own inadequacy in answering the most pressing questions of modernity' (Barr 2011,

p. 134). This explains at least in part why China's current geopolitical and economic ascendancy is seen as such a threat to the hegemony of the West, and why, increasingly, Western governments are taking up a hawkish stand against the emerging superpower. Talk is now rife about a comprehensive 'decoupling' of the US and China, forcing to undo the connectivity that has been established in decades of neoliberal globalization (that has been so powerfully lucrative for the global capitalist class, both in China and the West) (Johnson and Gramer 2020). Ironically, however, such a confrontational stance based on a wholesale demonization of China may only reinforce China's own adversarial global politics, potentially leading to a self-fulfilling prophecy and only hastening the so-called decline of the West, as Singaporean diplomat Kishori Mahbubani (2020) ominously warned in his book *Has China Won?*

Global geopolitical divisions and heightened superpower tension inevitably have corrosive social and cultural effects by enhancing mutual mistrust. Not surprisingly, recent surveys have shown a double escalation of anti-China sentiment in the US and of anti-US sentiment in China (Panda 2020, Pew Research Center 2020). Emotionally invested nationalist paranoia (Hage 2003) is being whipped up by political leaders not just in the US and China, but also in countries such as Australia, and it may be difficult to keep it in check, rekindling narratives of a racially tinged, real and imagined 'clash of civilizations' (Strand 2020), in which the world is no longer perceived as 'one', shared by a single humanity, but as separate geopolitical and ethno-cultural spheres locked into mutual suspicion and hostility.

This points to the complexities and multiplicities of racism as a divisive cultural force. In the context of worldwide struggles against white hegemony, it is important to realize that anti-Chinese racism today is not the same as, for example, anti-Muslim or anti-black racism. While in the latter the racialized other is devalued as worthless inferiors, anti-Chinese racism is, by contrast, motivated by a much more ambivalent anxiety: it entails not just cultural aversion and distrust, but also a sense of *awe* of China's power and astonishing 'rise' and a *fear* of the 'threat' it is projected to pose (Pan 2012). In this light, racism against Chinese (and against Asians who are mistaken for being Chinese) is more akin to anti-semitism, inviting a comparison of Chinese people with the Jews, which was already current in early twentieth-century colonial Southeast Asia, the region which has historically harboured the largest contingent of the Chinese diaspora (Chirot and Reid 1997). Similar to the Jews, in stereotypical western representations the Chinese are portrayed, as Franck Billé (2018, p. 18) has noted, as 'simultaneously maligned and admired, charged with both superior qualities and with despicable, inhuman traits', posing a threat to white racial supremacy. This resonates with notions of Asians as the 'model minority', as highly intelligent and technically brilliant but also calculating and ruthless – an image going back to the evil Fu Manchu, the popular fictional character in early twentieth-century Hollywood (Frayling 2014). The reinvigoration of such a polarized, racialized view of the world and its human inhabitants – risking the ostracization of millions of diasporic and mixed-race people whose creolized identities are a legacy of the global migrations of at least the past two centuries – is another dimension of the organic crisis we are currently experiencing, cutting across the cultural contradictions of neoliberalism in which, on the one hand, the significance of 'race' is disavowed in favour of 'colour-blind' individualist competition (in the case of black people), but where, on the other hand, 'race' is amplified as a signifier precisely of the unscrupulousness of that competition (in the case of Chinese), in which the fear is that whites might lose. In short, the rising geopolitical tensions we are seeing between China and the West today may also fuel the legitimization of a proverbial 'race war' by absolutizing the divide between the 'white' and 'yellow' 'races' – a world view that, troublingly, has already found fertile ground in China itself (Cheng 2019).

Circumventing the climate crisis

The loss of a sense of 'common humanity' is especially problematic in light of the most existential dimension of our contemporary predicament: climate change and the ecological crisis. Much Western environmental discourse tends to speak for or on behalf of an abstract 'humankind', a culturally and racially undifferentiated 'we', but the environmental movement has long been criticized for its lack of racial and ethnic diversity, with the implicit assumption of 'we' as white (and middle class), even in new radical groups such as Extinction Rebellion (Curnow and Helferty 2018, Nugent 2020). But it is obvious that this planetary crisis cannot be addressed without the participation of people of all racial and class backgrounds. Nor, for that matter, can it be done without the participation and cooperation of China, which is after all the home of one-sixth of the world's human population, as well as the rest of the world outside the privileged Euro-American centre (including Australasia). The fight for action to manage climate change – widely recognized as the single-most important 'slow emergency' facing us – highlights *par excellence* the necessity of a cosmopolitan sense of pan-human solidarity and cooperation.

But even in the politics of responding to climate change historically entrenched divisions play a formative role. International climate change governance is the unstable result of very complex negotiations at the global level, which has seen major divisions between rich, developed countries and poorer, developing countries. In such negotiations, consideration of normative issues of justice and equity are crucial, especially in relation to historical disparities in who caused the global warming we are seeing today, and structural inequalities in capacity to take on the actions required (Okereke and Conventry 2016). But, as has been observed in relation to the 2015 Paris Agreement, such ethical considerations have been largely evaded, replaced by an 'everyone is responsible' discourse and institutional framework that sidestep the disproportionate role of the rich and powerful developed world in triggering human-induced climate change (Ciplet and Timmons Roberts 2017). As Okereke and Conventry (2016, p. 846) remark, '[i]t is evident that the normative architecture of the global order remains hostile to solidarist concepts of justice'.

But it is difficult to determine what 'solidarity' can even mean in the context of the inevitability of climate change. In this regard, it is useful to consider Dipesh Chakrabarty's (2017) reflections on the tensions between globalization and global warming. In his view, a serious inclusion of the 'Global South' in our conversation about climate change requires a deep engagement with the real materiality, but also the intrinsic contradictions of the desire for modernization in the postcolonial, developing world. To take a mundane example, air-conditioning is an everyday cooling technology that is a taken for granted comfort in wealthy countries, but its acquisition is still a popular aspiration among the millions of ordinary people in India and elsewhere in poorer countries, especially now that the globe is getting warmer. There is an obvious irony here, as Chakrabarty observes: 'The very technology that can help to protect people from climate change also accelerates the rate of climate change' (2017, p. 270). For Chakrabarty, this dilemma posits the difficulty of being modern, and it confronts us with the limits of any exclusively human-centred notions of global politics. As he puts it:

> We knew that humans ... were also a biological species, *homo sapiens*, but the knowledge was of no special political import. But when the planet faces, for the first time in its entire history, the bleak prospect of a 'great extinction' driven by the activities of one biological species, us, the urgency of creating a sense of politics based on this second understanding of ourselves as a species dawns on us. But we don't know yet how to do that (Chakrabarty 2017, p. 281).

We could say that this is where we are at in our present condition: *we don't know*. We do not know how we should respond to the escalating crises – not just ecological but also economic, ideological and cultural – that intersect and converge to threaten to wipe us all out because we, as a species, are too internally divided to act as a unitive collective, as a 'single humanity'. Indeed, humanity's very lack of knowing how to unite is part and parcel of the current organic crisis: a crisis where the old is slowly but surely dying, but where the new cannot yet be born. In this transitional vacuum, it is disheartening to see how prevailing neoliberal principles of market-based solutions, private sector initiative and proprietary technological innovation, which thrive on competition and rivalry, are now widely accepted as privileged modes of climate action (Okereke and Conventry 2016). President Trump's decision to pull the United States out of the Paris climate agreement in 2017, based emphatically on the selfish neoliberal idea of 'America First', highlighted the magnitude of the challenges faced by humanity to overcome its ingrained and ubiquitous disagreements and divisions, which won't be overcome simply by Trump's salutary departure.

Beyond crisis: towards critical cosmopolitanization

In this paper, I have highlighted the pervasive human divisions which both buttress, and are exacerbated by, the multiplying crises affecting our societies at present, underpinned by a neoliberalized value system of competitive individualism and particularist self-interest. In the face of such historically entrenched and politically charged divisions – of race, class, nation and otherwise – the rhetoric of a 'common humanity' is powerless in efforts to attain a greater sense of human solidarity and the nurturing of an inclusive, common civic culture. How can we move beyond this political impasse, this social paralysis, this morbid interregnum?

To be sure, some authors are convinced that there is no future for modern civilization as we know it. Pablo Servigne and Raphael Stevens (2020, p. 88), for example, argue, in reference to the prevailing neoliberal capitalist system, that 'the ever more globalized, interconnected and locked-in structure of our civilization not only makes it highly vulnerable to the slightest internal or external disruption but now subjects it to processes of systemic collapse'. As spokespeople of the growing collapsology movement in France, Servigne and Stevens urge us to seriously prepare for this coming collapse. But for them 'collapse' is not the end, but the beginning of a new future: a future for the transition to which we can start working on right now. As they put it: 'The certainty is that we will never again be in the 'normal' situation that we have experienced over the past few decades' (Servigne & Stevens 2020, p. 178). Surely the pandemic has irrevocably brought this home to us: in post-pandemic life, things will never be the same again.

At the same time, however, we need to emphasize the profound *uncertainty* that this transitional epoch brings with it. This means taking seriously Gramsci's notion that an organic crisis constitutes a long-running historical process that ushers in 'a distinct phase of instability and uncertainty (and [is] not only … a transition between two stable periods)' (Babic 2020, p. 769). This is a period in which massive volatility, flux and insecurity is, for the time being, the new normal: we have no way of knowing what is going to happen next even as crisis events may accumulate in rapid succession (including, as scientists warn, new pandemics, more bushfires and other environmental disasters, as well as, all too possibly, further explosions of populist protest, the ascendancy of authoritarian leaders, and military clashes between China and the US). In this interregnum of transitional ambiguity, if not chaos, the best we could do is engage with the full complexity and difficulty of the present – what Donna Haraway (2016) has called 'staying with the trouble'. Haraway does not have a lot of time for those who revel in the inevitability of collapse, who say that 'the game is over, it's too late, there's no sense trying to make anything better' (2016, p. 3). Instead, she proposes that we attempt to 'stay with the trouble', by which she means that we face our predicament head on and work together on more modest possibilities of partial recuperation, in the recognition that 'we require each other in unexpected collaborations and combinations, ... we become with each other or not at all' (Haraway 2016, p. 3). In this regard, uncertainty is a positive, not a negative thing, because it keeps things open, and thus subject to action, as we respond to the unpredictabilities at hand.

The crises of 2020 have provided multiple examples of such partial recuperations, small positive changes that may, over time, add up to larger, more enduring transformation. The Covid-19 pandemic has allowed many to reassess their priorities, as they realize the importance of collective action (such as mask-wearing) for public health and reduce their attachment to the consumerist lifestyles promoted by neoliberal culture. At the same time, acts of solidarity have been numerous, not only in response to the bushfires but also during the Black Lives Matter protests, which were joined by many whites and diverse people of colour, including many people of Asian descent, who have been encouraged to see the heightened racism against them during the pandemic as part of the broader struggle against racial injustice (Lang 2020). Meanwhile, Chinese and western scientists continued to collaborate – including in research for a new vaccine – despite the deteriorating geopolitical tensions between China and the US (Lew 2020). And in relation to the environment, the experience of cleaner air, absence of traffic jams and massive decline in CO_2 emissions have raise people's awareness of the limitations of prevailing ways of life and the need to develop better ways of living together, as cities are fast-tracking the conversion of roads into bike lanes to promote a safe mode of urban transport that is also ecologically sound (Connolly 2020).

These are small but positive actions that respond to situated challenges at hand, generating 'nonutopian but positive futurities that can reactivate the world-making powers of society' (Masco 2017, p. S75). What they have in common, in different ways, is that they gesture towards a cosmopolitan horizon by working critically against the grain of self-interested divisions and particularist exclusions that still prevail. Here, cosmopolitanism should not be seen as an ideal condition or vision, but as a socially and politically grounded *process* of ongoing cosmopolitanization, which consists precisely in the continuing attempt to overcome the myriad differences and divisions that prevent sharing, cooperation and united action for a better future for all. The work of cosmopolitanization will never be done, because a universal common humanity will never be fully achieved (Ang 2014).

What we are also made to be aware of, however, is that cosmopolitanism is not enough if it remains solely focused on the unity of humanity. As difficult but important as it is to nurture and maintain a vision of one world and a single humankind against the myriad divisions and exclusions that ravage world society, as I have briefly (and only partially) sketched in this essay, cosmopolitanism must also reach beyond its own human horizon to address not just the global, but the planetary challenge facing us (Chakrabarty 2017). In other words, we must also reckon with the fact that we humans, as the dominant colonizer of the planet, are responsible for its impending destruction and the possible extinction not only of ourselves, but also of the many other species living on earth. This requires a cosmopolitan openness to difference that includes a critique of its own human biases.

Disclosure statement

No potential conflict of interest was reported by the author.

Further information

This Special Issue article has been comprehensively reviewed by the Special Issue editors, Associate Professor Ted Striphas and Professor John Nguyet Erni.

ORCID

Ien Ang ⓘ http://orcid.org/0000-0002-4877-0026

References

Anastasi, A., 2020. Crisis maneuvers. *Viewpoint Magazine*, 15 Apr https://www.viewpointmag.com/2020/04/15/crisis-maneuvers/.

Anderson, B., et al., 2019. Slow emergencies: temporality and the racialized biopolitics of emergency governance. *Progress in human geography*, 44 (4), 621–639.

Ang, I., 2014. Beyond unity in diversity: cosmopolitanizing identities in a globalizing world. *Diogenes*, 60 (1), 1–11.

Babic, M., 2020. Let's talk about the interregnum: Gramsci and the crisis of the liberal world order. *International affairs*, 96 (3), 767–786.

Baldwin, C. and Ross, H., 2020. Beyond a tragic fire season: a window of opportunity to address climate change? *Australasian journal of environmental management*, 27 (1), 1–5.

Barr, M., 2011. *Who's afraid of China?: The challenge of Chinese soft power*. London: Zed Books.

Berlant, L., 2011. *Cruel optimism*. Durham: Duke University Press.

Billé, F., 2018. Introduction. *In*: F. Billé and S. Urbansky, eds. *Yellow Perils: China narratives in the contemporary world*. Honolulu: University of Hawai'i Press. 1–34.

Billé, F. and Urbansky, S., eds., 2018. *Yellow Perils. China narratives in the contemporary world*. Honolulu: University of Hawai'i Press.

Boseley, S., 2020. US and UK "lead push against global patent pool for Covid-19 drugs". *The Guardian*, 17 May. https://www.theguardian.com/world/2020/may/17/us-and-uk-lead-push-against-global-patent-pool-for-covid-19-drugs.

Brown, W., 2015. *Undoing the demos. neoliberalism's stealth revolution*. New York: Zone Books.

Chakrabarty, D., 2017. Planetary crises and the difficulty of being modern. *Millennium: journal of international studies*, 46 (3), 259–282.

Cheng, Y., 2019. *Discourses of race and rising China*. Cham, Switzerland: Palgrave Macmillan.

Chirot, D. and Reid, A., eds., 1997. *Essential outsiders: Chinese and Jews in the modem transformation of southeast Asia and central Europe*. Seattle and London: University of Washington Press.

Ciplet, D. and Timmons Roberts, J., 2017. Climate change and the transition to neoliberal environmental governance. *Global environmental change*, 46, 148–156.

Connolly, K., 2020. "Cleaner and greener": Covid-19 prompts world's cities to free public space of cars. *The Guardian*, 18 May. https://www.theguardian.com/world/2020/may/18/cleaner-and-greener-covid-19-prompts-worlds-cities-to-free-public-space-of-cars.

Curnow, J. and Helferty, A., 2018. Contradictions of solidarity: whiteness, settler coloniality and the mainstream environmental movement. *Environment and society*, 9 (1), 145–163.

Daszak, P., 2020. We know disease X was coming. It's here now. *The New York Times*, 27 Feb. https://www.nytimes.com/2020/02/27/opinion/coronavirus-pandemics.html.

Duménil, G. and Lévy, D., 2011. *The crisis of neoliberalism*. Cambridge, MA: Harvard University Press.

Duru, M., 2020. Covid-19, a disease of the anthropocene and biodiversity. *Up' Magazine*, 4 May. https://up-magazine.info/en/planete/biodiversite/52859-covid-19-maladie-de-lanthropocene-et-de-la-biodiversite/.

Frayling, C., 2014. *The Yellow Peril: Dr Fu Manchu and the rise of chinaphobia*. London: Thames & Hudson.

Gibson-Graham, J.K., 2006. *A postcapitalist politics*. Minneapolis: University of Minnesota Press.

Gramsci, A., 1971. *Selections from the prison notebooks*. Eds and Trans Quintin Hoare and Geoffrey Nowell Smith. New York: International Publishers.

Hage, G., 2003. *Against paranoid nationalism*. Sydney: Pluto Press.

Haraway, D., 2016. *Staying with the trouble: making Kin in the Chthulucene*. Durham & London: Duke University Press.

Haynes, S., 2020. As coronavirus spreads, so does Xenophobia and anti-Asian racism. *Time*, 6 Mar. https://time.com/5797836/coronavirus-racism-stereotypes-attacks/.

Hira, A., 2009. The political economy of the global pharmaceutical industry: Why the poor lack access to medicine and what might be done about it. *International journal of development issues*, 8, 84–101.

Hohle, R., 2018. *Racism in the neoliberal era: a meta history of elite white power*. New York: Routledge.

Johnson, K. and Gramer, R., 2020. The great decoupling. *Foreign Policy*, 14 May. https://foreignpolicy.com/2020/05/14/china-us-pandemic-economy-tensions-trump-coronavirus-covid-new-cold-war-economics-the-great-decoupling/.

Klein, N., 2014. *This changes everything: capitalism vs. the climate*. New York: Simon & Schuster.

Lang, C., 2020. The Asian American response to black lives matter is part of a long, complicated history. *Time*, 26 June. https://time.com/5851792/asian-americans-black-solidarity-history/.

Lent, J., 2020. Coronavirus spells the end of the neoliberal era. What's next? *Open Democracy*, 12 Apr. https://www.opendemocracy.net/en/transformation/coronavirus-spells-the-end-of-the-neoliberal-era-whats-next/.

Levenson, Z., 2020. An organic crisis is upon us: when Gramsci goes viral. *Spectre Journal*, 20 Apr. https://spectrejournal.com/an-organic-crisis-is-upon-us/.

Lew, L., 2020. Coronavirus trumps poor US-China relations as scientific collaboration spikes, study shows. *South China Morning Post*, 23 July. https://www.scmp.com/news/china/diplomacy/article/3094423/coronavirus-trumps-poor-us-china-relations-scientific.

Lynteris, C., 2018. Yellow Peril epidemics: the political ontology of degeneration and emergence. *In*: F. Billé, and S. Urbansky, eds. *Yellow Perils. China narratives in the contemporary world*. Honolulu: University of Hawai'i Press, 35–59.

Mahbubani, K., 2020. *Has China won? The Chinese challenge to American primacy*. New York: Public Affairs.

Masco, J., 2017. The crisis in crisis. *Current anthropology*, 58 (Supplement 15), S65–S76.

Mason, P., 2015. *Postcapitalism: A guide to our future*. UK: Penguin Books.

McCarthy, S., 2020. Pandemics are an "Existential Threat" to us that we can prevent, Scientists say'. *Inkstone*, 11 Apr. https://www.inkstonenews.com/health/pandemics-are-existential-threat-us-we-can-prevent-scientists-say/article/3078751.

Munn, L., 2020. Angry by design: technical architectures and toxic communication. *Humanities and social sciences communications*, 7 (1), 1–11.

Nugent, C., 2020. A revolution's evolution: inside extinction rebellion's attempt to reform its climate activism. *Time*, 9 July. https://time.com/5864702/extinction-rebellion-climate-activism/.

Okereke, C. and Conventry, P., 2016. Climate justice and the international regime: before, during and after Paris. *WIRE's clim change*, 7, 834–851.

Öniş, Z. and Güven, A.B., 2011. The global economic crisis and the future of neoliberal globalization: rupture versus continuity'. *Global governance*, 17 (4), 469–488.

Oxfam International, 2020. Open letter: uniting behind a people's vaccine against COVID-19, 14 May. https://medium.com/@Oxfam/uniting-behind-a-peoples-vaccine-against-covid-19-87eec640976.

Pan, C., 2012. *Knowledge, desire and power in global politics: Western representations of China's rise*. Cheltenham, UK: Edward Elgar Publishing.

Panda, A., 2020. Survey: Chinese report less favorable views of US democracy. *The Diplomat*, 9 Apr. https://thediplomat.com/2020/04/survey-chinese-report-less-favorable-views-of-us-democracy/.

Parr, A., 2014. *The wrath of capital. neoliberalism and climate change politics*. New York: Columbia University Press.

Pew Research Center, 2020. U.S. views of China increasingly negative amid coronavirus outbreak, April. https://www.pewresearch.org/global/wp-content/uploads/sites/2/2020/04/PG_2020.04.21_U.S.-Views-China_FINAL.pdf.

Piketty, T., 2020. *Capital and ideology*. Trans. Arthur Goldhammer. Cambridge, MA: Harvard University Press.

Servigne, P. and Stevens, R., 2020. *How everything can collapse*. Trans. Andrew Brown. Cambridge: Polity Press.

Srnicek, N. and Williams, A., 2016. *Inventing the future. Postcapitalism and a world without work*. London: Verso.

Strand, D., 2020. The clash of civilizations has arrived. *Providence*, 8 Apr. https://providencemag.com/2020/04/clash-of-civilizations-arrived-china-coronavirus/.

Streeck, W., 2017. *How will capitalism end?* London: Verso.

The Guardian, 2020. There is such a thing as society, says Boris Johnson from bunker. 30 Mar. https://www.theguardian.com/politics/2020/mar/29/20000-nhs-staff-return-to-service-johnson-says-from-coronavirus-isolation.

The New Daily, 2020. "Covid parties": the wildly irresponsible trend that's killing people, 14 July. https://thenewdaily.com.au/news/coronavirus/2020/07/14/coronavirus-parties-trend/.

Venn, C., 2018. *After capital*. London: SAGE.

Index

Note: Figures are indicated by *italics*. Endnotes are indicated by the page number followed by 'n' and the endnote number e.g., 20n1 refers to endnote 1 on page 20.

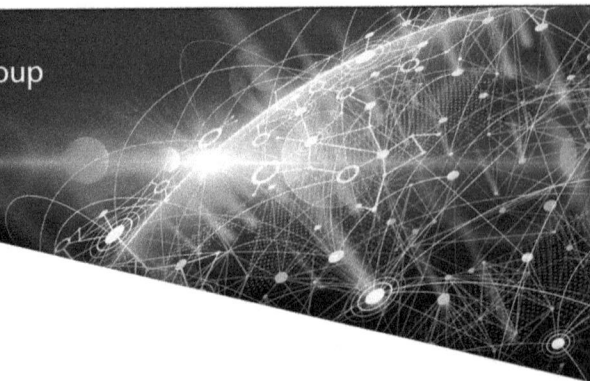

For Product Safety Concerns and Information please contact our EU
representative GPSR@taylorandfrancis.com
Taylor & Francis Verlag GmbH, Kaufingerstraße 24, 80331 München, Germany

www.ingramcontent.com/pod-product-compliance
Lightning Source LLC
Chambersburg PA
CBHW060745220326
41598CB00022B/2333